AF127114

Glaucoma: New Diagnostic and Therapeutic Approaches

Glaucoma: New Diagnostic and Therapeutic Approaches

Guest Editor

Da-Wen Lu

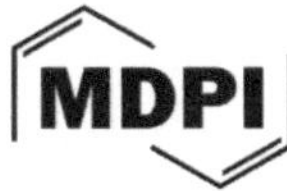

Basel • Beijing • Wuhan • Barcelona • Belgrade • Novi Sad • Cluj • Manchester

Guest Editor
Da-Wen Lu
Department of
Ophthalmology
Tri-Service General Hospital
National Defense Medical
Center
Taipei
Taiwan

Editorial Office
MDPI AG
Grosspeteranlage 5
4052 Basel, Switzerland

This is a reprint of the Special Issue, published open access by the journal *Biomedicines* (ISSN 2227-9059), freely accessible at: https://www.mdpi.com/journal/biomedicines/special_issues/FR2RE42UZ7.

For citation purposes, cite each article independently as indicated on the article page online and as indicated below:

Lastname, A.A.; Lastname, B.B. Article Title. *Journal Name* **Year**, *Volume Number*, Page Range.

ISBN 978-3-7258-3619-2 (Hbk)
ISBN 978-3-7258-3620-8 (PDF)
https://doi.org/10.3390/books978-3-7258-3620-8

Contents

About the Editor

Da-Wen Lu

Professor Da-Wen Lu is a Professor of Ophthalmology at Tri-Service General Hospital, Taiwan, and a member of the Glaucoma Research Society. He specializes in the medical treatment and surgical management of cataracts and glaucoma. His current research interests focus on novel pharmacological treatments for glaucoma, including the development of new rho kinase inhibitors, and the application of artificial intelligence (AI) in glaucoma management. His team contributed to the development of novel dual-targeted rho kinase inhibitor therapy in collaboration with Taiwan's Industrial Technology Research Institute (ITRI), which was recognized with a Gold Medal in the "Ophthalmic Innovation" category at the 2024 Edison Awards.

Preface

Glaucoma remains a leading cause of irreversible blindness worldwide, posing significant challenges to visual function and quality of life. This Reprint aims to present the latest advancements in glaucoma diagnostics and treatment, covering a wide range of topics from innovative diagnostic techniques to personalized therapeutic strategies, ultimately promoting clinical excellence and fostering interdisciplinary collaboration.

This Special Issue features research reflecting major breakthroughs in artificial intelligence, imaging technologies, genetics, immunology, surgical innovations, and novel therapies. Several studies explore the application of deep learning in glaucoma detection, including its role in diagnosing high myopia-associated glaucoma and integrating few-shot learning with optical coherence tomography angiography (OCTA) to enhance diagnostic accuracy. Additionally, papers highlight the incorporation of genetic factors into risk prediction models, improving the precision of disease progression monitoring and paving the way for personalized treatment approaches.

This Reprint also examines the systemic associations of glaucoma, particularly its relationship with type 2 diabetes (T2D). Innovative Mendelian randomization studies provide new insights into potential causal mechanisms. Furthermore, the role of immune system dysregulation in glaucoma pathogenesis is increasingly recognized, with studies indicating that retinal microvascular changes and immune dysfunction could serve as promising therapeutic targets.

Surgical innovations are another key focus of this Special Issue. Studies evaluate the long-term efficacy of endocyclophotocoagulation (ECP) combined with phacoemulsification, Ahmed valve implantation in complex glaucoma cases, and the impact of the Preserflo MicroShunt on microvascular flow, offering valuable evidence for future minimally invasive surgical applications. Additionally, emerging research highlights novel structural biomarkers for early diagnosis, the association between olfactory dysfunction and glaucoma as a neurodegenerative disease, and the potential of nicotinamide as a neuroprotective agent in glaucoma therapy.

This Reprint is intended for ophthalmologists, vision science researchers, biomedical engineers, pharmaceutical developers, medical educators, and all healthcare professionals interested in the latest advancements in glaucoma care. We extend our sincere gratitude to all of the internationally recognized experts who contributed to this Special Issue, covering a wide spectrum from basic science to clinical applications. We also appreciate the reviewers for their insightful feedback in enhancing manuscript quality and the editorial team for their professional assistance in ensuring the successful publication of this Special Issue.

By compiling these cutting-edge research findings, this Special Issue seeks to bridge the gap between academia and clinical practice, facilitate the adoption of innovative technologies, and ultimately improve treatment outcomes and visual health for glaucoma patients worldwide.

Da-Wen Lu
Guest Editor

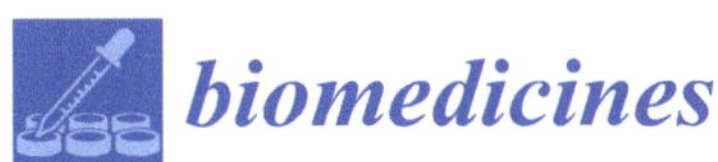

MDPI

Review

Olfactory Dysfunction and Glaucoma

Valeria Iannucci, Alice Bruscolini, Giannicola Iannella, Giacomo Visioli, Ludovico Alisi, Mauro Salducci, Antonio Greco and Alessandro Lambiase *

Department of Sense Organs, Sapienza University of Rome, Viale del Policlinico 155, 00161 Rome, Italy; valeria.iannucci@uniroma1.it (V.I.); alice.bruscolini@uniroma1.it (A.B.); giannicola.iannella@uniroma1.it (G.I.); giacomo.visioli@uniroma1.it (G.V.); ludovico.alisi@uniroma1.it (L.A.); mauro.salducci@uniroma1.it (M.S.); antonio.greco@uniroma1.it (A.G.)

* Correspondence: alessandro.lambiase@uniroma1.it; Tel.: +39-06-4997-5300

Abstract: Background: Olfactory dysfunction is a well-known phenomenon in neurological diseases with anosmia and hyposmia serving as clinical or preclinical indicators of Alzheimer's disease, Parkinson's disease, and other neurodegenerative disorders. Since glaucoma is a neurodegenerative disease of the visual system, it may also entail alterations in olfactory function, warranting investigation into potential sensory interconnections. Methods: A review of the current literature of the last 15 years (from 1 April 2008 to 1 April 2023) was conducted by two different authors searching for topics related to olfaction and glaucoma. Results: three papers met the selection criteria. According to these findings, patients with POAG appear to have worse olfaction than healthy subjects. Furthermore, certain predisposing conditions to glaucoma, such as pseudoexfoliation syndrome and primary vascular dysregulation, could possibly induce olfactory changes that can be measured with the Sniffin Stick test. Conclusions: the scientific literature on this topic is very limited, and the pathogenesis of olfactory changes in glaucoma is not clear. However, if the results of these studies are confirmed by further research, olfactory testing may be a non-invasive tool to assist clinicians in the early diagnosis of glaucoma.

Keywords: smell; olfaction; olfactory test; hyposmia; neurodegeneration; glaucoma; retinal ganglion cells; pseudoexfoliation syndrome; olfactory dysfunction; olfactory disorders

Citation: Iannucci, V.; Bruscolini, A.; Iannella, G.; Visioli, G.; Alisi, L.; Salducci, M.; Greco, A.; Lambiase, A. Olfactory Dysfunction and Glaucoma. *Biomedicines* **2024**, *12*, 1002. https://doi.org/10.3390/biomedicines12051002

Academic Editor: Da-Wen Lu

Received: 28 March 2024
Revised: 27 April 2024
Accepted: 29 April 2024
Published: 2 May 2024

1. Introduction

The sense of smell is one of the human senses that enables the perception of odors or scents in the environment. Although often neglected in medical practice, an olfactory dysfunction significantly impacts the quality of life [1]. Hyposmia or anosmia reduces the enjoyment of food, social relationships, and work skills. In addition, alterations in the sense of smell can expose people to the risk of damage from fumes, toxic substances, and spoiled food.

In recent years it has been shown that olfactory dysfunction may be an early sign of major neurodegenerative diseases such as Parkinson's and Alzheimer's [2–4]. In addition, it seems that the deterioration of olfactory function could be associated with the progression of these neurodegenerative disease and early cognitive impairment [1,5]. According to this evidence, Knight and colleagues reported that better olfactory performance is associated with a lower risk of progression of cognitive impairment and is a predictor of longevity [6].

The retina and optic nerve are highly specialized neural structures and direct extensions of the central nervous system. The interdependence of the brain, optic nerve, and retinal tropism has been well documented [7], and thinning of the retinal nerve fiber layer (RNFL), assessed with optical coherence tomography (OCT), has been confirmed in many neurodegenerative diseases, such as Alzheimer's [8,9], Parkinson's [10], and multiple sclerosis [11].

Glaucoma is an optic neuropathy characterized by visual field defects and changes in the optic nerve head and nerve fiber layer; it is the leading cause of irreversible bilateral blindness, affecting approximately 80 million people worldwide [12].

Glaucoma shares some common pathogenetic mechanisms, particularly with Alzheimer's disease, such as mitochondrial dysfunction, neuroinflammation, and oxidative stress [13–16]. Over the years, evidence has shown that glaucoma should not be considered a purely ophthalmologic disease because it damages not only the optic nerve but also other brain structures involved in vision [17,18].

Could glaucoma, as a neurodegenerative disease of the visual system, be associated with early neurological olfactory damage, as well as Alzheimer's and Parkinson's diseases?

This review analyzed this medical hypothesis and reported the current scientific evidence on these two potentially related topics.

2. Smell Dysfunction Causes

Several clinical conditions can cause olfactory dysfunction [1].

- Upper respiratory infections;
- Nasal and sinus conditions such as sinusitis, nasal polyps, or inflammation of the nasal passages can interfere with the ability to smell by blocking airflow or affecting olfactory receptors;
- Head trauma, including injuries to the head, especially to the frontal lobes or the area around the nose, can damage the olfactory nerves and cause loss of smell;
- Aging: as people age, there may be a natural decline in the sense of smell due to changes in the olfactory system;
- Medications: some medications, including certain antibiotics, antidepressants, and antihypertensives, can cause olfactory dysfunction as a side effect;
- Toxic chemical exposure: exposure to certain chemicals or toxins, such as solvents, pollutants, or heavy metals, can damage the olfactory system and cause loss of smell;
- Genetic factors: in rare cases, genetic conditions can affect a person's ability to smell.
- Neurological conditions: neurological diseases, such as Alzheimer's, Parkinson's, multiple sclerosis, or epilepsy, can affect the sense of smell.

The association between neurodegenerative diseases and smell issues is well established in the literature [2–5,11,19–27]. It is estimated to be present in 90% of patients with early Parkinson's disease (PD) and 85% of patients with early Alzheimer's disease (AD) [28]. Olfactory dysfunction has been reported as a prodromal symptom, which is often given little clinical relevance. Hyposmia is already present in mild cognitive impairment and tends to worsen as the disease progresses; odor identification is the most impaired among the olfactory functions in these patients [3,5,19,29].

In PD, hyposmia is one of the first non-motor signs of the disease [28,30,31], and olfactory hallucinations (phantosmia) are reported in up to 21% of cases [32]. In addition, the olfactory threshold has been proposed as a test to differentiate Lewy bodies dementia (LBD) from Parkinson's dementia, as patients with LBD have a much lower olfactory threshold [33].

Although olfaction is compromised in both AD and PD, Rahayel and colleagues note that olfactory identification and discrimination, which require higher cognitive functions, are more impaired in AD. In contrast, the olfactory threshold is lower in PD [27].

The pathophysiology of olfactory dysfunction in neurodegenerative diseases is unclear.

In an immunocytochemical study, Brozetti et al. found that molecules classically associated with neurodegeneration, such as α-synuclein, β-amyloid, and hyperphosphorylated tau, were present in the olfactory neuroepithelia of healthy subjects. The researchers hypothesize that these proteins are misfolded in response to an unknown stimulus and then transported to the olfactory bulb, gradually forming pathological aggregates. This process would cause the early olfactory impairment observed in diseases such as Alzheimer's and Parkinson's [34].

Furthermore, smell is not only impaired in AD and PD. In multiple sclerosis, olfactory dysfunction has a prevalence of 27.2% [11], and there appears to be a correlation between olfactory bulb volume reduction and hyposmia [35]. According to several meta-analyses, many other neuropsychiatric disorders affect the sense of smell (Table 1). Specifically, olfactory discrimination, impaired in schizophrenia but not in frontotemporal dementia, may contribute to the differential diagnosis between these two disorders [36].

Table 1. Smell function involvement in neuropsychiatric diseases.

Alzheimer's disease and Mild cognitive impairment	Jung et al. 2019 [5]. Roalf et al. 2017 [19]. Rahayel et al. 2012 [27]. Kotecha et al. 2018 [3]. Mesholam et al. 1998 [2].
Parkinson's disease	Mesholam et al. 1998 [2]. Rahayel et al. 2012 [27] Sui et al. 2019 [4]. Lyu et al. 2021 [23]. Alonso et al. 2021 [20] Trentin et al. 2022 [21]
Multiple sclerosis	Mirmosayyeb et al. 2022 [11]
Epilepsy	Khurshid et al. 2019 [22]
Rapid Eye Movement Sleep Behavior Disorder	Lyu et al. 2021 [23].
Autism-spectrum disorders	Crow et al. 2020 [24]
Obsessive–Compulsive Disorder	Crow et al. 2020 [24]
Severe anorexia nervosa	Mai et al. 2020 [25]
Schizophrenia	Carnemolla et al. 2020 [36]
Frontotemporal dementia	Carnemolla et al. 2020 [36] Kamath et al. 2019 [26]

Olfactory Dysfunction Evaluation

Different tests have been developed to test olfactory function. Electrophysiological tests (olfactory evoked potentials, OEPs) are mainly used for research and legal purposes [37]. In clinical practice, the sense of smell can be assessed with relatively simple, non-invasive, and inexpensive tests.

The most widely used and established tests in clinical practice are the Sniffing Stick Test (SST) and the University of Pennsylvania Smell Identification Test (UPSIT) [38].

The SST is a pen-like odor delivery device, designed and developed by Kobal and Hummel [39,40]. This test assesses all three components of olfactory function, expressed in a final score (threshold, discrimination, and identification Score, TDI score).

Odor identification tests ask the patient to identify a series of odors, one at a time, by answering a multiple-choice questionnaire. Odor discrimination tests the individual's ability to identify which of the three odors presented is different from the other two. The odor threshold is a measure of the lowest concentration of an odorant substance that the subject can detect using serial dilutions [41,42].

The UPSIT (University of Pennsylvania Smell Identification Test) is a standardized test to evaluate the olfactory function. It is a scratch-and-sniff test that presents various odors in a multiple-choice format to identify the type of smell.

The UPSIT is widely used in clinical settings to assess the ability to identify different smells and to detect changes or deficiencies in the sense of smell. It helps in diagnosing various conditions related to olfactory dysfunction, such as anosmia (complete loss of smell), hyposmia (reduced sensitivity to smell), or specific smell disorders (Table 2).

Table 2. Smell dysfunctions [43].

Term	Definition
Dysosmia	General term for smell dysfunction
Quantitative smell dysfunction	
Anosmia	Sense of smell is absent or almost absent, with an impact on daily life activity
Hyposmia	Composite TDI score* < 10th percentile
Normosmia	Composite TDI score* > 10th percentile
Hyperosmia	Composite TDI score* > 90th percentile
Qualitative smell dysfunction	
Olfactory intolerance	Intolerance to common odors, unconfirmed with smell tests.
Parosmia	Olfactory dysperception in the presence of a real odor stimulus
Phantosmia	Olfactory dysperception in the absence of a real odor stimulus

* TDI-score: Threshold Discrimination Identification score.

This test provides a quantitative measure of olfactory function, aiding doctors in determining the degree of impairment and monitoring the olfactory dysfunction of smell over time.

3. Glaucoma and Neurodegeneration

Glaucoma is a heterogeneous group of diseases clinically characterized by specific patterns of visual field loss and optic nerve head damage. Diffuse damage to highly specialized neural structures and an insidious onset that causes noticeable symptoms only in the late stages of the disease, make glaucoma the leading cause of irreversible blindness worldwide [12]. Glaucoma is often associated with high intraocular pressure (IOP), which is one of the major risk factors for developing the disease and the only therapeutic target for medical and surgical treatment. For this reason, glaucoma has traditionally been considered a purely ophthalmologic disease. Today, there is increasing evidence [17,18,44–46] that glaucoma should be considered a multifaceted neurodegenerative disease in which IOP is only one piece in a complex mosaic.

Specifically, apoptosis of the retinal ganglion cell (RGC) is the hallmark of glaucoma, but it has been widely shown that other brain structures associated with vision are also involved [17,47].

The RGC is a highly specialized neuron whose cell soma is located in the inner layers of the retina. The axons of these cells converge to form the optic nerve, the chiasm (where they partially cross over), and the optic tract and then form synapses in the lateral geniculate nucleus. The primary visual pathway then continues through optic radiation to the primary cerebral cortex, providing the conscious experience of vision.

Along the retino–geniculo–cortical pathways, visual stimuli are divided into two main systems: the magnocellular and parvocellular systems. The magnocellular system has a faster response time and seems to be specialized for visuospatial perception, motion, and stereopsis, allowing for rapid detection and localization of a moving object in the visual field. The parvocellular system, on the other hand, has a slower response time and provides discriminative cues such as the shape, color, and contrast of the observed object. This allows the object to be examined, recognized, and categorized [17,18]. This topographic map is present in the retina, is replicated in the lateral geniculate nucleus, and is maintained all the way to the visual cortex.

There is evidence in both animal models and humans that glaucoma damages both the parvocellular and magnocellular pathways, but there is no agreement on which one is more impaired [17,18].

Loss of RGCs and their axons causes atrophy of the optic nerve head and inner retinal layers, which can be detected by clinical examination and optical coherence tomography (OCT), and also appears to affect the posterior brain structures of the visual system.

Damage to the posterior visual pathways is suggested by increased latency and reduction of the electrical signal as measured by visual evoked potentials (VEPs) [47].

This widespread cerebral damage has been confirmed by nuclear magnetic resonance (MRI) imaging studies. MRI morphometric analyses have documented that neurodegeneration in glaucoma patients affects not only the optic nerve, chiasm, and optic tract, as might be expected, but also the lateral geniculate nucleus of the thalamus, the optic radiations, and the visual cortex [45,46] Specifically, in glaucoma, trophism and function of the primary visual cortex, as assessed by functional MRI, correlate with both RNFL thickness and perimetric defect [44].

This evidence suggests that the trophism of neurons involved in visual pathways is interdependent, as has been demonstrated in other neurodegenerative diseases, and that atrophy in glaucoma spreads to all the cerebral structures involved in vision. This would be true both from the retina to the brain (anterograde neurodegeneration) and vice versa, from the brain to the retina (retrograde neurodegeneration), via trans-synaptic degeneration [18].

The causes of RGCs loss are not fully understood.

According to the mechanical theory, ocular hypertension is thought to disrupt axoplasmic transport by mechanically compressing the optic nerve bundle through the pores of the lamina cribrosa, [48] inducing apoptosis in RGCs. The lamina cribrosa is a diaphragm between the intraocular and subarachnoid compartments, and the delta between intraocular and intracranial pressure, called the translaminar cribrosa pressure (TLCP) gradient, appears to be involved in the pathogenesis of glaucoma. Thus, not only increased IOP but also decreased cerebrospinal fluid pressure can mechanically deform the lamina cribrosa [48] and damage the optic nerve head.

As highly specialized neurons, RGCs are particularly susceptible to hypoxic injury. Therefore, the ischemic theory suggests that impaired blood flow may promote neurodegeneration in glaucoma; accordingly, increased expression of hypoxia-induced factor 1alpha (HIF-1alpha) has been found in retinal areas corresponding to perimetric scotomas [49]. In addition to the mechanical and ischemic theories, excitotoxicity, oxidative stress, and neuroinflammation also play a role in neurodegeneration [48].

In excitotoxicity, there is an alteration in synaptic homeostasis with excessive glutamate release from the presynaptic neuron and calcium ion accumulation at the postsynaptic neuron. Excess calcium would activate lytic enzymes (lipase, endonuclease, and protease) and nitric oxide synthetase, which would induce cell apoptosis.

Mitochondrial dysfunction and the reduction of antioxidant enzymes also appear to play a role in glaucoma, as does neuroinflammation mediated by astrocytes, microglia, and Müller cells [48].

Glaucoma has a multifactorial complex etiology, and the above pathogenetic mechanisms have been described in other neurodegenerative diseases, particularly Alzheimer's disease [13–15]. In fact, cohort studies have shown an overlap between the risk of developing glaucoma and Alzheimer's disease (Bayer et al. showed a 25.9% prevalence of glaucoma in AD) [50].

Apoptosis is the common step that leads to loss of function, mainly affecting the limbic system in AD and the visual pathways in glaucoma [13].

In line with these data, glaucoma therapy has now fully embraced neuroprotective molecules, such as citicoline [7,51,52], that have been used in Alzheimer's disease therapy [53,54], and other neurotrophins have been studied in glaucoma research [55–57].

As previously mentioned, glaucoma is classically associated with ocular hypertension, one of the main risk factors for developing the disease.

However, the relevance of primary neurodegeneration is particularly evident in cases of normal tension glaucoma (NTG), where the intraocular pressure (IOP) lies within the normal range, but the visual field loss often progresses independently, suggesting a pressure-independent mechanism of neurodegeneration.

The pathogenesis of NTG remains unclear, but several mechanisms have been proposed, including ischemic theory and increased TLCP gradient, which may contribute significantly to neurodegeneration in these patients [58,59].

Specifically, microvascular endothelial dysfunction and abnormal vasoreactivity in response to the sympathetic autonomic nervous system (PVD, primary vascular dysregulation, according to Flammer and colleagues) have been observed, supported by an imbalance between nitric oxide (NO, vasodilator) and endothelin-1 (ET-1, vasoconstrictor) [60]. Reynaud's phenomenon, migraine, and silent cardiovascular and cerebrovascular diseases are often associated with normal tension glaucoma [58,59]. Accordingly, Takahashi et al. found a correlation between abnormal nailfold and optic disc vasoconstriction in response to the cold-water provocation test in NTG patients [61].

NTG appears to be even more related to Alzheimer's disease than glaucoma associated with ocular hypertension. In fact, Tamura et al. found a high prevalence of glaucoma (23.8%) in AD compared to healthy subjects ($p = 0.0002$), with no differences in intraocular pressure [62]. In a 13-year retrospective cohort study, Chen et al. found an increased risk of Alzheimer's disease in normal tension glaucoma (Hazard Ratio 1.52) in the Taiwanese population, supporting the link between these diseases [63].

Another shared feature between glaucoma and AD is the abnormal deposition of proteinaceous aggregates [13]. Plaques of beta-amyloid and tangles of hyperphosphorylated tau protein are the hallmarks of Alzheimer's disease, and pseudoexfoliative glaucoma (PXG) is associated with diffuse deposition of proteinaceous material (pseudoexfoliation syndrome, PXS).

In PXS, these fibrillar deposits can be found in ocular and extraocular tissues, such as the vascular endothelium, skin, heart, liver, lungs, kidneys, meninges, and gallbladder. The ocular complications of PXS include glaucoma and zonular weakness with possible lens dislocation following trauma or surgery [64].

According to the literature, pseudoexfoliation syndrome may be a marker of neurodegeneration and share features with Alzheimer's disease [65]. In fact, both PXS and AD are age-related disorders and involve abnormal protein misfolding and aggregation [13,64]. Furthermore, apolipoprotein E (APOE) and amyloid, which play a key role in the pathogenesis of Alzheimer's disease [13,15,63], were also found in the fibrillar material of PXS [64].

Glaucoma and Alzheimer's are very different diseases, and their pathogeneses are still unclear, but their common features have attracted the attention of researchers.

Could there be a common pathogenetic mechanism that affects both the olfactory and visual systems at the same time, causing glaucoma patients to experience early loss of smell as described in other neurodegenerative diseases?

4. Smell Function and Glaucoma

Unfortunately, this topic has not been widely studied and reported in the literature.

After a literature search, just three articles analyzing glaucoma and olfactory dysfunction were identified and considered (Table 3).

Mozaffarieh and colleagues investigated olfaction in normal tension glaucoma (NTG) [66]. Thirty-six patients with NTG and 36 healthy controls matched for age and sex were enrolled; in both groups, half of the subjects had signs compatible with vasospasm, such as migraine, tinnitus, hypotension, and cold extremities. Olfaction was assessed by self-report and SST. Subjects with vasospasm were significantly better at identifying odors than the others, either by self-report or SST ($p < 0.001$), whether they were glaucomatous or healthy subjects. The difference remained statistically significant even after the results were adjusted for age. This study only uses the 12-item identification test in the olfactory dysfunction evaluation. This is a substantial limitation. The authors speculate that subjects with PVD, who would already have differential gene expression of ATP-binding cassette (ABC) proteins [67], may also have a different gene expression of odorant-binding proteins, which would result in increased odor perception.

Table 3. Smell function and glaucoma.

Authors	*n*	Smell Test	Outcomes
Mozaffarieh, M. et al. (2010) [66]	36 NTG patients and 36 healthy controls; half participants in both groups had PVD.	SST	In both groups, subjects with PVD had better smell outcomes ($p < 0.001$)
Gugleta, K. et al. (2010) [68]	30 POAG patients	SST	Olfactory threshold was significantly lower in POAG than healthy controls ($p = 0.01$)
Dikmetas, O. et al. (2022) [69]	20 POAG patients 20 PXG patients 20 PXS patients	SST	Complex olfactory abnormalities that affected threshold, discrimination, and identification differently in each group. The PXG group showed the worst TDI score.

NTG = normal tension glaucoma; POAG = primary open-angle glaucoma; PXG = pseudoexfoliative glaucoma; PXS = pseudoexfoliative syndrome; PVD = primary vascular dysregulation; SST = Sniffin Stick test; TDI score = threshold discrimination identification score.

Subsequently, Gugleta et al. enrolled 30 patients with primary open-angle glaucoma (POAG) and compared olfactory performance with a healthy control group [68]. While the TDI score did not differ significantly between the two groups, the olfactory threshold was significantly lower in POAG than in healthy controls ($p = 0.01$). Again, patients with evidence of vasospasm, as assessed by a cold extremity and nail capillaroscopy, had a better olfactory threshold compared to POAG patients without vasospasm ($p = 0.036$).

In a cross-sectional study published in 2022, Dikmetas and colleagues investigated olfactory function in POAG and PXG [69]. The researchers included 20 patients with POAG, 20 with PXG, and 20 subjects with PXS without glaucoma. Olfactory performance was assessed using the SST, and significant differences were found between the groups.

Specifically, odor identification was significantly lower in POAG compared to the control group ($p = 0.01$) and in PXG compared to all others ($p < 0.000$ for POAG and PXS $p < 0.02$ for healthy subjects).

Odor discrimination was significantly impaired in subjects with PXG compared to the others ($p < 0.000$ for each group).

Finally, patients with POAG and PXG had a statistically significant impairment in olfactory threshold compared to healthy controls ($p = 0.033$ and $p = 0.001$, respectively).

According to the TDI score, smell function was more compromised in PXG. Olfactory sensitivity was also impaired in POAG compared to healthy subjects and in PXS compared to POAG and healthy subjects.

These data may support that, in glaucoma, as in other neurodegenerative diseases, complex olfactory abnormalities mainly affect odor sensitivity. Furthermore, different types of glaucoma appear to be associated with different olfactory dysfunctions. The authors hypothesize that a possible link between olfactory dysfunction and glaucoma may be related to abnormal accumulation of tau protein, which has been demonstrated in both murine models of Parkinson's disease with olfactory dysfunction [70] and murine models of glaucoma [71].

5. Discussion

The olfactory function has been studied in many neurodegenerative diseases, mainly Alzheimer's and Parkinson's. However, there is little data on olfaction in glaucoma, a neurodegenerative disease of the visual system. Nevertheless, the available data are interesting.

First, not all types of glaucoma affect olfactory function similarly. Mozaffarieh and Gugleta found hyperosmia in their sample, while Dikmetas found reduced olfactory function in patients with PXG compared with PAOG and in POAG compared with the healthy control group [66,68,69].

PXG develops in the context of a PXS, and NTG is often associated with blood-flow abnormalities in response to stimulation of the sympathetic nervous system (PVD, primary vascular dysregulation, according to Flammer and colleagues) [60].

The significance of hyperosmia in patients with primary vascular dysregulation and its possible association with NTG can only be cautiously speculated. The available data suggest that patients with PVD are more likely to experience hyperosmia and may be more prone to develop NTG, and a possible link between hyperosmia, vasospasm, and neurodegeneration should be further investigated.

To summarize the results of these studies, certain predisposing conditions to glaucoma, such as pseudoexfoliation syndrome and primary vascular dysregulation, may possibly induce olfactory changes that can be measured with the Sniffin Stick test.

However, when the olfactory performance of PXS patients is compared with those who developed glaucoma, the latter have worse olfactory function.

In addition, patients with POAG appear to have worse olfaction than healthy subjects, although this is less pronounced than in people with PXG.

More evidence is needed to update clinical practice and incorporate olfactory testing into glaucoma management, as these studies have some limitations. All three studies have small sample sizes. Mozaffarieh and Gugleta focused on PVD, while Dikmetas studied PXG, so the results of the three studies are not fully comparable. None of the studies correlated olfactory function with the visual field, and the possible effects of glaucoma medical therapy on olfaction are not explained. Finally, although the results of these studies are statistically significant, there are no clear hypotheses to justify them. It could be speculated that olfactory neural pathways may be particularly susceptible to non-specific neurodegeneration. This may explain the evidence of olfactory dysfunction in a wide range of neuropsychiatric disorders and possibly in glaucoma.

Although there are few studies on this topic, the possibility that olfaction may be impaired in glaucoma remains attractive and is based on two well-established data in the literature, namely olfactory dysfunction is an early marker in a variety of neurodegenerative diseases, and glaucoma is not limited to the eye but is a complex neurodegenerative disease of the visual system.

Expansion of the sample size and refinement of the protocol may overcome this lack of evidence. If these speculations are confirmed in further research, olfactory testing may be useful in the future to facilitate early diagnosis of glaucoma, e.g., by screening patients with PXS and patients with Raynaud's phenomenon or nail capillaroscopy alterations.

The SST can quantitatively measure olfactory dysfunction. In glaucoma, there appear to be complex olfactory modifications that may alter the olfactory threshold, discrimination, and identification to variable degrees. The TDI score gives an idea of the overall olfactory dysfunction but also provides a precise characterization of each of the olfactory functions. This, combined with the quick administration (15–20 min), makes the SST the most interesting test to assess olfactory function in glaucoma.

As olfactory testing is inexpensive and non-invasive, and glaucoma has a high social burden, it may be worthwhile to investigate further the possible links between the visual and olfactory systems. It may be interesting to assess whether there is a correlation between visual, cognitive, and olfactory function. Furthermore, recent works have correlated pseudoexfoliation syndrome with neurosensory hearing loss [72] and possibly glaucoma [73]. These data suggest that PXS may correlate with multisensory impairment (hyposmia, glaucoma, and hearing loss), opening the possibility of a multidisciplinary approach to screening for sense-organ disorders, which would likely have a positive impact on the quality of life of these patients.

Author Contributions: V.I. conception, planning, literature search, and drafting; A.B., G.V., L.A. and M.S.: drafting and editing (ophthalmology); G.I. and A.G. drafting and editing (otolaryngology); A.G. critical review of the manuscript; A.L. critical review and final supervision of the manuscript. All authors have read and agreed to the published version of the manuscript.

Funding: This publication has been co-funded by the European Union—ESF REACT-EU, PON Research and Innovation 2014–2020.

Institutional Review Board Statement: Not applicable.

Informed Consent Statement: Not applicable.

Data Availability Statement: No new data were created or analyzed in this study. Data sharing is not applicable to this article.

Acknowledgments: V.I. sincerely thanks Antonella Falace for her precious assistance in consulting the literature.

Conflicts of Interest: The authors declare no conflicts of interest.

References

1. Cha, H.; Kim, S.; Seo, M.s.; Kim, H.s. Effects of olfactory stimulation on cognitive function and behavior problems in older adults with dementia: A systematic literature review. *Geriatr. Nurs.* **2021**, *42*, 1210–1217. [CrossRef] [PubMed]
2. Mesholam, R.I.; Moberg, P.J.; Mahr, R.N.; Doty, R.L. Olfaction in Neurodegenerative Disease: A Meta-analysis of Olfactory Functioning in Alzheimer's and Parkinson's Diseases. *Arch. Neurol.* **1998**, *55*, 84. [CrossRef]
3. Kotecha, A.; Corrêa, A.; Fisher, K.; Rushworth, J. Olfactory Dysfunction as a Global Biomarker for Sniffing out Alzheimer's Disease: A Meta-Analysis. *Biosensors* **2018**, *8*, 41. [CrossRef]
4. Sui, X.; Zhou, C.; Li, J.; Chen, L.; Yang, X.; Li, F. Hyposmia as a Predictive Marker of Parkinson's Disease: A Systematic Review and Meta-Analysis. *BioMed Res. Int.* **2019**, *2019*, 3753786. [CrossRef]
5. Jung, H.J.; Shin, I.; Lee, J. Olfactory function in mild cognitive impairment and Alzheimer's disease: A meta-analysis. *Laryngoscope* **2019**, *129*, 362–369. [CrossRef]
6. Knight, J.E.; Yoneda, T.; Lewis, N.A.; Muniz-Terrera, G.; Bennett, D.A.; Piccinin, A.M. Transitions Between Mild Cognitive Impairment, Dementia, and Mortality: The Importance of Olfaction. *J. Gerontol. Ser. A* **2023**, *78*, 1284–1291. [CrossRef] [PubMed]
7. Parisi, V.; Coppola, G.; Centofanti, M.; Oddone, F.; Angrisani, A.M.; Ziccardi, L.; Ricci, B.; Quaranta, L.; Manni, G. Evidence of the neuroprotective role of citicoline in glaucoma patients. In *Progress in Brain Research*; Elsevier: Amsterdam, The Netherlands, 2008; Volume 173, pp. 541–554. [CrossRef]
8. Coppola, G.; Di Renzo, A.; Ziccardi, L.; Martelli, F.; Fadda, A.; Manni, G.; Barboni, P.; Pierelli, F.; Sadun, A.A.; Parisi, V. Optical Coherence Tomography in Alzheimer's Disease: A Meta-Analysis. *PLoS ONE* **2015**, *10*, e0134750. [CrossRef] [PubMed]
9. Trebbastoni, A.; D'antonio, F.; Bruscolini, A.; Marcelli, M.; Cecere, M.; Campanelli, A.; Imbriano, L.; de Lena, C.; Gharbiya, M. Retinal nerve fibre layer thickness changes in Alzheimer's disease: Results from a 12-month prospective case series. *Neurosci. Lett.* **2016**, *629*, 165–170. [CrossRef]
10. Lee, Y.W.; Lim, M.N.; Lee, J.Y.; Yoo, Y.J. Central retina thickness measured with spectral-domain optical coherence tomography in Parkinson disease: A meta-analysis. *Medicine* **2023**, *102*, e35354. [CrossRef]
11. Mirmosayyeb, O.; Ebrahimi, N.; Barzegar, M.; Afshari-Safavi, A.; Bagherieh, S.; Shaygannejad, V. Olfactory dysfunction in patients with multiple sclerosis; A systematic review and meta-analysis. *PLoS ONE* **2022**, *17*, e0266492. [CrossRef]
12. Tham, Y.C.; Li, X.; Wong, T.Y.; Quigley, H.A.; Aung, T.; Cheng, C.Y. Global Prevalence of Glaucoma and Projections of Glaucoma Burden through 2040. *Ophthalmology* **2014**, *121*, 2081–2090. [CrossRef] [PubMed]
13. Saccà, S.C.; Paluan, F.; Gandolfi, S.; Manni, G.; Cutolo, C.A.; Izzotti, A. Common aspects between glaucoma and brain neurodegeneration. *Mutat. Res. Rev. Mutat. Res.* **2020**, *786*, 108323. [CrossRef] [PubMed]
14. Zheng, C.; Liu, S.; Zhang, X.; Hu, Y.; Shang, X.; Zhu, Z.; Huang, Y.; Wu, G.; Xiao, Y.; Du, Z.; et al. Shared genetic architecture between the two neurodegenerative diseases: Alzheimer's disease and glaucoma. *Front. Aging Neurosci.* **2022**, *14*, 880576. [CrossRef] [PubMed]
15. Sen, S.; Saxena, R.; Tripathi, M.; Vibha, D.; Dhiman, R. Neurodegeneration in Alzheimer's disease and glaucoma: Overlaps and missing links. *Eye* **2020**, *34*, 1546–1553. [CrossRef] [PubMed]
16. Chan, J.W.; Chan, N.C.; Sadun, A.A. Glaucoma as Neurodegeneration in the Brain. *EB* **2021**, *13*, 21–28. [CrossRef]
17. Yücel, Y.; Gupta, N. Glaucoma of the brain: A disease model for the study of transsynaptic neural degeneration. In *Progress in Brain Research*; Elsevier: Amsterdam, The Netherlands, 2008; Volume 173, pp. 465–478. [CrossRef]
18. You, M.; Rong, R.; Zeng, Z.; Xia, X.; Ji, D. Transneuronal Degeneration in the Brain During Glaucoma. *Front. Aging Neurosci.* **2021**, *13*, 643685. [CrossRef] [PubMed]
19. Roalf, D.R.; Moberg, M.J.; Turetsky, B.I.; Brennan, L.; Kabadi, S.; Wolk, D.A.; Moberg, P.J. A quantitative meta-analysis of olfactory dysfunction in mild cognitive impairment. *J. Neurol. Neurosurg. Psychiatry* **2017**, *88*, 226–232. [CrossRef]

20. Alonso, C.C.G.; Silva, F.G.; Costa, L.O.P.; Freitas, S.M.S.F. Smell tests can discriminate Parkinson's disease patients from healthy individuals: A meta-analysis. *Clin. Neurol. Neurosurg.* **2021**, *211*, 107024. [CrossRef] [PubMed]
21. Trentin, S.; Fraiman de Oliveira, B.S.; Ferreira Felloni Borges, Y.; de Mello Rieder, C.R. Systematic review and meta-analysis of Sniffin Sticks Test performance in Parkinson's disease patients in different countries. *Eur. Arch. Otorhinolaryngol.* **2022**, *279*, 1123–1145. [CrossRef]
22. Khurshid, K.; Crow, A.J.D.; Rupert, P.E.; Minniti, N.L.; Carswell, M.A.; Mechanic-Hamilton, D.J.; Kamath, V.; Doty, R.L.; Moberg, P.J.; Roalf, D.R. A Quantitative Meta-analysis of Olfactory Dysfunction in Epilepsy. *Neuropsychol. Rev.* **2019**, *29*, 328–337. [CrossRef]
23. Lyu, Z.; Zheng, S.; Zhang, X.; Mai, Y.; Pan, J.; Hummel, T.; Hähner, A.; Zou, L. Olfactory impairment as an early marker of Parkinson's disease in REM sleep behaviour disorder: A systematic review and meta-analysis. *J. Neurol. Neurosurg. Psychiatry* **2021**, *92*, 271–281. [CrossRef] [PubMed]
24. Crow, A.J.D.; Janssen, J.M.; Vickers, K.L.; Parish-Morris, J.; Moberg, P.J.; Roalf, D.R. Olfactory Dysfunction in Neurodevelopmental Disorders: A Meta-analytic Review of Autism Spectrum Disorders, Attention Deficit/Hyperactivity Disorder and Obsessive–Compulsive Disorder. *J. Autism. Dev. Disord.* **2020**, *50*, 2685–2697. [CrossRef] [PubMed]
25. Mai, Y.; Zhang, X.; Li, Z.; Wu, X.; Zeng, B.; Fang, Y.; Zou, L.; Zhao, J.; Hummel, T. Olfaction is a Marker of Severity but Not Diagnosis in Anorexia Nervosa: A Systematic Review and Meta-Analysis. *Neuropsychol. Rev.* **2020**, *30*, 251–266. [CrossRef]
26. Kamath, V.; Chaney, G.A.S.; DeRight, J.; Onyike, C.U. A meta-analysis of neuropsychological, social cognitive, and olfactory functioning in the behavioral and language variants of frontotemporal dementia. *Psychol. Med.* **2019**, *49*, 2669–2680. [CrossRef] [PubMed]
27. Rahayel, S.; Frasnelli, J.; Joubert, S. The effect of Alzheimer's disease and Parkinson's disease on olfaction: A meta-analysis. *Behav. Brain Res.* **2012**, *231*, 60–74. [CrossRef] [PubMed]
28. Dan, X.; Wechter, N.; Gray, S.; Mohanty, J.G.; Croteau, D.L.; Bohr, V.A. Olfactory dysfunction in aging and neurodegenerative diseases. *Ageing Res. Rev.* **2021**, *70*, 101416. [CrossRef] [PubMed]
29. Silva, M.d.M.e.; Mercer, P.B.S.; Witt, M.C.Z.; Pessoa, R.R. Olfactory dysfunction in Alzheimer's disease Systematic review and meta-analysis. *Dement. Neuropsychol.* **2018**, *12*, 123–132. [CrossRef]
30. Bang, Y.; Lim, J.; Choi, H.J. Recent advances in the pathology of prodromal non-motor symptoms olfactory deficit and depression in Parkinson's disease: Clues to early diagnosis and effective treatment. *Arch. Pharm. Res.* **2021**, *44*, 588–604. [CrossRef]
31. Fatuzzo, I.; Niccolini, G.F.; Zoccali, F.; Cavalcanti, L.; Bellizzi, M.G.; Riccardi, G.; de Vincentiis, M.; Fiore, M.; Petrella, C.; Minni, A.; et al. Neurons, Nose, and Neurodegenerative Diseases: Olfactory Function and Cognitive Impairment. *Int. J. Mol. Sci.* **2023**, *24*, 2117. [CrossRef]
32. Toh, W.L.; Yolland, C.; Gurvich, C.; Barnes, J.; Rossell, S.L. Non-visual hallucinations in Parkinson's disease: A systematic review. *J. Neurol.* **2023**, *270*, 2857–2889. [CrossRef]
33. Fogue, C.; Lemdani, M.; Huart, C. Nasal chemosensory tests: Biomarker between dementia with Lewy bodies and Parkinson disease dementia. *J. Rhinol.* **2020**, *58*, 605–609. [CrossRef] [PubMed]
34. Brozzetti, L.; Sacchetto, L.; Cecchini, M.P.; Avesani, A.; Perra, D.; Bongianni, M.; Portioli, C.; Scupoli, M.; Ghetti, B.; Monaco, S.; et al. Neurodegeneration-Associated Proteins in Human Olfactory Neurons Collected by Nasal Brushing. *Front. Neurosci.* **2020**, *14*, 145. [CrossRef] [PubMed]
35. Goektas, O.; Schmidt, F.; Bohner, G.; Erb, K.; Ludemann, L.; Dahlslett, B.; Harms, L.; Fleiner, F. Olfactory bulb volume and olfactory function in patients with multiple sclerosis. *Rhin.* **2011**, *49*, 221–226. [CrossRef] [PubMed]
36. Carnemolla, S.E.; Hsieh, J.W.; Sipione, R.; Landis, B.N.; Kumfor, F.; Piguet, O.; Manuel, A.L. Olfactory dysfunction in frontotemporal dementia and psychiatric disorders: A systematic review. *Neurosci. Biobehav. Rev.* **2020**, *118*, 588–611. [CrossRef] [PubMed]
37. Simmen, D.; Briner, H.R. Olfaction in rhinology—Methods of assessing the sense of smell. *Rhinology* **2006**, *44*, 98–101. [PubMed]
38. Saltagi, A.K.; Saltagi, M.Z.; Nag, A.K.; Wu, A.W.; Higgins, T.S.; Knisely, A.; Ting, J.Y.; Illing, E.A. Diagnosis of Anosmia and Hyposmia: A Systematic Review. *Allergy Rhinol.* **2021**, *12*, 21526567211026568. [CrossRef] [PubMed]
39. Hummel, T.; Sekinger, B.; Wolf, S.R.; Pauli, E.; Kobal, G. 'Sniffin' Sticks': Olfactory Performance Assessed by the Combined Testing of Odour Identification, Odor Discrimination and Olfactory Threshold. *Chem. Senses* **1997**, *22*, 39–52. [CrossRef]
40. Kobal, G.; Klimek, L.; Wolfensberger, M.; Gudziol, H.; Temmel, A.; Owen, C.M.; Seeber, H.; Pauli, E.; Hummel, T. Multicenter investigation of 1,036 subjects using a standardized method for the assessment of olfactory function combining tests of odor identification, odor discrimination, and olfactory thresholds. *Eur. Arch. Oto-Rhino-Laryngol.* **2000**, *257*, 205–211. [CrossRef] [PubMed]
41. Rumeau, C.; Nguyen, D.T.; Jankowski, R. How to assess olfactory performance with the Sniffin' Sticks test ®. *Eur. Ann. Otorhinolaryngol. Head Neck Dis.* **2016**, *133*, 203–206. [CrossRef]
42. Doty, R.L.; Shaman, P.; Dann, M. Development of the university of pennsylvania smell identification test: A standardized microencapsulated test of olfactory function. *Physiol. Behav.* **1984**, *32*, 489–502. [CrossRef]
43. Hernandez, A.K.; Landis, B.; Altundag, A.; Fjaeldstad, A.W.; Gane, S.; Holbrook, E.H.; Huart, C.; Konstantinidis, I.; Lechner, M.; Macchi, A.; et al. Olfactory Nomenclature: An Orchestrated Effort to Clarify Terms and Definitions of Dysosmia, Anosmia, Hyposmia, Normosmia, Hyperosmia, Olfactory Intolerance, Parosmia, and Phantosmia/Olfactory Hallucination. *ORL* **2023**, *85*, 312–320. [CrossRef] [PubMed]
44. Yu, L.; Xie, L.; Dai, C.; Xie, B.; Liang, M.; Zhao, L.; Yin, X.; Wang, J. Progressive Thinning of Visual Cortex in Primary Open-Angle Glaucoma of Varying Severity. *PLoS ONE* **2015**, *10*, e0121960. [CrossRef] [PubMed]

45. Chen, W.W.; Wang, N.; Cai, S.; Fang, Z.; Yu, M.; Wu, Q.; Tang, L.; Guo, B.; Feng, Y.; Jonas, J.B.; et al. Structural Brain Abnormalities in Patients with Primary Open-Angle Glaucoma: A Study with 3T MR Imaging. *Investig. Ophthalmol. Vis. Sci.* **2013**, *54*, 545. [CrossRef] [PubMed]
46. Zhou, W.; Muir, E.R.; Chalfin, S.; Nagi, K.S.; Duong, T.Q. MRI Study of the Posterior Visual Pathways in Primary Open Angle Glaucoma. *J. Glaucoma* **2017**, *26*, 173–181. [CrossRef]
47. Parisi, V. Neural conduction in the visual pathways in ocular hypertension and glaucoma. *Graefes Arch. Clin. Exp. Ophthalmol.* **1997**, *235*, 136–142. [CrossRef] [PubMed]
48. Mastropasqua, L. *Ophthalmology Up-to-Date*; Fabiano: Asti, Italy, 2023; Volume 1, ISBN 9788831256575.
49. Tezel, G. Hypoxia-Inducible Factor 1α in the Glaucomatous Retina and OpticNerve Head. *Arch. Ophthalmol.* **2004**, *122*, 1348. [CrossRef] [PubMed]
50. Bayer, A.U.; Ferrari, F.; Erb, C. High Occurrence Rate of Glaucoma among Patients with Alzheimer's Disease. *Eur. Neurol.* **2002**, *47*, 165–168. [CrossRef]
51. Rossetti, L.; Iester, M.; Tranchina, L.; Ottobelli, L.; Coco, G.; Calcatelli, E.; Ancona, C.; Cirafici, P.; Manni, G. Can Treatment With Citicoline Eyedrops Reduce Progression in Glaucoma? The Results of a Randomized Placebo-controlled Clinical Trial. *J. Glaucoma* **2020**, *29*, 513–520. [CrossRef]
52. Rossetti, L.; Goni, F.; Montesano, G.; Stalmans, I.; Topouzis, F.; Romano, D.; Galantin, E.; Delgado-Gonzales, N.; Giammaria, S.; Coco, G.; et al. The effect of citicoline oral solution on quality of life in patients with glaucoma: The results of an international, multicenter, randomized, placebo-controlled cross-over trial. *Graefes Arch. Clin. Exp. Ophthalmol.* **2023**, *261*, 1659–1668. [CrossRef]
53. Bonvicini, M.; Travaglini, S.; Lelli, D.; Antonelli Incalzi, R.; Pedone, C. Is Citicoline Effective in Preventing and Slowing Down Dementia?—A Systematic Review and a Meta-Analysis. *Nutrients* **2023**, *15*, 386. [CrossRef]
54. Piamonte, B.L.C.; Espiritu, A.I.; Anlacan, V.M.M. Effects of Citicoline as an Adjunct Treatment for Alzheimer's Disease: A Systematic Review. *JAD* **2020**, *76*, 725–732. [CrossRef] [PubMed]
55. Mallone, F.; Sacchetti, M.; Bruscolini, A.; Scuderi, L.; Marenco, M.; Lambiase, A. Neurotrophic Factors in Glaucoma and Innovative Delivery Systems. *Appl. Sci.* **2020**, *10*, 9015. [CrossRef]
56. Oddone, F.; Roberti, G.; Micera, A.; Busanello, A.; Bonini, S.; Quaranta, L.; Agnifili, L.; Manni, G. Exploring Serum Levels of Brain Derived Neurotrophic Factor and Nerve Growth Factor Across Glaucoma Stages. *PLoS ONE* **2017**, *12*, e0168565. [CrossRef] [PubMed]
57. Lambiase, A.; Aloe, L.; Centofanti, M.; Parisi, V.; Bao, S.N.; Mantelli, F.; Colafrancesco, V.; Manni, G.L.; Bucci, M.G.; Bonini, S.; et al. Experimental and clinical evidence of neuroprotection by nerve growth factor eye drops: Implications for glaucoma. *Proc. Natl. Acad. Sci. USA* **2009**, *106*, 13469–13474. [CrossRef] [PubMed]
58. Fan, N.; Wang, P.; Tang, L.; Liu, X. Ocular Blood Flow and Normal Tension Glaucoma. *BioMed Res. Int.* **2015**, *2015*, 308505. [CrossRef] [PubMed]
59. Leung, D.Y.L.; Tham, C.C. Normal-tension glaucoma: Current concepts and approaches—A review. *Clin. Exp. Ophthalmol.* **2022**, *50*, 247–259. [CrossRef] [PubMed]
60. Flammer, J.; Konieczka, K.; Flammer, A.J. The primary vascular dysregulation syndrome: Implications for eye diseases. *EPMA J.* **2013**, *4*, 14. [CrossRef] [PubMed]
61. Takahashi, N.; Kiyota, N.; Kunikata, H.; Yamazaki, M.; Nishimura, T.; Shiga, Y.; Aoyagi, H.; Shidomi, M.; Tsuda, T.; Ohtsuka, T.; et al. Vasoreactivity of the optic nerve head, nailfold, and facial skin in response to cold provocation in normal-tension glaucoma patients. *BMC Ophthalmol.* **2023**, *23*, 316. [CrossRef] [PubMed]
62. Tamura, H.; Kawakami, H.; Kanamoto, T.; Kato, T.; Yokoyama, T.; Sasaki, K.; Izumi, Y.; Matsumoto, M.; Mishima, H.K. High frequency of open-angle glaucoma in Japanese patients with Alzheimer's disease. *J. Neurol. Sci.* **2006**, *246*, 79–83. [CrossRef]
63. Chen, Y.Y.; Lai, Y.J.; Yen, Y.F.; Shen, Y.C.; Wang, C.Y.; Liang, C.Y.; Lin, K.H.; Fan, L.W. Association between normal tension glaucoma and the risk of Alzheimer's disease: A nationwide population-based cohort study in Taiwan. *BMJ Open* **2018**, *8*, e022987. [CrossRef]
64. Padhy, B.; Alone, D.P. Is pseudoexfoliation glaucoma a neurodegenerative disorder? *J. Biosci.* **2021**, *46*, 97. [CrossRef]
65. Jeong, W.C.; Min, J.Y.; Kang, T.G.; Bae, H. Association between pseudoexfoliation and Alzheimer's disease-related brain atrophy. *PLoS ONE* **2023**, *18*, e0286727. [CrossRef] [PubMed]
66. Mozaffarieh, M.; Hauenstein, D.; Schoetzau, A.; Konieczka, K.; Flammer, J. Smell perception in normal tension glaucoma patients. *Mol. Vis.* **2010**, *16*, 506–510. [PubMed]
67. Wunderlich, K.; Zimmerman, C.; Gutmann, H.; Teuchner, B.; Flammer, J.; Drewe, J. Vasospastic persons exhibit differential expression of ABC-transport proteins. *Mol. Vis.* **2003**, *9*, 756–761. [PubMed]
68. Gugleta, K.; Kochkorov, A.; Katamay, R.; Husner, A.; Welge-Lüssen, A.; Flammer, J.; Orgül, S. Olfactory Function in Primary Open-Angle Glaucoma Patients. *Klin. Monatsbl. Augenheilkd.* **2010**, *227*, 277–279. [CrossRef] [PubMed]
69. Dikmetas, O.; Aygün, O.; Kocabeyoglu, S.; Süslü, A.E.; Kilic, B.; Karakaya, J.; Iester, M.; Irkec, M. Smell Sensitivity in Primary Open-angle Glaucoma and Pseudoexfoliation Glaucoma. *J. Glaucoma* **2022**, *31*, 300–304. [CrossRef]
70. Chiasseu, M.; Cueva Vargas, J.L.; Destroismaisons, L.; Vande Velde, C.; Leclerc, N.; Di Polo, A. Tau Accumulation, Altered Phosphorylation, and Missorting Promote Neurodegeneration in Glaucoma. *J. Neurosci.* **2016**, *36*, 5785–5798. [CrossRef]
71. Beauchamp, L.C.; Chan, J.; Hung, L.W.; Padman, B.S.; Vella, L.J.; Liu, X.M.; Coleman, B.; Bush, A.I.; Lazarou, M.; Hill, A.F.; et al. Ablation of tau causes an olfactory deficit in a murine model of Parkinson's disease. *Acta Neuropathol. Commun.* **2018**, *6*, 57. [CrossRef]

72. Shih, M.C.; Gordis, T.M.; Lambert, P.R.; Nguyen, S.A.; Meyer, T.A. Hearing Loss in Exfoliation Syndrome: Systematic Review and Meta-Analysis. *Laryngoscope* **2023**, *133*, 1025–1035. [CrossRef]
73. Meliante, L.A.; Piccotti, G.; Tanga, L.; Giammaria, S.; Manni, G.; Coco, G. Glaucoma, Pseudoexfoliation and Hearing Loss: A Systematic Literature Review. *J. Clin. Med.* **2024**, *13*, 1379. [CrossRef]

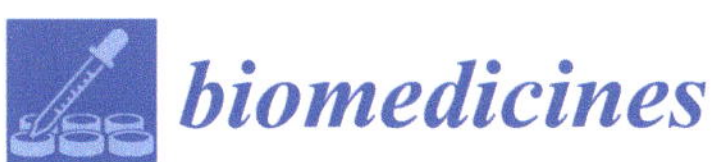 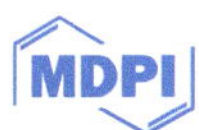

Article

Immune Analysis Using Vitreous Optical Coherence Tomography Imaging in Rats with Steroid-Induced Glaucoma

Maria J. Rodrigo [1,2,3], Manuel Subías [1,2,4], Alberto Montolío [5,6], Teresa Martínez-Rincón [1,2], Alba Aragón-Navas [7,8,9], Irene Bravo-Osuna [7,8,9], Luis E. Pablo [1,2,3,4], Jose Cegoñino [5,6], Rocío Herrero-Vanrell [7,8,9], Elena Garcia-Martin [1,2,3,*] and Amaya Pérez del Palomar [5,6]

1 Department of Ophthalmology, Miguel Servet University Hospital, 50009 Zaragoza, Spain; mariajesusrodrigo@hotmail.es (M.J.R.); manusubias@gmail.com (M.S.); teresamrincon@gmail.com (T.M.-R.); lpablo@unizar.es (L.E.P.)
2 Miguel Servet Ophthalmology Research Group (GIMSO), Aragon Health Research Institute (IIS Aragon), University of Zaragoza, 50009 Zaragoza, Spain
3 National Ocular Researcha Network RD21/0002/0050, RICORS Red de Enfermedades Inflamatorias (RD21/0002), Carlos III Health Institute, 28220 Madrid, Spain
4 Biotech Vision, Instituto Oftalmologico Quiron, 50012 Zaragoza, Spain
5 Biomaterials Group, Aragon Engineering Research Institute (I3A), University of Zaragoza, 50018 Zaragoza, Spain; amontolio@unizar.es (A.M.); jcegoni@unizar.es (J.C.); amaya@unizar.es (A.P.d.P.)
6 Department of Mechanical Engineering, University of Zaragoza, 50018 Zaragoza, Spain
7 Innovation, Therapy and Pharmaceutical Development in Ophthalmology (InnOftal) Research Group, UCM 920415, Department of Pharmaceutics and Food Technology, Faculty of Pharmacy, Complutense University of Madrid, 28040 Madrid, Spain; albarago@ucm.es (A.A.-N.); ibravo@ucm.es (I.B.-O.); rociohv@ucm.es (R.H.-V.)
8 Health Research Institute of the San Carlos Clinical Hospital (IdISSC), 28040 Madrid, Spain
9 University Institute of Industrial Pharmacy (IUFI), School of Pharmacy, Complutense University of Madrid, 28040 Madrid, Spain
* Correspondence: egmvivax@yahoo.com; Tel.: +34-976765558; Fax: +34-976566234

Citation: Rodrigo, M.J.; Subías, M.; Montolío, A.; Martínez-Rincón, T.; Aragón-Navas, A.; Bravo-Osuna, I.; Pablo, L.E.; Cegoñino, J.; Herrero-Vanrell, R.; Garcia-Martin, E.; et al. Immune Analysis Using Vitreous Optical Coherence Tomography Imaging in Rats with Steroid-Induced Glaucoma. *Biomedicines* **2024**, *12*, 633. https://doi.org/10.3390/biomedicines12030633

Academic Editor: James A. Marrs

Received: 3 February 2024
Revised: 24 February 2024
Accepted: 1 March 2024
Published: 13 March 2024

Abstract: Glaucoma is a multifactorial pathology involving the immune system. The subclinical immune response plays a homeostatic role in healthy situations, but in pathological situations, it produces imbalances. Optical coherence tomography detects immune cells in the vitreous as hyperreflective opacities and these are subsequently characterised by computational analysis. This study monitors the changes in immunity in the vitreous in two steroid-induced glaucoma (SIG) animal models created with drug delivery systems (microspheres loaded with dexamethasone and dexamethasone/fibronectin), comparing both sexes and healthy controls over six months. SIG eyes tended to present greater intensity and a higher number of vitreous opacities ($p < 0.05$), with dynamic fluctuations in the percentage of isolated cells (10 μm^2), non-activated cells (10–50 μm^2), activated cells (50–250 μm^2) and cell complexes (>250 μm^2). Both SIG models presented an anti-inflammatory profile, with non-activated cells being the largest population in this study. However, smaller opacities (isolated cells) seemed to be the first responder to noxa since they were the most rounded (recruitment), coinciding with peak intraocular pressure increase, and showed the highest mean Intensity (intracellular machinery), even in the contralateral eye, and a major change in orientation (motility). Studying the features of hyperreflective opacities in the vitreous using OCT could be a useful biomarker of glaucoma.

Keywords: optical coherence tomography; vitreous body; glaucoma; animal models; inflammation

1. Introduction

Chronic glaucoma is a leading cause of irreversible blindness in the world [1]. Increase in intraocular pressure (IOP) is a risk factor strongly associated with the onset and progression of this optic neuropathy. However, several studies have indicated that the pathogenesis of the disease is multifactorial, and the immune perspective seems to be of great relevance [2]. Residential glial cells are found to become activated in the early stages of glaucoma. Elevated IOP triggers secondary responses responsible for retinal ganglion cell (RGC) degeneration. Although the primary response may be favourable in protecting the eye, the subsequent events that lead to long-lasting activation of glial cells and adaptive immune responses can be destructive [3]. RGC death results in irreversible visual field impairment [4,5] that is only detectable once 25–30% of RGCs is lost, leading to delayed diagnosis. It is therefore essential to develop new tools and markers to enable earlier detection. Furthermore, the association between autoimmunity and progressive neuron loss in glaucoma may also allow the development of novel therapeutic interventions that eventually offer a cure for the disease.

Immune cells present different morphologies based on their state of activation [6–8]. Soma size, analysed by in vivo fluorescence imaging, was proposed as a significant marker of immune activation in the brain [6] and retina of glaucomatous mice [9]. Microglial activation (Iba1+ staining) appears to be the earliest detectable change in the retina [10] that strongly correlates with and predicts the severity of glaucomatous neurodegeneration [11]. Very few studies, however, have extensively analysed the vitreous in entities with parainflammation [12]. Hyalocytes [13] are resident vitreous cells that participate in immune regulation by means of phagocytic activity and their contractile properties. In response to noxa, they are replaced and increase their mitotic activity. All these changes are postulated as early biomarkers of value for diagnosing ocular diseases [14].

Optical coherence tomography (OCT) is an objective, fast and cost-efficient technology that allows in vivo acquisition of high-resolution cross-sectional images micrometres from the eye structures. Latest-generation OCT systems allow non-invasive evaluation of the vitreous in acute and chronic inflammatory processes under standard clinical conditions. They also allow evaluation of the changes that occur after treatment [15–17]. In our previous paper on the use of computational OCT image analysis, we demonstrated that hyalocyte-like Iba1+ cells were observed as hyperreflective opacities and described their behaviour in the active/non-active state by characterising them in terms of size, intensity, eccentricity and orientation in two chronic glaucoma models in rats with ocular hypertension (OHT) [18].

This paper aims to corroborate the reliability of using computational OCT image analysis of hyperreflective opacities in the vitreous as a biomarker of vitreous immunity, in this case in two chronic steroid-induced glaucoma (SIG) rat models previously developed by our research group by injecting biodegradable microspheres (Ms) loaded with dexamethasone (MsDx) and a combination of dexamethasone and fibronectin (MsDxF) (with sustained release of the active compounds) into the anterior chamber of the eye [19,20]. Chronic exposure to glucocorticoids can raise IOP and is known to exert a negative effect in the form of maladaptive glial cell alterations and neuron damage or loss [21], leading to SIG [22]. We corroborate and validate the computational analysis of the individual hyperreflective opacities as a better technique than the overall relative measure of immunity using OCT. The study of eccentricity, intensity and orientation characteristics of vitreous opacities using OCT is a reproducible and reliable method of non-invasive assessment of SIG.

2. Materials and Methods

2.1. Data Collection

The dataset comprised images of the vitreoretinal interface obtained using OCT (HR-OCT Spectralis, Heidelberg® Engineering, Heidelberg, Germany) in two previous interventional studies on the generation of steroid-induced glaucoma models (MsDx and MsDxF) [19,20], which detail the methodology followed. The experiment was previously approved by the Ethics Committee for Animal Research (PI34/17) of the University of Zaragoza (Spain) and was carried out in strict accordance with the Association for

Research in Vision and Ophthalmology's Statement on the Use of Animals. The MsDx model was generated by injecting a 2-microlitre suspension (10% w) of biodegradable PLGA microspheres [23] loaded with dexamethasone into the anterior chamber of Long–Evans rats' right eyes at 0 and 4 weeks [19]. The second model (MsDxF) was generated by administering a 2-microlitre suspension (10% w) of biodegradable PLGA microspheres co-loaded with dexamethasone and fibronectin at baseline in a single injection [20]. The left eyes did not undergo intervention. IOP (using a Tonolab® rebound tonometer) measurement and OCT scans of both eyes were performed at 0, 2, 4, 6, 8, 12, 18 and 24 weeks. A cohort that did not undergo intervention served as the control and was scanned at 0, 12 and 24 weeks.

2.2. Image Analysis

Images were acquired using a high-resolution OCT device with a plane power polymethylmethacrylate contact lens (thickness 270 μm, diameter 5.2 mm) (Cantor+Nissel®, Northamptonshire, Northampton, UK) adapted to the rat cornea [24]. The retinal posterior pole protocol with automatic segmentation, eye-tracking software and a tracking application were used to ensure that the same points were re-scanned throughout this study. "Enhance depth imaging" mode was disabled in all cases.

The raw OCT images were exported in Audio Video Interleave (AVI) format. In the rodent version of this OCT device, the videos were composed of cross-sectional images acquired from 61 3 mm long B-scans centred on the optic nerve. These cross-sectional images had a resolution of 3 μm/pixel and an area of 2.906 mm^2 (1536 × 496 pixels). Therefore, each pixel had an area of 3.815 μm^2. These videos were analysed using a custom program implemented in MatLab (version R218a, MathWorks Inc., Natick, MA, USA). The imaging data were analysed by a masked reader. Two different researchers, likewise masked, performed OCT segmentation to verify reproducibility.

In order to measure the immune response, relative intensity in the vitreous/retinal pigment epithelium (VIT/RPE) was quantified [15,25,26]. Our customised program segments the vitreous and RPE by locating the inner limiting membrane (ILM) and the inner and outer layers of the RPE using greyscale conversion (Figure 1). VIT/RPE intensity was calculated as the mean of the pixel intensity in each region, giving VIT/RPE relative intensity in each cross-sectional image. VIT/RPE relative intensity in each eye is the mean of all B-scans.

The vitreous opacities in each cross-sectional image were analysed as they are closely related to the immune cells. OCT analysis of hyperreflective opacities in the vitreoretinal interface does not require a correction factor for histological correlation [27] and ensures the characterisation of the actual opacity. These opacities were classified according to size based on previous morphological analyses of retinal microglia and histological analyses of hyalocytes [28]. Soma size can be used to discriminate between non-activated and activated cells, as the morphology of microglia varies according to their state of activation: the smallest cells (corresponding to early growth) have a rounded or amoeboid morphology; resting (non-activated) cells have a thin cell body with branched cellular processes; and reactive (activated) cells have a larger somatic size and exhibit phagocytic activity and motility [6,7].

Our custom program automatically measured hyperreflective opacities and classified them into groups according to their size: isolated cells (<10 μm^2), non-activated cells (10–50 μm^2), activated cells (50–250 μm^2) and cell complexes (>250 μm^2). The size of the opacities was calculated according to the number of pixels in each opacity. Background intensity is lower than opacity intensity; therefore, background speckle noise was removed to ensure the measurement of hyperreflective opacities (see Figure 1). In this way, the physiological ocular phenomena were eliminated [29].

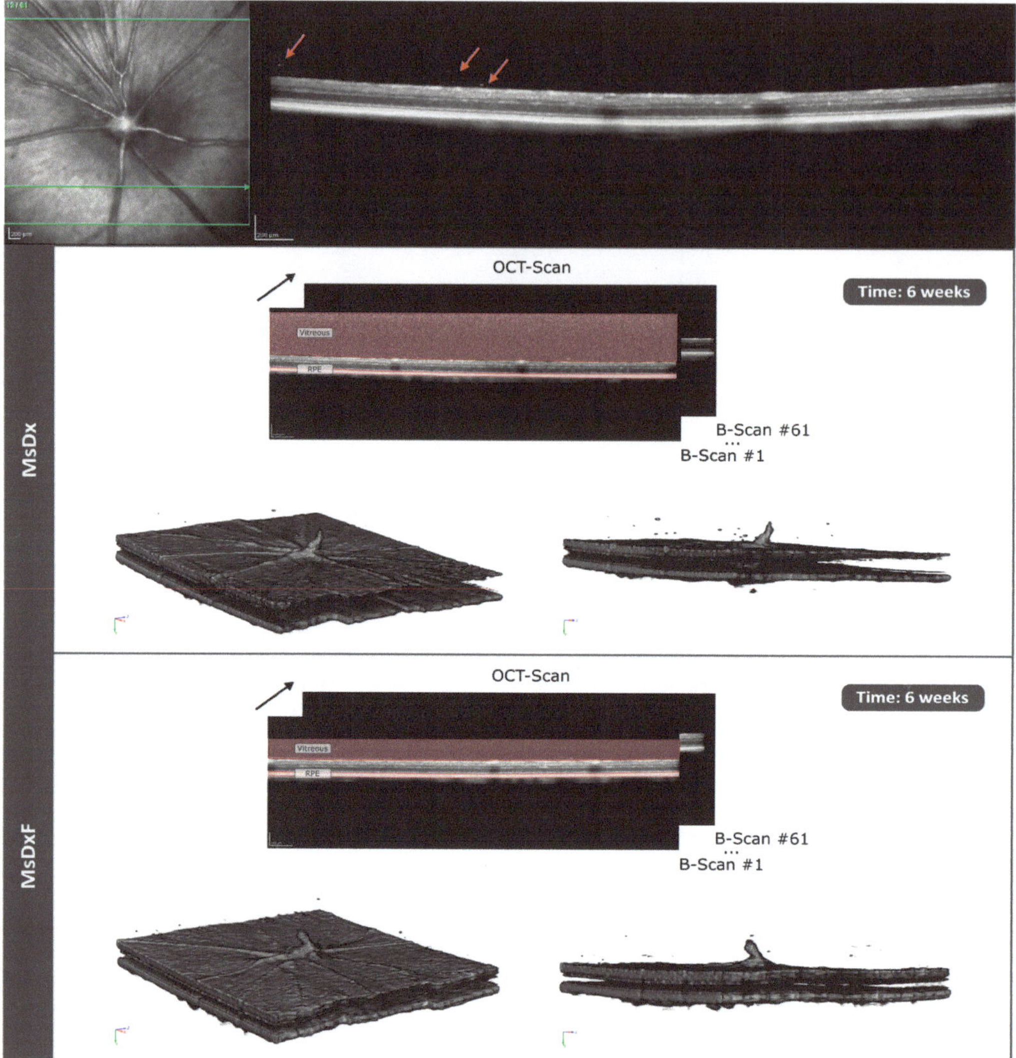

Figure 1. OCT scan and 3D reconstruction of 61 right-eye B-scans in two models of steroid-induced glaucoma at 6 weeks' follow-up. The black arrow indicates image sequencing by optical coherence tomography (serial slices). Abbreviations: MsDx: cohort with microspheres loaded with dexamethasone; MsDxF: cohort with microspheres loaded with dexamethasone and fibronectin injected into the anterior chamber; OCT: optical coherence tomography; RPE: retinal pigment epithelium. Red arrows show the vitreous opacities.

Several parameters can be calculated for each opacity. The total cell area, calculated by the number of opacities and the area of each opacity, represented the overall immune response to the induced glaucoma model. The mean number of opacities was an indicator of immunity to noxa over time, allowing analysis of in situ resident immune cellularity and intra- or extra-ocular recruitment [30–33]. The mean area of opacities was calculated for all cells and for each group according to cell size, attaining reliable cell soma reproducibility.

The changing proportion between the activated and non-activated cell populations was analysed by quantifying the cell percentage for each group.

Opacity/cell intensity, calculated as the mean of the intensity of each pixel in the opacity, is related to immune activation because it implies gene–protein expression prior to soma remodelling. Eccentricity was also calculated: values close to 1 indicate linear, elongated or flat cell morphology, while values close to 0 represent a rounded shape. Opacity/cell orientation was used as an indirect parameter of motility or active displacement of immunity towards the damage [7,9,11,34,35].

2.3. Statistical Analysis

All data were recorded in an Excel database and statistical analysis was performed using SPSS software version 20.0 (SPSS Inc., Chicago, IL, USA). The variables under study were eyes (intervened right eye versus non-intervened left eye), sex (male versus female), type of steroid-induced glaucoma model (MsDx versus MsDxF) and control, number of injections, IOP and vitreous signal features using OCT (VIT/RPE relative intensity, total area, mean number of opacities, mean area of opacities, opacity percentage and opacity eccentricity, intensity and orientation).

After checking for variable normality with the Kolmogorov–Smirnov test, we performed a parametric test using multiple ANOVA comparisons and correlations with Pearson's P test. All values were expressed as mean ± standard deviations. Values of $p < 0.05$ were considered to indicate statistical significance, and the Bonferroni correction for multiple comparisons was calculated to avoid a high false-positive rate. In Figures 2 and 3, statistically significant differences are indicated as follows: A (MsDx–MsDxF), B (MsDx–control), C (MsDxF–control). Figures 4–9 show isolated cells (<10 μm^2; group 1), non-activated cells (10–50 μm^2; group 2), activated cells (50–250 μm^2; group 3) and cell complexes (>250 μm^2; group 4). Statistically significant differences ($p < 0.05$) are indicated with alphabetic markers as follows: a (group 1–group 2), b (group 1–group 3), c (group 1–group 4), d (group 2–group 3), e (group 2–group 4) and f (group 3–group 4).

3. Results

3.1. Microsphere Characterisation

Both microsphere formulations (MsDx and MsDxF) were spherical and had a mean particle size of approximately 14 µm and a unimodal particle size distribution. The microspheres' surface was influenced by the production method: those prepared via evaporation solvent from a simple emulsion (MsDx) had non-porous surfaces, according to scanning electron microscopy (SEM), while the use of the double-emulsion technique (MsDxF) produced small surface pores in the microspheres. Dexamethasone loading was approximately 60 µg DX/mg Ms for the MsDx and approximately 72 µg DX/mg Ms for the MsDxF. In both cases, sustained release of the active compounds was observed for several weeks. For a more detailed description of these results, see previous studies published by the research group [19,20,36].

3.2. Ophthalmological Analysis

A total of 280 OCT videos, obtained from 120 rats (60% females/40% males) at different times of study follow-up, were analysed. MsDx (n = 43 rats): 49 videos from the right eye (RE)/49 videos from the left eye (LE); MsDxF (n = 44): 44 RE/50 LE; healthy controls (n = 32): 31 RE/57 LE. IOP progressively increased in both SIG models and differences were found between the sexes. Glaucomatous and healthy males had higher IOP levels than females throughout the study (data extracted from [19,20,37]) (Figure 2).

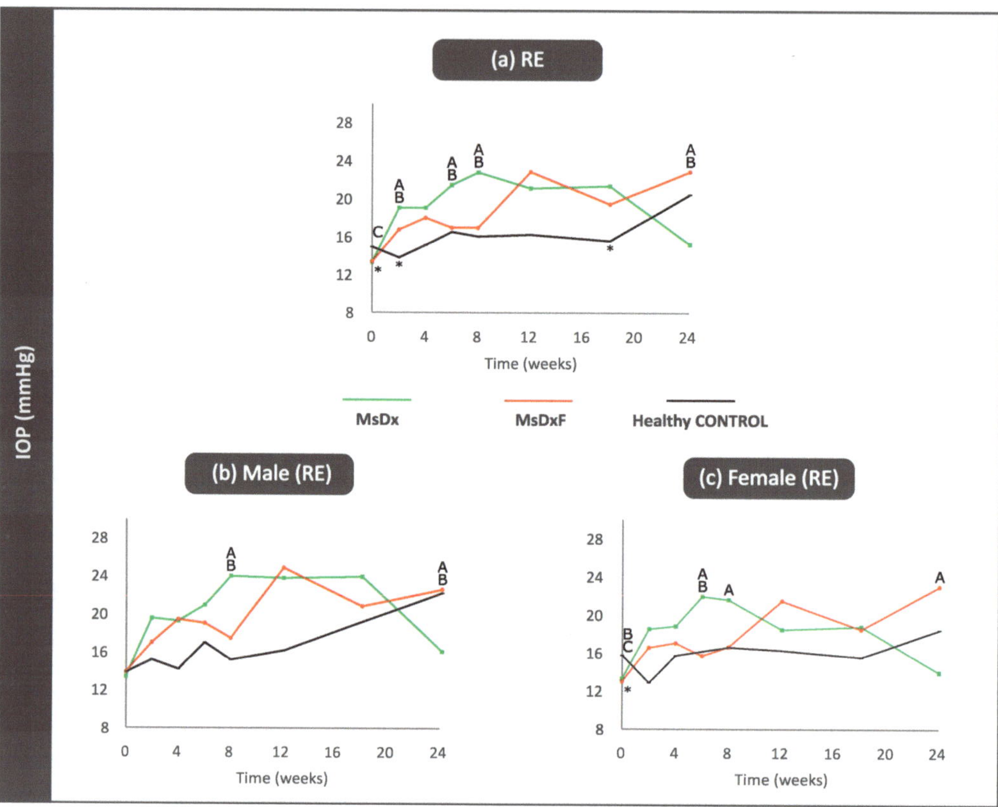

Figure 2. Intraocular pressure curves (right eyes) in two steroid-induced glaucoma models and healthy controls for all right eyes (**a**), for the right eyes of the males (**b**) and for the right eyes of the females (**c**). Abbreviations: MsDx: cohort with microspheres loaded with dexamethasone; MsDxF: cohort with microspheres loaded with dexamethasone and fibronectin injected into the anterior chamber; IOP: intraocular pressure (data extracted from [37,38]). *: statistical significance ($p < 0.05$) between glaucoma models and healthy controls (ANOVA); A: significant differences between MsDx and MsDxF; B: significant differences between MsDx and healthy controls; C: significant differences between MsDxF and healthy controls.

3.3. *Computational Analysis*

3.3.1. VIT/RPE Intensity

OCT analysis of the vitreous detected slightly higher VIT/RPE intensities in the injected right eyes in both SIG models in the final stages of this study ($p > 0.05$). The MsDx model generated with two injections showed a higher VIT/RPE signal than the MsDxF model generated with a single injection throughout the study; however, after the first injection (week 2), both SIG models showed similar VIT/RPE intensities to healthy controls (Figure 3a). Non-injected left eyes showed a slight increase in vitreous signal intensity versus healthy controls (Figure 3b). Healthy control animals' IOP and vitreous signal intensity measurements were lower than those of both SIG animals (Figures 2 and 3). Lastly, the influence of sex was analysed. In general, females with SIG showed slightly higher VIT/RPE OCT intensity than males and their healthy female counterparts. Healthy control males showed increased vitreous intensity at week 12 (16 weeks of life), after which vitreous intensity declined (Figure 3c,d).

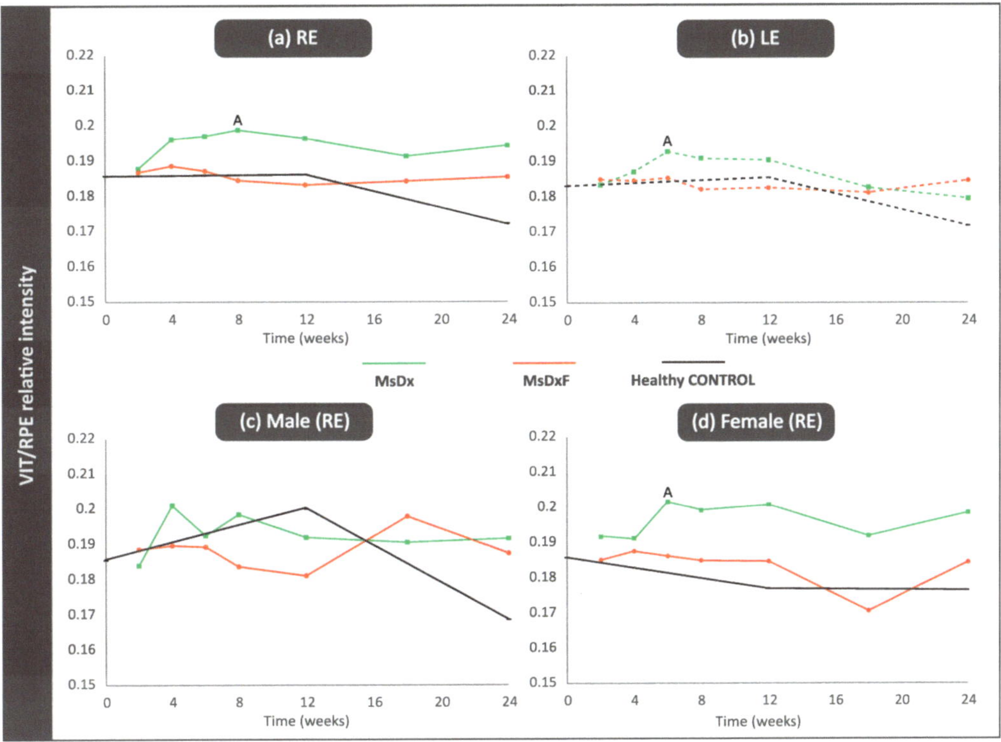

Figure 3. VIT/RPE signal intensity. (**a**) Right eye from both sexes; (**b**) Left eye from both sexes; (**c**) males; (**d**) females. Abbreviations: RE: right eye; LE: left eye; MsDx: cohort with microspheres loaded with dexamethasone (green); MsDxF: cohort with microspheres loaded with dexamethasone and fibronectin injected into the anterior chamber (red); healthy CONTROL: cohort of healthy animals non intervented (black); VIT: vitreous; RPE: retinal pigment epithelium. A: significant differences between MsDx and MsDxF.

3.3.2. Correlation Analysis

A correlation study was performed with the aim of evaluating the influence of the model on the VIT/RPE intensity. Both SIG models are induced by intraocular injections, which involve rupture of the eye barrier and induce anterior chamber-associated immune deviation (ACAID) [39,40]. However, no strong statistically significant correlations between either injections or intensities analysed by OCT were found in any SIG model or in the healthy cohort, which implies a lower level of immune involvement. The most relevant results and correlations are shown in bold in Table 1.

MsDx cohort: Both sexes presented an inverse correlation between IOPs at different times, which was moderate in females (IOP 0 w/6 w in the right eye and IOP 2 w/18 w in the left eye) and strong in males (IOP 2 w/12 w; r = −0.825, p = 0.012). Eyes with initially lower IOPs were more likely to present higher IOPs at later times [18]. Furthermore, IOP at early stages (2 and 4 w) correlated directly with OCT intensity at the final stages (24 w in the right eye and 18 w in the left eye). This suggests a greater anti-inflammatory effect exerted by dexamethasone in the injected right eye, delaying the IOP/OCT intensity correlation in both sexes (males IOP 2 w/OCT 24 w; r = 0.999, p = 0.029, and females IOP 8 w/OCT 18 w; r = 0.999, p = 0.012). The inverse correlation (possibly reflecting the protective effect of dexamethasone) was observed in males at week 6 (IOP 6 w/OCT 6 w; r = −0.999, p = 0.030) and in females at week 8 (IOP 2 w/OCT 8 w; r = −0.999, p = 0.019). This protection was lost later when a direct correlation was found in males at week 8 (IOP 8 w/OCT 8 w; r = 0.999, *p* = 0.028) and in females at week 18 (IOP 8 w/OCT 18 w; r = 0.999, *p* = 0.012). This suggests earlier loss of anti-inflammatory action due to dexamethasone in males since a direct IOP/OCT correlation was found earlier in this sex.

Table 1. Correlations in both steroid-induced glaucoma and healthy control animals. Abbreviations: RE: right eye; LE: left eye; IOP: intraocular pressure; OCT: optical coherence tomography; w: weeks; MsDx: cohort with microspheres loaded with dexamethasone; MsDxF: cohort with microspheres loaded with dexamethasone and fibronectin injected into the anterior chamber; HC: healthy controls; im: inverse moderate correlation; m: moderate correlation. In bold: statistically significant correlations.

	Right Eye			**Left Eye**		
	MsDx	**MsDxF**	**HC**	**MsDx**	**MsDxF**	**HC**
IOP/IOP	4 w/6 w(m)	6 w/12 w (m)	**4 w/8 w** (r = 0.934, *p* = 0.020)	2 w/18 w (im)	2 w/4 w (m) 4 w/6-8-24 w (m)	
IOP/OCT	**2 w/24 w** (r = 0.988, *p* = 0.002) **4 w/24 w** (r = 0.896, *p* = 0.040)		**18 w/24 w** (r = 0.854, *p* = 0.031)	**4 w/18 w** (r = 0.889, *p* = 0.043)	**0 w/8 w** (r = 0.882, *p* = 0.020) **0 w/12 w** (r = −0.851, *p* = 0.032) **6 w/8 w** (r = 0.813, *p* = 0.049)	24 w/24 w (im)

MsDxF cohort: Females also presented a moderate inverse correlation (IOP 0 w/18 w) and a direct correlation (IOP 0 w/12 w), supporting the more progressive and delayed IOP increase in right eyes. This was also the case in left eyes (IOP 4 w/24 w; r = 0.919, *p* = 0.010). However, males showed a strong direct correlation earlier (IOP 2 w/8 w; r = 0.841, *p* = 0.002), which seems to imply a predisposition for an earlier IOP increase in males in this model. No IOP/OCT correlations were found in the injected right eye. However, male left eyes showed a strong inverse correlation at 12 w (IOP 0 w/OCT 12 w; r = −0.851, *p* = 0.032) and a direct correlation at 8 w (IOP 0 w/OCT 8 w; r = 0.882, *p* = 0.020, and IOP 6 w/OCT 8 w; r = 0.813, *p* = 0.049) and at 18 w (IOP 2 w/OCT 18 w; r = 0.999, *p* = 0.022).

Healthy control cohort: An early and positive IOP correlation (IOP 4 w/IOP 8 w; r = 0.934, *p* = 0.020) was observed in both sexes. Females showed an inverse correlation according to IOP at early stages (IOP 0 w/6 w; r = −0.999, *p* = 0.021) and a direct IOP/OCT correlation at the intermediate (IOP 12 w/OCT 12 w; r = 0.997, *p* = 0.049, in the left eye) and late stages (IOP 18 w/OCT 24 w; r = 0.854, *p* = 0.031, in the right eye). In females, the age-related degenerative process [41,42] produces higher vitreous OCT intensity (reflex of immune involvement and/or activation) correlated with ocular normotension. But males showed a moderate inverse correlation at the end of this study (IOP 24 w/OCT 24 w).

3.3.3. In Vivo Analysis of Vitreous Immunity

In our previous paper, we showed that the hyperreflective opacities in the vitreous corresponded to hyalocyte-like Iba1+ cells [18,43] and that hypertensive eyes revealed many hyalocyte-like cells surrounding the ciliary body, some of which migrated from the ciliary body, crossing to the vitreous cavity [14]. In this study, the characteristics and behaviour of the hyperreflective opacities were analysed individually using OCT image processing.

As a representation of total immune response [6,9], the total area of opacities/cells was quantified. In both SIG models, induced eyes showed significantly increased total areas (MsDx > MsDxF) versus healthy control animals (Figure 4a). To find out if the increase in total cell area was because of an increased number or cell size, and thus an increase in activated cells, the mean number of opacities was quantified over the study period. A constant number of opacities (10–20) was found in the healthy control cohort, in contrast to a higher and fluctuating number of opacities found in both SIG cohorts (approximately 45–35 opacities/cells in MsDx and MsDxF, respectively). Both SIG cohorts showed an initial increase, coinciding with the first intraocular injection and with OHT levels (Figure 4b). The results of these two in-depth analyses concur with previous findings [18,26].

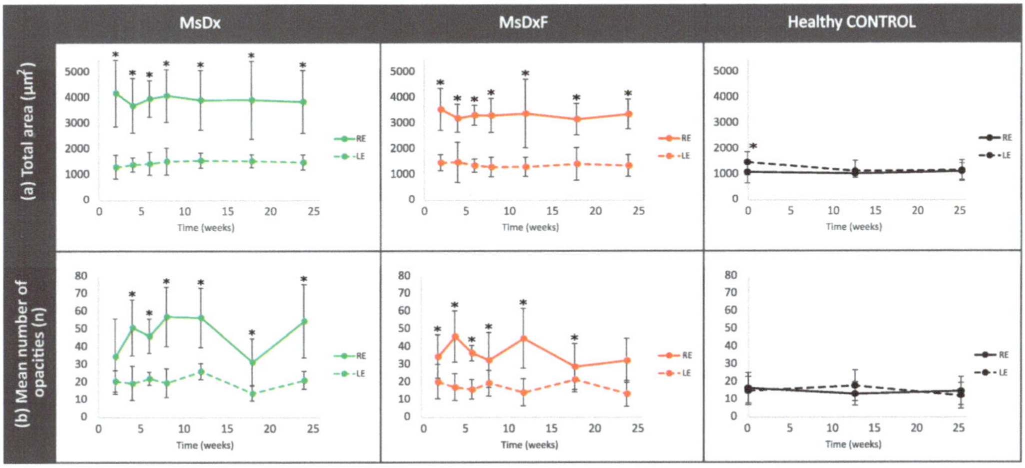

Figure 4. Changes in total immune response (**a**) and cellular quantification (**b**) in both steroid-induced glaucoma and healthy control animals. Abbreviations: RE: right eye; LE: left eye; MsDx: cohort with microspheres loaded with dexamethasone; MsDxF: cohort with microspheres loaded with dexamethasone and fibronectin injected into the anterior chamber; n: number; *: statistical significance ($p < 0.05$), using ANOVA test.

To assess the reproducibility and reliability of the measurement, the hyperreflective opacities or vitreous cell populations were divided, as we carried out previously in [18], into isolated cells (<10 μm^2), non-activated cells (10–50 μm^2), activated cells (50–250 μm^2) and cell complexes (>250 μm^2) [6,9] (Figure 5). This division based on size was possible because the study of the vitreoretinal interface does not require a correction factor and consequently can be measured directly.

Cell populations maintain similar sizes over time, implying reliability of measurement. Complexes > 250 μm^2 undergo the biggest variations, with peaks at the onset of damage. Statistically significant differences ($p < 0.05$) were highlighted with alphabetic markers as follows: a (group 1–group 2), b (group 1–group 3), c (group 1–group 4), d (group 2–group 3), e (group 2–group 4) and f (group 3–group 4).

Percentage of Opacities/Cells by Size

Changes in the proportion in the non-activated and activated state in both SIG cohorts versus healthy eyes are shown in Figure 6. The healthy controls and both SIG cohorts showed a population ratio ordered from lowest to highest as follows: isolated cells (less than 10 μm^2) < complexes (more than 250 μm^2) < activated cells (50–250 μm^2) < non-activated cells (10–50 μm^2). A specular response was found between opacities of 10–50 μm^2 (non-activated cells) and 50–250 μm^2 (activated cells) and between opacities of 50–250 μm^2 (activated cells) and opacities > 250 μm^2 (complexes). Dynamic fluctuations were observed in both SIG cohorts, but on average, opacities 10–50 μm^2 in size (non-activated cells) comprised approximately 40–50%. Both SIG cohorts maintained an anti-inflammatory profile throughout the study, with the MsDx model exhibiting a lower proportion of activated cells and higher cumulative intraocular dexamethasone release. This contrasts with the non-steroid glaucoma models, which had a higher percentage of opacities 50–250 μm^2 in size (activated cells) [18].

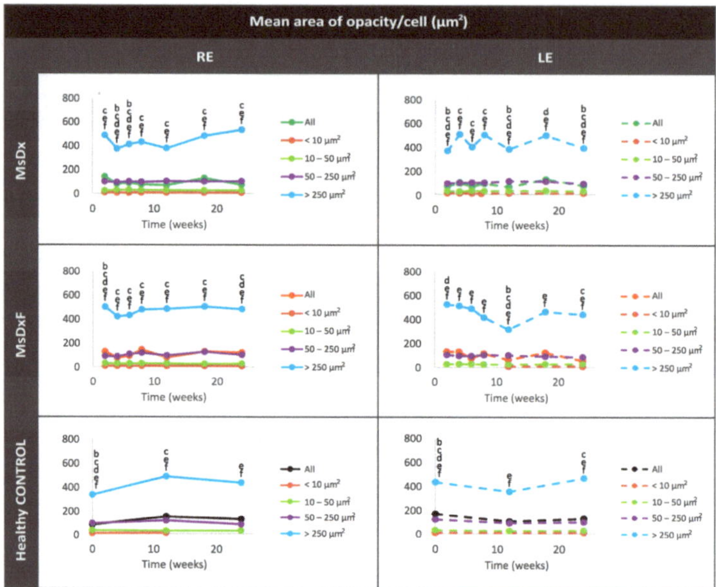

Figure 5. Cell subdivisions based on the mean area of vitreous opacities measured using OCT. Statistically significant differences ($p < 0.05$) were highlighted with alphabetic markers as follows: a (group 1–group 2), b (group 1–group 3), c (group 1–group 4), d (group 2–group 3), e (group 2–group 4) and f (group 3–group 4). Abbreviations: MsDx: cohort with microspheres loaded with dexamethasone; MsDxF: cohort with microspheres loaded with dexamethasone and fibronectin injected into the anterior chamber; isolated cells: < 10 μm^2 (group 1); non-activated cells: 10–50 μm^2 (group 2); activated cells: 50–250 μm^2 (group 3); cell complexes: >250 μm^2 (group 4).

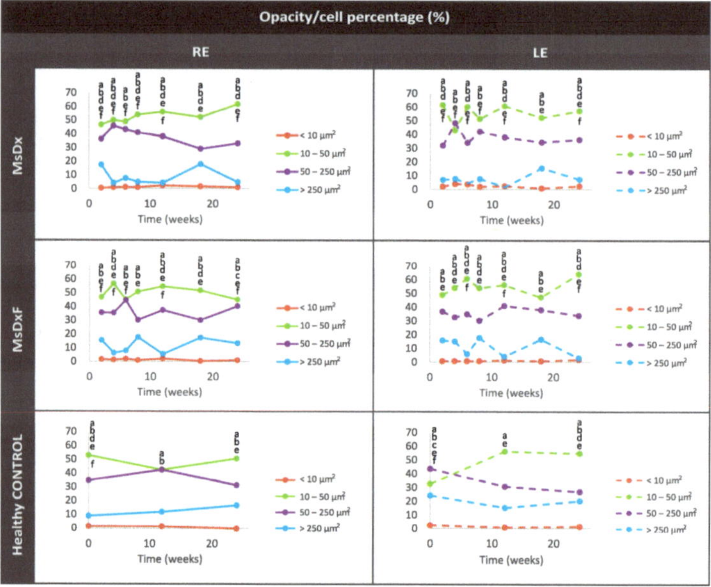

Figure 6. Changes in the vitreous immune population (opacities) in both steroid-induced glaucoma and healthy control animals throughout 6 months. Abbreviations: MsDx: cohort with microspheres

loaded with dexamethasone; MsDxF: cohort with microspheres loaded with dexamethasone and fibronectin injected into the anterior chamber; isolated cells: opacities < 10 μm^2 (group 1); non-activated cells: 10–50 μm^2 (group 2); activated cells: 50–250 μm^2 (group 3); cell complexes: >250 μm^2 (group 4). Data represented as percentages. Statistically significant differences ($p < 0.05$) were highlighted with alphabetic markers as follows: a (group 1–group 2), b (group 1–group 3), c (group 1–group 4), d (group 2–group 3), e (group 2–group 4) and f (group 3–group 4).

Average Eccentricity of the Opacities/Cells

This analysis enhanced the characterisation of cell morphology as rounded morphology (eccentricity close to 0) versus linear or flat morphology (eccentricity close to 1). In healthy controls and both SIG cohorts, isolated opacities/cells (<10 μm^2) presented the most rounded or amoeboid morphology (eccentricity 0.85) as opposed to opacities/cells with progressively larger sizes of 10–50 μm^2 (non-activated), followed by those measuring 50–250 μm^2 (activated cells) and <250 μm^2 (cell complexes), these being increasingly flat (eccentricity 0.95–1). However, both SIG cohorts showed higher roundness in isolated cells (0.4–0.7) than in healthy cells (0.8) (Figure 7). In both SIG cohorts, the lower eccentricities coincided with increases in OHT in the MsDx model at week 4 (both sexes) (Figure 2a) and week 18 (in males) (Figure 2b), and in the MsDxF model at week 4 (both sexes) and week 24 (higher in females) (Figure 2c). The MsDx model with the highest IOP levels showed the lowest eccentricities at those times. The higher roundness of the isolated cells is related to recruitment to the noxa. Our findings were in accordance with a previous study showing that the number of intravitreal cells was higher in adult mice with experimentally elevated IOP [10].

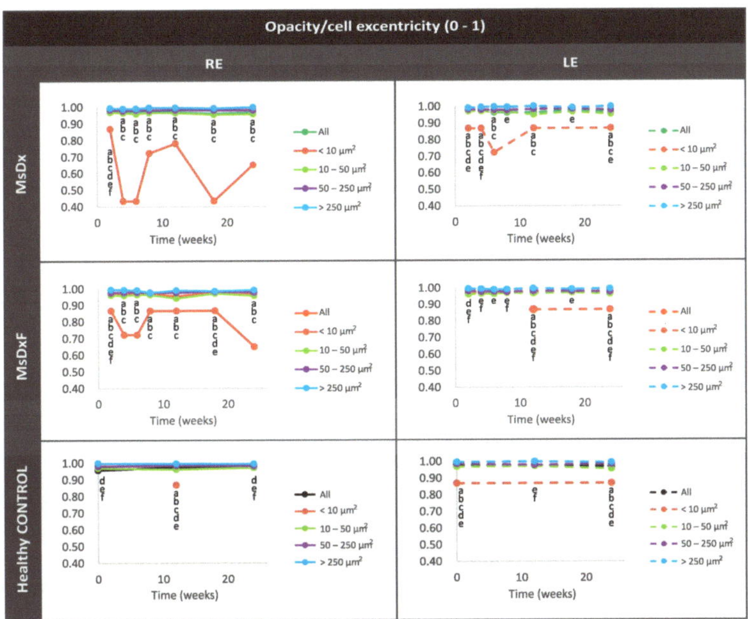

Figure 7. Mean eccentricity of vitreous opacity detected using in vivo OCT, according to size, in both steroid-induced glaucoma and healthy control animals. Indirect study of cell soma morphology. Abbreviations: MsDx: cohort with microspheres loaded with dexamethasone; MsDxF: cohort with microspheres loaded with dexamethasone and fibronectin injected into anterior chamber; isolated cells: opacities < 10 μm^2 (group 1); non-activated cells: 10–50 μm^2 (group 2); activated cells: 50–250 μm^2 (group 3); cell complexes: >250 μm^2 (group 4). Statistically significant differences ($p < 0.05$) were highlighted with alphabetic markers as follows: a (group 1–group 2), b (group 1–group 3), c (group 1–group 4), d (group 2–group 3), e (group 2–group 4) and f (group 3–group 4).

Mean Intensity of Opacities/Cells

Under physiological conditions, the lowest intensity was quantified in isolated opacities/cells (<10 μm^2) and progressively increased with size: opacities of 10–50 μm^2 (non-activated cells) followed by opacities of 50–250 μm^2 (activated cells). However, in both SIG cohorts, the greatest change in intensity was quantified in the smallest opacities/cells (<10 μm^2) (Figure 8) as a manifestation of activation of intracellular machinery and coinciding with the increase in size. As soma size increased (activated cells with pseudopod formation) [13,28,44,45], there was a relative decrease in mean intensity.

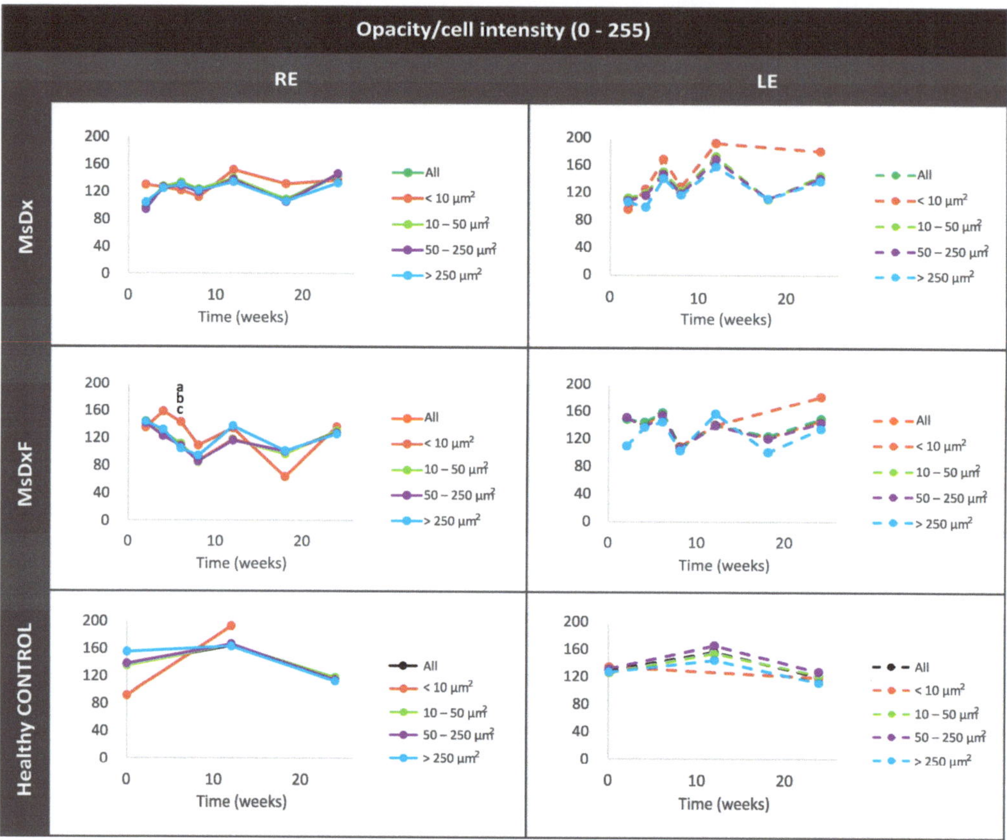

Figure 8. Mean intensity of opacities/cells based on size in both steroid-induced glaucoma and healthy control animals. Abbreviations: MsDx: cohort with microspheres loaded with dexamethasone; MsDxF: cohort with microspheres loaded with dexamethasone and fibronectin injected into the anterior chamber; isolated cells: opacities < 10 μm^2; non-activated cells: 10–50 μm^2; activated cells: 50–250 μm^2; cell complexes: >250 μm^2. Statistically significant differences ($p < 0.05$) were highlighted with alphabetic markers as follows: a (group 1–group 2), b (group 1–group 3) and c (group 1–group 4). Mean Orientation of the Opacities/Cells.

Orientation was analysed to measure an active shift (change in mean orientation) of immunity towards the damage [11,14,34,46]. The healthy control cohort did not experience any change. However, both SIG cohorts (MsDxF > MsDx) showed a change in orientation of the smallest opacities (<10 μm^2: isolated ovoid cells) around 12 weeks (Figure 9), when both SIG cohorts experienced an increase in neuroretinal thickness, as found in our previous studies with these same models (Supplementary Figure S1) [19,20].

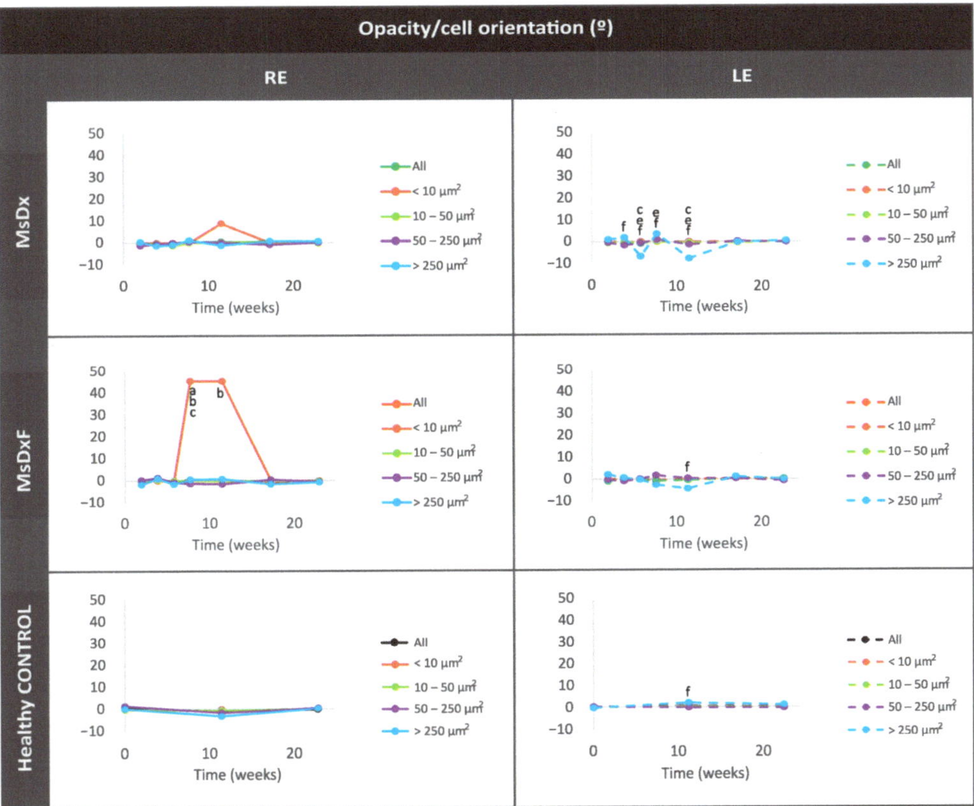

Figure 9. Mean orientation of vitreous opacity detected using OCT, according to size, in both steroid-induced glaucoma and healthy control animals. In vivo analysis for motility. Abbreviations: MsDx: cohort with microspheres loaded with dexamethasone; MsDxF: cohort with microspheres loaded with dexamethasone and fibronectin injected into the anterior chamber; isolated cells: opacities < 10 µm^2 (group 1); non-activated cells: 10–50 µm^2 (group 2); activated cells: 50–250 µm^2 (group 3); cell complexes: >250 µm^2 (group 4). Statistically significant differences ($p < 0.05$) were highlighted with alphabetic markers as follows: a (group 1–group 2), b (group 1–group 3), c (group 1–group 4), e (group 2–group 4) and f (group 3–group 4).

4. Discussion

Glaucoma is a multifactorial pathology in which immunity seems to be an early and important factor [47]. Elevated IOP triggers an innate immune response involving resident immune cells, such as microglia, and the infiltration of macrophages/monocytes and other secondary responses are responsible for RGC degeneration in glaucoma [7]. The primary response may be initially favourable in protecting the eye; it restores tissue equilibrium and promotes tissue cleaning, healing and functionality. If there is a defect in immune response pathways due to accumulating risk factors, prolonged and sustained or restrained inflammatory stimulation, or "neo-antigens" generated with ageing, the physiological homeostasis may be disrupted and the regulatory mechanisms are altered [48], thereby converting beneficial immunity into a neurodestructive autoimmune process [49]. Proinflammatory markers [50] and early cytokine dysregulation have been demonstrated independently and prior to the detection of RGC and axonal loss [7,51]. The subsequent events that lead to long-lasting activation of glial cells and adaptive immune responses become destructive, disrupting the homeostasis of the retina and resulting in the dysfunction of the immune-privileged status of the eye [3].

A possible therapeutic target for alleviating non-IOP-dependent factors could be modulating immunity. Controlling immune activation reduced optic nerve damage and reactive microglia-mediated neuroprotection in mouse retina, but eliminating it proved disadvantageous [7,52,53]. This study shows concordant results. Both SIG models showed lower vitreous signal intensities and lower counts of hyperreflective opacities (Figures 3 and 4) than those found in previous non-steroid glaucoma models [18], but computational analysis of vitreous hyperreflective opacities revealed similar behaviour (Figures 6–9). However, these SIG models developed significant neuroretinal damage with worse electroretinographic functionality, reduced structural thickness and lower RGC counts [19]. In other words, the presence of the steroid, which a priori could be thought to exert a protective anti-inflammatory effect, did not; rather, it produced and worsened the glaucomatous damage, as occurs in corticosteroid-induced glaucoma in humans [54]. Recent studies suggest that the immunity activated in glaucoma may not be counterbalanced by efficient immune suppression, and a greater stimulation response is characterised by increased proliferation and proinflammatory cytokine secretion. The potent anti-inflammatory effect of dexamethasone is well known. However, in this paper, it was used to generate two SIG models via sustained release from biodegradable Ms. Dexamethasone exerts a beneficial protective effect in a situation of overt and active inflammation [55], but in our study, we started from animals with no acute inflammation to counteract, sustainedly creating a potential imbalance in the delicate equilibrium of ocular immune privilege. Resident immunity may have been altered by overriding ocular immune inhibitors [56], and the balance tipped towards proinflammation with significant neuroretinal damage in both models.

Several research groups have tried to study immunity in vivo, but the need for genetically modified animals or the development of highly complex technology was prohibitive [48], and also ex vivo with dead animals as a result [57]. Enabled by the ability of light to pass through different optical densities, OCT is a fast, non-invasive device that provides in vivo scans of the neuroretinal structure and measurement of the retinal layers [58,59]. However, OCT has the handicap of not being able to differentiate among cell types within the neuroretinal thickness from glial, supporting or vascular cells. In the retina [9], in vivo microglia tracking using cSLO imaging has been reported [60]. This technique requires the use of animals genetically modified to express fluorescence, and thus, it cannot be used on humans. Analysis of the vitreoretinal interface using OCT, however, is nowadays a standard technique employed in ophthalmological clinics. Our group recently demonstrated that vitreous immune cells can be detected as hyperreflective opacities at the vitreoretinal interface and monitored using OCT imaging [18] in healthy and glaucomatous animals, coinciding with another group, who also confirmed it by confocal immunofluorescence in retinal vascular disease [61]. In the first phase, we focused on VIT/RPE relative intensity after a positive correlation with clinical vitreous turbidity was demonstrated [62] and validated under different conditions [17,26,63]. In the second phase, deeper computational analysis was performed to characterise the hyperreflective opacities that were confirmed by histology as hyalocyte-like Iba1+ cells (a microglial marker). Microglia and macrophages undergo characteristic morphological changes with their function. In an inactive situation, they are branched to sense changes in the microenvironment. The vitreous medium's high water content makes it ideal for the transmission of soluble molecules, meaning that hyalocytes can easily and rapidly detect changes in the microenvironment [64] to target the noxa. Dexamethasone is a soluble molecule that was injected into the anterior chamber. It could target the vitreous chamber and modify the vitreous microenvironment, causing both SIG cohorts to maintain an anti-inflammatory profile since a higher proportion of non-activated cells were counted throughout the study (Figure 6). Furthermore, when damaged, hyalocytes [13] are activated and change shape (the number/size of intracellular organelles and, thus, the membrane content increase, facilitating detection by OCT imaging as hyperreflectivity), proliferate and migrate. These cells were associated with areas of retinal nerve fibre layer degeneration in glaucomatous patients [46], and a study using OCT detected a higher density of vitreous opacities close to areas of cell death [25].

Our previous paper on vitreous analysis in glaucoma detected increased intensity (onset of intracellular machinery) in the smallest opacities and a change in orientation (onset of displacement) as indicators of activation [18]. It suggested that the smallest opacities would be the first detected changes and could serve as an early marker of immune activation in the vitreous. This study of SIG corroborates these results. Eccentricity and intensity seem to be related to the increase in IOP (Figures 2a and 7), while the change in orientation seems to be related to the increase in retinal thickness (Figure 9 and Supplementary Figure S1). Orientation is particularly relevant in the MsDxF cohort, which showed a marked change (Figure 9), indicating cells are oriented towards a certain point (retinal damage). This change in orientation coincided with an increase in the mean number of opacities (Figure 4b), suggesting that more cells were directed to the same retinal area. At later stages, the mean orientation returns to 0, which suggests that there could be more neuroretinal areas damaged in different areas and, therefore, more orientations to be adopted by the cells, nullifying the summation effect of the mean orientation. This hypothesis was confirmed by the results observed at later stages in the MsDx cohort. MsDx showed a further increase in cells (Figure 4b) but no change in orientation was observed, suggesting that these cells took several orientations and cancelled out their effect, which coincided with the increased neuroretinal damage evidenced by low RGC counts in our previous study [19]. It is possible that the return to 0 orientation of the opacities/hyalocytes in the two models could indicate "ageing or motility damage" because of the accumulation, repetition and chronicity of oxidative stress [35].

In this SIG study, the ocular barrier is altered in both Ms models by means of an intraocular injection in the anterior chamber that triggers an inflammatory response (ACAID response) [65]. In contrast to previous hypertensive models such as those induced by episcleral vein sclerosis or unloaded microspheres, no direct correlation was found between inducing injections, vitreous intensity or vitreous microglial or hyalocyte response [10]. This suggests that the pro-inflammatory effect of the intraocular injection was partly counteracted by the anti-inflammatory effect of the initial release of dexamethasone. As with non-SIG models [18], those animals with the lowest initial IOP had the highest IOP after the application of hypertensive stimuli, and in the MsDx cohort, higher IOP at week 2 correlated with higher vitreous signals detected by OCT at week 24 ($r = 0.988$, $p = 0.002$). Similarly, in left eyes, an inverse correlation was found between baseline IOP levels and vitreous OCT at week 12 ($r = -0.851$, $p = 0.032$), reflecting possible higher late contralateral inflammatory vitreous activation in the more hypotensive (susceptible) non-induced eyes. In this sense, different studies of glaucoma models have demonstrated stable, lower-intensity immune activation in the retina [66] and vitreous of the contralateral eye after OHT induction [18]. In this study, no increase in the number of opacities was observed in contralateral eyes, which means the hyalocytes were resident (without recruitment), but changes were detected in cell populations, eccentricity and intensity. Characterisation of hyperreflective opacities/immune cells (hyalocyte-like Iba1+ cells) in the healthy control cohort was explored in depth in our previous paper [18,61]. In summary, healthy rats showed a higher proportion of vitreous opacities in OCT, coinciding with sizes corresponding to non-activated cells, consistent with an anti-inflammatory or steady state [61] of the eye and immune inhibitory privilege [56,65]. A variable number of opacities corresponding to cells activated to maintain homeostasis was also quantified [11].

Limitations and future perspectives: There is still a long way to fully achieve the understanding of immune cell actions and cascades in both healthy and glaucomatous eyes. The authors are aware that there remain many aspects and unknowns to resolve. The obtained results could not be easily extrapolated to humans and more data are needed regarding the effectiveness of this study. The limitations in the histologic phenotyping of our study meant it could not clarify the paradigm of the infiltrative origin [67] of the increased vitreous opacities, although previous groups demonstrated the involvement of blood-derived inflammatory cells [61]. It would be beneficial to perform a computational study correlating the changes in the parameters of eccentricity, intensity and orientation of the vitreous opacities with neuroretinal changes, and to corroborate our topographic hypothesis of a change in orientation of those vitreous cells towards the RGC damage cluster by means of whole-mount histological studies or with new in vivo damage detection techniques [68,69]. Glaucoma therapies based on neuro-immunomodulatory targeting are emerging and immune cells could be important candidates [35].

5. Conclusions

Our method of analysing vitreous opacities/hyalocytes using OCT could serve as a promising imaging biomarker to detect immunity in the eye. It could help in the early diagnosis of disease onset and progression applicable to glaucoma and, potentially, in other multifactorial neurodegenerative diseases [70,71]. This study supports the previous evidence that simple, non-invasive in vivo analysis of glaucoma from the immune perspective is possible. We corroborate and validate the computational analysis of the individual hyperreflective opacities as a better technique than the overall relative measure of immunity using VIT/RPE by OCT. A clear example is the MsDxF cohort, which hardly exhibited any difference in vitreous signal intensity compared to the healthy control cohort, but in which subsequent detailed analysis showed higher cell counts and the study of eccentricity, intensity and orientation characteristics using OCT coincided with the clinical milestones of increased IOP or neuroretinal change. In view of the above, we believe that the individualised study of vitreous opacities is a reproducible and reliable method and offers information that can be correlated with clinical data, which could serve as a non-invasive biomarker in glaucoma diagnosis.

Supplementary Materials: The following supporting information can be downloaded at: https://www.mdpi.com/article/10.3390/biomedicines12030633/s1, Supplementary Figure S1: Retinal thickness measured with OCT. Abbreviations: MsDx: cohort with microspheres loaded with dexamethasone; MsDxF: cohort with microspheres loaded with dexamethasone and fibronectin injected into the anterior chamber; RE: right eye; LE: left eye; w: weeks. Data extracted from [19,20] (CYB license).

Author Contributions: Conceptualization, M.J.R., A.M. and A.P.d.P.; methodology, A.M., M.S., T.M.-R., A.A.-N. and A.P.d.P.; software, M.S., A.M., J.C. and A.P.d.P.; validation, A.P.d.P.; formal analysis, M.J.R., A.M. and E.G.-M.; investigation, M.S., A.M., T.M.-R., J.C. and A.A.-N.; resources, E.G.-M., L.E.P., R.H.-V., J.C. and A.P.d.P.; data curation, A.M.; writing—original draft preparation, M.J.R., A.M., A.P.d.P., I.B.-O. and R.H.-V.; writing—review and editing, M.J.R., A.M., A.P.d.P., I.B.-O. and R.H.-V.; visualization, M.J.R. and A.M.; supervision, M.J.R., I.B.-O., R.H.-V., E.G.-M. and L.E.P.; project administration, R.H.-V., E.G.-M. and L.E.P.; funding acquisition, M.J.R., E.G.-M., A.P.d.P. and L.E.P. All authors have read and agreed to the published version of the manuscript.

Funding: This research was funded by Grants M17/00213, JR22/00057, PI17/01726, PI17/01946 and PI20/00437 (Carlos III Health Institute), and by MAT2017-83858-C2-1, MAT2017-83858-C2-2, MCIN/AEI/10.13039/501100011033. PID2020-113281RB-C2-2 was funded by MCIN/AEI/10.13039/501100011033 and by "ERDF A way of making Europe". This study has been funded by Instituto de Salud Carlos III (ISCIII) through the project "RD21/0002/0050" and co-funded by the European Union "NextGenerationEU/PRTR". This study has been funded by the Government of Aragon through the research group "B23_23R". A.A.N. is supported by grant PRE2018-083951 funded by "ESF Investing in your future".

Institutional Review Board Statement: The animal study protocol was approved by the Institutional Review Board Ethics Committee for Animal Research (PI34/17) of the University of Zaragoza (Spain) (20 July 2017) for studies involving animals.

Informed Consent Statement: Not applicable.

Data Availability Statement: The authors confirm that the data supporting the findings of this study are available within the article and its Supplementary Materials. Derived data supporting the findings of this study are available from the corresponding author on request.

Acknowledgments: The authors would like to acknowledge the use of Servicio General a la Investigación-SAI, Universidad de Zaragoza.

Conflicts of Interest: Authors L.E.P. and M.S. were employed by the company Biotech Vision SLP (Spin-Off Company). The remaining authors declare that the research was conducted in the absence of any commercial or financial relationships that could be construed as potential conflicts of interest. The funders had no role in the design of the study; in the collection, analyses, or interpretation of data; in the writing of the manuscript; or in the decision to publish the results.

References

1. Quigley, H.; Broman, A.T. The number of people with glaucoma worldwide in 2010 and 2020. *Br. J. Ophthalmol.* **2006**, *90*, 262–267. [CrossRef]
2. Yang, X.; Zeng, Q.; Göktaş, E.; Gopal, K.; Al-Aswad, L.; Blumberg, D.M.; Cioffi, G.A.; Liebmann, J.M.; Tezel, G. T-Lymphocyte Subset Distribution and Activity in Patients With Glaucoma. *Investig. Ophthalmol. Vis. Sci.* **2019**, *60*, 877–888. [CrossRef] [PubMed]
3. Jiang, S.; Kametani, M.; Chen, D.F. Adaptive Immunity: New Aspects of Pathogenesis Underlying Neurodegeneration in Glaucoma and Optic Neuropath. *Front. Immunol.* **2020**, *11*, 65. [CrossRef]
4. Jonas, J.B.; Aung, T.; Bourne, R.R.; Bron, A.M.; Ritch, R.; Panda-Jonas, S. Glaucoma. *Lancet* **2017**, *390*, 2183–2193. [CrossRef]
5. Lau, L.I.; Liu, C.J.L.; Chou, J.C.K.; Hsu, W.M.; Liu, J.H. Patterns of visual field defects in chronic angle-closure glaucoma with different disease severity. *Ophthalmology* **2003**, *110*, 1890–1894. [CrossRef] [PubMed]
6. Kozlowski, C.; Weimer, R.M. An Automated Method to Quantify Microglia Morphology and Application to Monitor Activation State Longitudinally In Vivo. *PLoS ONE* **2012**, *7*, e31814. [CrossRef] [PubMed]
7. Wei, X.; Cho, K.-S.; Thee, E.F.; Jager, M.J.; Chen, D.F. Neuroinflammation and microglia in glaucoma: Time for a paradigm shift. *J. Neurosci. Res.* **2019**, *97*, 70–76. [CrossRef]
8. Kettenmann, H.; Hanisch, U.-K.; Noda, M.; Verkhratsky, A.; Microglia, P.O. Physiology of Microglia. *Physiol. Rev.* **2011**, *91*, 461–553. [CrossRef]
9. Bosco, A.; Romero, C.O.; Ambati, B.K.; Vetter, M.L. In Vivo Dynamics of Retinal Microglial Activation During Neurodegeneration: Confocal Ophthalmoscopic Imaging and Cell Morphometry in Mouse Glaucoma. *J. Vis. Exp.* **2015**, *2015*, e52731. [CrossRef]
10. Kezic, J.M.; Chrysostomou, V.; Trounce, I.A.; McMenamin, P.G.; Crowston, J.G. Effect of anterior chamber cannulation and acute IOP elevation on retinal macrophages in the adult mouse. *Investig. Ophthalmol. Vis. Sci.* **2013**, *54*, 3028–3036. [CrossRef]
11. Bosco, A.; Romero, C.O.; Breen, K.T.; Chagovetz, A.A.; Steele, M.R.; Ambati, B.K.; Vetter, M.L. Neurodegeneration severity can be predicted from early microglia alterations monitored in vivo in a mouse model of chronic glaucoma. *Dis. Model. Mech.* **2015**, *8*, 443–455. [CrossRef]
12. Boehm, M.R.R.; Oellers, P.; Thanos, S. Inflammation and immunology of the vitreoretinal compartment. *Inflamm. Allergy Drug Targets* **2011**, *10*, 283–309. [CrossRef]
13. Sakamoto, T.; Ishibashi, T. Hyalocytes: Essential cells of the vitreous cavity in vitreoretinal pathophysiology? *Retina* **2011**, *31*, 222–228. [CrossRef]
14. Vagaja, N.N.; Chinnery, H.R.; Binz, N.; Kezic, J.M.; Rakoczy, E.P.; McMenamin, P.G. Changes in murine hyalocytes are valuable early indicators of ocular disease. *Investig. Ophthalmol. Vis. Sci.* **2012**, *53*, 1445–1451. [CrossRef]
15. Keane, P.A.; Karampelas, M.; Sim, D.A.; Sadda, S.R.; Tufail, A.; Sen, H.N.; Nussenblatt, R.B.; Dick, A.D.; Lee, R.W.; Murray, P.I.; et al. Objective measurement of vitreous inflammation using optical coherence tomography. *Ophthalmology* **2014**, *121*, 1706–1714. [CrossRef]
16. Uji, A.; Yoshimura, N. Microarchitecture of the Vitreous Body: A High-Resolution Optical Coherence Tomography Study. *Am. J. Ophthalmol.* **2016**, *168*, 24–30. [CrossRef]
17. Sreekantam, S.; Macdonald, T.; Keane, P.A.; Sim, D.A.; Murray, P.I.; Denniston, A.K. Quantitative analysis of vitreous inflammation using optical coherence tomography in patients receiving sub-Tenon's triamcinolone acetonide for uveitic cystoid macular oedema. *Br. J. Ophthalmol.* **2017**, *101*, 175–179. [CrossRef]
18. Rodrigo, M.J.; Subías, M.; Montolío, A.; Méndez-Martínez, S.; Martínez-Rincón, T.; Arias, L.; García-Herranz, D.; Bravo-Osuna, I.; Garcia-Feijoo, J.; Pablo, L.; et al. Analysis of Parainflammation in Chronic Glaucoma Using Vitreous-OCT Imaging. *Biomedicines* **2021**, *9*, 1792. [CrossRef]
19. Rodrigo, M.J.; Garcia-Herranz, D.; Aragón-Navas, A.; Subias, M.; Martinez-Rincón, T.; Mendez-Martínez, S.; Cardiel, M.J.; García-Feijoo, J.; Ruberte, J.; Herrero-Vanrell, R.; et al. Long-term corticosteroid-induced chronic glaucoma model produced by intracameral injection of dexamethasone-loaded PLGA microspheres. *Drug Deliv.* **2021**, *28*, 2427–2446. [CrossRef]
20. Aragón-Navas, A.; Rodrigo, M.J.; Garcia-Herranz, D.; Martinez, T.; Subias, M.; Mendez, S.; Ruberte, J.; Pampalona, J.; Bravo-Osuna, I.; Garcia-Feijoo, J.; et al. Mimicking chronic glaucoma over 6 months with a single intracameral injection of dexamethasone/fibronectin-loaded PLGA microspheres Mimicking chronic glaucoma over 6 months with a single intracameral injection of dexamethasone/fibronectin-loaded PLGA microspheres. *Drug Deliv.* **2022**, *2022*, 2357–2374. [CrossRef]

21. Vyas, S.; Rodrigues, A.J.; Silva, J.M.; Tronche, F.; Almeida, O.F.X.; Sousa, N.; Sotiropoulos, I. Chronic Stress and Glucocorticoids: From Neuronal Plasticity to Neurodegeneration. *Neural Plast.* **2016**, *2016*, 1–15. [CrossRef]
22. Razeghinejad, M.R.; Katz, L.J. Steroid-induced iatrogenic glaucoma. *Ophthalmic Res.* **2012**, *47*, 66–80. [CrossRef]
23. Garcia-Herranz, D.; Rodrigo, M.J.; Subias, M.; Martinez-Rincon, T.; Mendez-Martinez, S.; Bravo-Osuna, I.; Bonet, A.; Ruberte, J.; Garcia-Feijoo, J.; Pablo, L.; et al. Novel Use of PLGA Microspheres to Create an Animal Model of Glaucoma with Progressive Neuroretinal Degeneration. *Pharmaceutics* **2021**, *13*, 237. [CrossRef] [PubMed]
24. Liu, X.; Wang, C.-H.; Dai, C.; Camesa, A.; Zhang, H.F.; Jiao, S. Effect of Contact Lens on Optical Coherence Tomography Imaging of Rodent Retina. *Curr. Eye Res.* **2013**, *38*, 1235. [CrossRef] [PubMed]
25. Korot, E.; Comer, G.; Steffens, T.; Antonetti, D.A. Algorithm for the Measure of Vitreous Hyperreflective Foci in Optical Coherence Tomographic Scans of Patients With Diabetic Macular Edema. *JAMA Ophthalmol.* **2016**, *134*, 15–20. [CrossRef] [PubMed]
26. Rodrigo, M.J.; del Palomar, A.P.; Montolío, A.; Mendez-Martinez, S.; Subias, M.; Cardiel, M.J.; Martinez-Rincon, T.; Cegoñino, J.; Fraile, J.M.; Vispe, E.; et al. Monitoring New Long-Lasting Intravitreal Formulation for Glaucoma with Vitreous Images Using Optical Coherence Tomography. *Pharmaceutics* **2021**, *13*, 217. [CrossRef] [PubMed]
27. Chu, C.J.; Herrmann, P.; Carvalho, L.S.; Liyanage, S.E.; Bainbridge, J.W.B.; Ali, R.R.; Dick, A.D.; Luhmann, U.F.O. Assessment and In Vivo Scoring of Murine Experimental Autoimmune Uveoretinitis Using Optical Coherence Tomography. *PLoS ONE* **2013**, *8*, e63002. [CrossRef] [PubMed]
28. Ogawa, K. Scanning electron microscopic study of hyalocytes in the guinea pig eye. *Arch. Histol. Cytol.* **2002**, *65*, 263–268. [CrossRef]
29. Liba, O.; Lew, M.D.; Sorelle, E.D.; Dutta, R.; Sen, D.; Moshfeghi, D.M.; Chu, S.; De La Zerda, A. Speckle-modulating optical coherence tomography in living mice and humans. *Nat. Commun.* **2017**, *8*, 15845. [CrossRef]
30. London, A.; Itskovich, E.; Benhar, I.; Kalchenko, V.; Mack, M.; Jung, S.; Schwartz, M. Neuroprotection and progenitor cell renewal in the injured adult murine retina requires healing monocyte-derived macrophages. *J. Exp. Med.* **2011**, *208*, 23–39. [CrossRef]
31. Jacobs, A.H.; Tavitian, B. Noninvasive Molecular Imaging of Neuroinflammation. *J. Cereb. Blood Flow. Metab.* **2012**, *32*, 1393–1415. [CrossRef] [PubMed]
32. Ajami, B.; Bennett, J.L.; Krieger, C.; Tetzlaff, W.; Rossi, F.M.V. Local self-renewal can sustain CNS microglia maintenance and function throughout adult life. *Nat. Neurosci.* **2007**, *10*, 1538–1543. [CrossRef]
33. Ajami, B.; Bennett, J.L.; Krieger, C.; McNagny, K.M.; Rossi, F.M.V. Infiltrating monocytes trigger EAE progression. but do not contribute to the resident microglia pool. *Nat. Neurosci.* **2011**, *14*, 1142–1150. [CrossRef] [PubMed]
34. Damisah, E.C.; Hill, R.A.; Rai, A.; Chen, F.; Rothlin, C.V.; Ghosh, S.; Grutzendler, J. Astrocytes and microglia play orchestrated roles and respect phagocytic territories during neuronal corpse removal in vivo. *Sci. Adv.* **2020**, *6*, eaba3239. [CrossRef] [PubMed]
35. Tay, T.L.; Béchade, C.; D'Andrea, I.; St-Pierre, M.K.; Henry, M.S.; Roumier, A.; Tremblay, M.E. Microglia gone rogue: Impacts on psychiatric disorders across the lifespan. *Front. Mol. Neurosci.* **2018**, *10*, 421. [CrossRef]
36. Rodrigo, M.J.; Bravo-Osuna, I.; Subias, M.; Montolío, A.; Cegoñino, J.; Martinez-Rincón, T.; Mendez-Martinez, S.; Aragón-Navas, A.; Garcia-Herranz, D.; Pablo, L.E.; et al. Tunable degrees of neurodegeneration in rats based on microsphere-induced models of chronic glaucoma. *Sci. Rep.* **2022**, *12*, 20622. [CrossRef] [PubMed]
37. Rodrigo, M.J.; Martinez-Rincon, T.; Subias, M.; Mendez-Martinez, S.; Luna, C.; Pablo, L.E.; Polo, V.; Garcia-Martin, E. Effect of age and sex on neurodevelopment and neurodegeneration in the healthy eye: Longitudinal functional and structural study in the Long–Evans rat. *Exp. Eye Res.* **2020**, *200*, 108208. [CrossRef]
38. Rodrigo, M.J.; Martinez-Rincon, T.; Subias, M.; Mendez-Martinez, S.; Garcia-Herranz, D.; Garcia-Feijoo, J.; Herrero-Vanrell, R.; Pablo, L.; Bravo-Osuna, I.; Munuera, I.; et al. Influence of sex on chronic steroid-induced glaucoma: 24-Weeks follow-up study in rats. *Exp. Eye Res.* **2023**, *238*, 109736. [CrossRef]
39. Forrester, J.V.; Xu, H. Good news–bad news: The Yin and Yang of immune privilege in the eye. *Front. Immunol.* **2012**, *3*, 338. [CrossRef]
40. Medawar, P.B. Immunity to homologous grafted skin; the fate of skin homografts. *Br. J. Exp. Pathol.* **1948**, *29*, 58–69.
41. Kehlet, S.N.; Willumsen, N.; Armbrecht, G.; Dietzel, R.; Brix, S.; Henriksen, K.; Karsdal, M.A. Age-related collagen turnover of the interstitial matrix and basement membrane: Implications of age- and sex-dependent remodeling of the extracellular matrix. *PLoS ONE* **2018**, *13*, e0194458. [CrossRef] [PubMed]
42. Perez, V.L.; Caspi, R.R. Immune mechanisms in inflammatory and degenerative eye disease. *Trends Immunol.* **2015**, *36*, 354–363. [CrossRef] [PubMed]
43. Zhu, M.; Provis, J.M.; Penfold, P.L. The human hyaloid system: Cellular phenotypes and inter-relationships. *Exp. Eye Res.* **1999**, *68*, 553–563. [CrossRef] [PubMed]
44. Noda, Y.; Hata, Y.; Hisatomi, T.; Nakamura, Y.; Hirayama, K.; Miura, M.; Nakao, S.; Fujisawa, K.; Sakamoto, T.; Ishibashi, T. Functional properties of hyalocytes under PDGF-rich conditions. *Investig. Ophthalmol. Vis. Sci.* **2004**, *45*, 2107–2114. [CrossRef] [PubMed]
45. Qiao, H.; Hisatomi, T.; Sonoda, K.H.; Kura, S.; Sassa, Y.; Kinoshita, S.; Nakamura, T.; Sakamoto, T.; Ishibashi, T. The characterisation of hyalocytes: The origin. phenotype, and turnover. *Br. J. Ophthalmol.* **2005**, *89*, 513–517. [CrossRef] [PubMed]
46. Castanos, M.V.; Zhou, D.B.; Linderman, R.E.; Allison, R.; Milman, T.; Carroll, J.; Migacz, J.; Rosen, R.B.; Chui, T.Y.P. Imaging of Macrophage-Like Cells in Living Human Retina Using Clinical OCT. *Investig. Ophthalmol. Vis. Sci.* **2020**, *61*, 48. [CrossRef] [PubMed]

47. Geyer, O.; Levo, Y. Glaucoma is an autoimmune disease. *Autoimmun. Rev.* **2020**, *19*, 102535. [CrossRef]
48. Ramírez, A.I.; Fernández-Albarral, J.A.; de Hoz, R.; López-Cuenca, I.; Salobrar-García, E.; Rojas, P.; Valiente-Soriano, F.J.; Avilés-Trigueros, M.; Villegas-Pérez, M.P.; Vidal-Sanz, M.; et al. Microglial changes in the early aging stage in a healthy retina and an experimental glaucoma model. In *Progress in Brain Research*; Elsevier B.V.: Amsterdam, The Netherlands, 2020; pp. 125–149. [CrossRef]
49. Tezel, G. The immune response in glaucoma: A perspective on the roles of oxidative stress. *Exp. Eye Res.* **2011**, *93*, 178–186. [CrossRef]
50. Sapienza, A.; Raveu, A.-L.; Reboussin, E.; Roubeix, C.; Boucher, C.; Dégardin, J.; Godefroy, D.; Rostène, W.; Goazigo, A.R.-L.; Baudouin, C.; et al. Bilateral neuroinflammatory processes in visual pathways induced by unilateral ocular hypertension in the rat. *J. Neuroinflamm.* **2016**, *13*, 44. [CrossRef]
51. Russo, R.; Varano, G.P.; Adornetto, A.; Nucci, C.; Corasaniti, M.T.; Bagetta, G.; Morrone, L.A. Retinal ganglion cell death in glaucoma: Exploring the role of neuroinflammation. *Eur. J. Pharmacol.* **2016**, *787*, 134–142. [CrossRef]
52. Tsai, T.; Reinehr, S.; Maliha, A.M.; Joachim, S.C. Immune Mediated Degeneration and Possible Protection in Glaucoma. *Front. Neurosci.* **2019**, *13*, 931. [CrossRef]
53. Todd, L.; Palazzo, I.; Suarez, L.; Liu, X.; Volkov, L.; Hoang, T.V.; Campbell, W.A.; Blackshaw, S.; Quan, N.; Fischer, A.J. Reactive microglia and IL1β/IL-1R1-signaling mediate neuroprotection in excitotoxin-damaged mouse retina. *J. Neuroinflamm.* **2019**, *16*, 118. [CrossRef]
54. Roberti, G.; Oddone, F.; Agnifili, L.; Katsanos, A.; Michelessi, M.; Mastropasqua, L.; Quaranta, L.; Riva, I.; Tanga, L.; Manni, G. Steroid-induced glaucoma: Epidemiology; pathophysiology; clinical management. *Surv. Ophthalmol.* **2020**, *65*, 458–472. [CrossRef] [PubMed]
55. Couret, C.; Poinas, A.; Volteau, C.; Riche, V.P.; Le Lez, M.L.; Errera, M.H.; Creuzot-Garcher, C.; Baillif, S.; Kodjikian, L.; Ivan, C.L.M.; et al. Comparison of two techniques used in routine care for the treatment of inflammatory macular oedema, subconjunctival triamcinolone injection and intravitreal dexamethasone implant: Medical and economic importance of this randomized controlled trial. *Trials* **2020**, *21*, 159. [CrossRef] [PubMed]
56. Taylor, A.W.; Ng, T.F. Negative regulators that mediate ocular immune privilege. *J. Leukoc. Biol.* **2018**, *103*, 1179–1187. [CrossRef] [PubMed]
57. Choi, S.; Hill, D.; Guo, L.; Nicholas, R.; Papadopoulos, D.; Cordeiro, M.F. Automated characterisation of microglia in ageing mice using image processing and supervised machine learning algorithms. *Sci. Rep.* **2022**, *12*, 1806. [CrossRef] [PubMed]
58. Staurenghi, G.; Sadda, S.; Chakravarthy, U.; Spaide, R.F. Proposed lexicon for anatomic landmarks in normal posterior segment spectral-domain optical coherence tomography: The IN•OCT consensus. *Ophthalmology* **2014**, *121*, 1572–1578. [CrossRef]
59. Choudhry, N.; Duker, J.S.; Freund, K.B.; Kiss, S.; Querques, G.; Rosen, R.; Sarraf, D.; Souied, E.H.; Stanga, P.E.; Staurenghi, G.; et al. Classification and Guidelines for Widefield Imaging: Recommendations from the International Widefield Imaging Study Group. *Ophthalmol. Retin.* **2019**, *3*, 843–849. [CrossRef]
60. Liu, S.; Li, Z.; Weinreb, R.N.; Xu, G.; Lindsey, J.D.; Ye, C.; Yung, W.; Pang, C.-P.; Lam, D.S.C.; Leung, C.K. Tracking Retinal Microgliosis in Models of Retinal Ganglion Cell Damage. *Investig. Opthalmol. Vis. Sci.* **2012**, *53*, 6254. [CrossRef] [PubMed]
61. Rajesh, A.; Droho, S.; Lavine, J.A. Macrophages in close proximity to the vitreoretinal interface are potential biomarkers of inflammation during retinal vascular disease. *J. Neuroinflamm.* **2022**, *19*, 203. [CrossRef]
62. Keane, P.A.; Balaskas, K.; Sim, D.A.; Aman, K.; Denniston, A.K.; Aslam, T.; Aslam, T. Automated analysis of vitreous inflammation using spectral-domain optical coherence tomography. *Transl. Vis. Sci. Technol.* **2015**, *4*, 4. [CrossRef]
63. Zarranz-Ventura, J.; Keane, P.A.; Sim, D.A.; Llorens, V.; Tufail, A.; Sadda, S.R.; Dick, A.D.; Lee, R.W.; Pavesio, C.; Denniston, A.K.; et al. Evaluation of Objective Vitritis Grading Method Using Optical Coherence Tomography: Influence of Phakic Status and Previous Vitrectomy. *Am. J. Ophthalmol.* **2016**, *161*, 172–180.e4. [CrossRef]
64. Gordon, S.; Plüddemann, A.; Estrada, F.M. Macrophage heterogeneity in tissues: Phenotypic diversity and functions. *Immunol. Rev.* **2014**, *262*, 36–55. [CrossRef]
65. Jiang, L.Q.; Streilein, J.W. Immune Privilege Extended to Allogeneic Tumor Cells in the Vitreous Cavity. *Investig. Ophthalmol. Vis. Sci.* **1991**, *32*, 224–228.
66. Ramírez, A.I.; de Hoz, R.; Fernández-Albarral, J.A.; Salobrar-Garcia, E.; Rojas, B.; Valiente-Soriano, F.J.; Avilés-Trigueros, M.; Villegas-Pérez, M.P.; Vidal-Sanz, M.; Triviño, A.; et al. Time course of bilateral microglial activation in a mouse model of laser-induced glaucoma. *Sci. Rep.* **2020**, *10*, 4890. [CrossRef]
67. O'Koren, E.G.; Mathew, R.; Saban, D.R. Fate mapping reveals that microglia and recruited monocyte-derived macrophages are definitively distinguishable by phenotype in the retina. *Sci. Rep.* **2016**, *6*, 20636. [CrossRef] [PubMed]
68. Cordeiro, M.F.; Guo, L.; Luong, V.; Harding, G.; Wang, W.; Jones, H.E.; Moss, S.E.; Sillito, A.M.; Fitzke, F.W. Real-time imaging of single nerve cell apoptosis in retinal neurodegeneration. *Proc. Natl. Acad. Sci. USA* **2004**, *101*, 13352–13356. [CrossRef] [PubMed]
69. Cordeiro, M.F.; Normando, E.M.; Cardoso, M.J.; Miodragovic, S.; Jeylani, S.; Davis, B.M.; Guo, L.; Ourselin, S.; A'Hern, R.; Bloom, P.A. Real-time imaging of single neuronal cell apoptosis in patients with glaucoma. *Brain* **2017**, *140*, 1757–1767. [CrossRef] [PubMed]

70. Coric, D.; Ometto, G.; Montesano, G.; Keane, P.A.; Balk, L.J.; Uitdehaag, B.M.J.; Petzold, A.; Crabb, D.P.; Denniston, A.K. Objective quantification of vitreous haze on optical coherence tomography scans: No evidence for relationship between uveitis and inflammation in multiple sclerosis. *Eur. J. Neurol.* **2020**, *27*, 144-e3. [CrossRef] [PubMed]
71. Nichols, M.R.; St-Pierre, M.K.; Wendeln, A.C.; Makoni, N.J.; Gouwens, L.K.; Garrad, E.C.; Sohrabi, M.; Neher, J.J.; Tremblay, M.E.; Combs, C.K. Inflammatory Mechanisms in Neurodegeneration. *J. Neurochem.* **2019**, *149*, 562. [CrossRef] [PubMed]

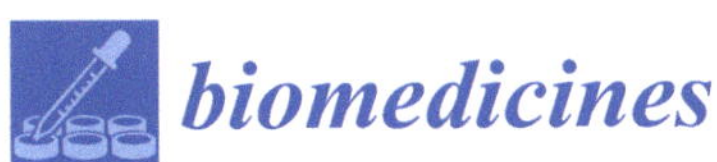

MDPI

Review

Unveiling Novel Structural Biomarkers for the Diagnosis of Glaucoma

Yu-Chien Tsai [1,2], Hsin-Pei Lee [1], Ta-Hsin Tsung [1], Yi-Hao Chen [1] and Da-Wen Lu [1,*]

1 Department of Ophthalmology, Tri-Service General Hospital, National Defense Medical Center, Taipei 114, Taiwan
2 Department of Ophthalmology, Taoyuan Armed Forces General Hospital, Taoyuan 325, Taiwan
* Correspondence: ludawen@yahoo.com; Tel.: +886-2-8792-3311

Abstract: Glaucoma, a leading cause of irreversible blindness, poses a significant global health burden. Early detection is crucial for effective management and prevention of vision loss. This study presents a collection of novel structural biomarkers in glaucoma diagnosis. By employing advanced imaging techniques and data analysis algorithms, we now can recognize indicators of glaucomatous progression. Many research studies have revealed a correlation between the structural changes in the eye or brain, particularly in the optic nerve head and retinal nerve fiber layer, and the progression of glaucoma. These biomarkers demonstrate value in distinguishing glaucomatous eyes from healthy ones, even in the early stages of the disease. By facilitating timely detection and monitoring, they hold the potential to mitigate vision impairment and improve patient outcomes. This study marks an advancement in the field of glaucoma, offering a promising avenue for enhancing the diagnosis and possible management.

Keywords: diagnosis; structural; image; biomarkers; glaucoma

Citation: Tsai, Y.-C.; Lee, H.-P.; Tsung, T.-H.; Chen, Y.-H.; Lu, D.-W. Unveiling Novel Structural Biomarkers for the Diagnosis of Glaucoma. *Biomedicines* **2024**, *12*, 1211. https://doi.org/10.3390/biomedicines12061211

Academic Editor: Biancamaria Longoni

Received: 29 April 2024
Revised: 21 May 2024
Accepted: 28 May 2024
Published: 29 May 2024

1. Introduction

Glaucoma stands as a pivotal concern in ophthalmology and is renowned for being a leading cause of irreversible blindness globally. It impacted an estimated 80 million people worldwide in 2020 and is still increasing till now, imposing a tremendous financial burden on both the individual and society [1,2]. It is a group of chronic and progressive retinal and optic neuropathies, characterized by irreversible morphological changes at the optic nerve head (ONH) and the inner retinal layers and visual field defects, which are associated with retinal ganglion cell (RGC) loss and an elevation of intraocular pressure (IOP) [3]. Glaucoma may not have any symptoms in the early stages and the optic nerve injury is already quite advanced when the patient presents with initial visual field defects, which makes it "the silent thief of sight" [4]. In most cases, the central vision is the last to be affected. As a consequence, glaucoma may remain undetected until it reaches a moderate or severe stage, thereby causing treatment and diagnosis delays and resulting in unaltered visual acuity change. A person may develop a heightened propensity for incidents involving falls and collisions with objects while walking, as well as encounter challenges while driving, by that juncture. This underscores the critical importance of early detection and vigilant monitoring to thwart visual disability associated with this condition. In this pursuit, the exploration and identification of glaucoma biomarkers have opened new horizons for early diagnosis, understanding risk profiles, pinpointing damage progression, and monitoring treatment response, with a hope of revolutionizing glaucoma management [5].

Diving deeper, the article unfolds the role of structural biomarkers in enhancing the specificity and sensitivity of glaucoma diagnosis [5]. It proposes innovative methodologies such as optical coherence tomography (OCT) and magnetic resonance imaging (MRI) in glaucoma research, showcasing how these methods complement traditional diagnostic approaches to offer a fuller, more accurate picture of the disease [6,7]. While elucidating the challenges faced and proposing future directions, this narrative is set against the backdrop of the newest findings in structural biomarker research, promising to significantly advance the field of glaucoma diagnosis [5,7].

2. Traditional Diagnostic Methods

Diagnosing glaucoma involves a comprehensive assessment of various ocular parameters to identify signs of optic nerve damage and associated vision loss [8]. The initial step often includes measuring intraocular pressure (IOP) through tonometry, as elevated IOP is a primary risk factor for glaucoma. However, the IOP is often influenced by corneal properties such as corneal thickness, corneal curvature, and elastic properties; thus, additional examination of the cornea or using specific equations for modified-IOP calculation is very important [9,10]. Among the glaucoma patients, almost one-third of the eyes have normal IOP, underscoring the necessity of conducting further diagnostic imaging instead of relying on the IOP readings [11]. Fundus photography allows for visualization of the optic nerve head and adjacent tissue, enabling clinicians to detect structural abnormalities indicative of glaucomatous damage like enlargement of the cup, disc hemorrhages, pallor of the disc, neuroretinal rim thinning, and neovascularization. OCT uses laser beams to provide high-resolution images in evaluating the ocular structures including the thickness of the retinal nerve fiber layer and neuroretinal rim of the optic nerve head [12]. Perimetry assesses peripheral vision and aids in identifying the characteristic patterns of visual field loss associated with glaucoma such as nasal step, temporal wedge defect, classic arcuate defect, generalized constriction, or tunnel vision defect with temporal crescent sparing [13]. Additionally, gonioscopy assesses the drainage angle of the eye, which is crucial in determining the risk of angle-closure glaucoma, and pachymetry for measuring central cornea thickness plays an important role in glaucoma diagnosis [14].

However, the limitation of current methods for diagnosing glaucoma is the incapacity to definitively diagnose the condition prior to significant glaucomatous damage. While RGC apoptosis has been recognized as the initial stage of cellular demise in glaucoma, it is approximated that a significant proportion of RGCs are lost prior to the detection of visual field abnormalities by conventional clinical examinations. The progress and incorporation of many diagnostic methods, such as imaging technology and functional tests, improve the accuracy of early glaucoma diagnosis and allow prompt management to maintain visual function [15].

3. Emerging Structural Diagnostic Biomarkers

In the quest for early and accurate diagnosis of glaucoma, structural biomarkers have emerged as a pivotal area of research. These biomarkers offer a promising avenue for detecting glaucoma at its nascent stage, potentially revolutionizing the approach to managing this vision-threatening condition. In diagnosing and tracking the progression of glaucoma, direct examination of the optic nerve and retinal nerve fiber layer is critical. The progression of damage to the optic disc and retina are an extremely reliable predictor of glaucoma-related functional impairment. Other ocular structures, including the scleral spur, also play a role in the development of glaucoma. Nevertheless, a few patients present with glaucomatous change, and a mere structural assessment fails to provide a sufficient diagnosis [15]. The advancement of imaging devices has facilitated improved visualization of the ganglion cell layer, nerve fiber layer, and optic disk head as potential diagnostic biomarkers. And using a combination of different parameters, structural and functional exams possess the capacity to enhance the early recognition and diagnosis of glaucoma. A summary of the biomarkers and their utility for glaucoma diagnosis are shown in Table 1.

Table 1. Summary of the biomarkers and their utility for glaucoma diagnosis.

Structural Biomarkers	Findings	Limitations	Utility for Glaucoma Detection
Scleral spur length	Shorter scleral spur length of POAG eyes than the healthy	The increase of IOP cannot be attributed only to the Schlemm's canal and scleral spur	Low
GCL/IPL thickness *	Decreased IPL and GCIPL thickness Less affected by the degree of myopia and myopia-related optic disc change than RNFL thickness	Still may be affected by highly myopic eyes (GCIPL hemifield test provides a superior diagnostic ability)	High
Vessel density and flow index	Decrease of vessel density and flow density in deep retinal vascular plexus and the whole retina	Superficial layer of retinal vasculature to obscure the deeper vessels of the retina Artifacts Ocular vascular changes in specific conditions including smoking, cardiovascular disease, hypoxia, and hyperoxia	Moderate
FAZ-related parameters * (perimeter and circularity index)	Higher FAZ perimeter Lower circularity index		Low
BMO-MRW *	Better determination of the borders of the neuroretinal rim Useful in myopic eyes	Affected by the diversity of disc size and retinal blood vessels	Moderate
BMO-MRA *	Useful in different disc size	Might not reflect the actual minimum area	
Lamina cribrosa morphology	Decreased laminar thickness Posterior displacement of the laminar insertion Greater lamina cribrosa curvature index	Need for prospective studies evaluating lamina cribrosa changes over time	Low–Moderate
Cortical thickness of the visual cortex	Thinning cortex was majorly found in the primary visual cortex	High cost; time consuming	Low
Fractional anisotropy (FA) values and mean diffusivity (MD)	Elevated MD and reduced FA in relation to the optic nerve and optic radiation	High cost; time consuming	Low

* GCL/IPL = ganglion cell layer (GCL) and inner plexiform layer (IPL). * FAZ = foveal avascular zone. * BMO-MRW/MRA = Bruch's membrane opening–minimum rim width (BMO-MRW) and minimum rim area (MRA).

3.1. *Anterior Segment*

Scleral Spur Length

Prior research has demonstrated that most of the resistance to the aqueous outflow is situated within the internal region of Schlemm's canal (SC) [16] and the scleral spur may also play a significant role in maintaining the diameter of the SC lumen. To maintain the SC lumen, the ciliary muscle's force makes the scleral spur displace backward thus stretching the trabecular meshwork and inner wall of the SC and widening the lumen [17,18]. An additional finding was that the average length of the scleral spur was notably reduced in eyes with POAG when compared to healthy eyes of the same age [19]. This suggests that a shorter scleral spur could potentially serve as a risk factor in the advancement of POAG, as it would lack the capacity to sustain the lumen of SC. Mu et al. reported using swept-source optical coherence tomography (SS-OCT) to conduct observations and make comparisons between the SC and scleral spur length of POAG and healthy individual eyes [20]. The study revealed a significantly shorter scleral spur length of the POAG eyes than the healthy eyes, and also a narrowing scleral spur opening in the POAG eyes. The length of the scleral spur demonstrated a strong diagnostic capacity in distinguishing eyes with primary open-angle glaucoma (POAG) from healthy eyes [20]. Meanwhile, there were other variables that might potentially contribute to the increase in intraocular pressure (IOP) associated with glaucoma. Therefore, it cannot be attributed only to the SC and scleral spur.

3.2. *Optical Coherence Tomography (OCT)*

Optical coherence tomography (OCT) imaging is crucial for the detection and management of glaucoma [21–23]. OCT enables precise and non-invasive measurement of alterations in important eye structures related to the diagnosis and the disease nature of glaucoma, ranging from the front part of the eye like the anterior chamber angle to the back part, which includes the macula area, optic nerve head (ONH) and retinal nerve fiber layer (RNFL) [24]. Innovative high-resolution imaging instruments have been developed, leading to notable enhancements in scanning speed, decreased acquisition duration, elevated image clarity, enhanced precision in segmentation, and diagnostic algorithms. These advancements have led to more precise and consistent measures for early detection and better surveillance of glaucoma [25]. Furthermore, OCT technical advancement has significantly improved the visibility of deeper structures within the ONH, which are considered crucial in understanding glaucoma etiology.

Among these supplementary imaging instruments, spectral-domain optical coherence tomography (SD-OCT) and swept-source OCT (SS-OCT) tend to be the most frequently implemented. Assessing the peripapillary RNFL thickness, optic nerve head, and macular ganglion cell–inner plexiform layer (GCIPL), SD-OCT permits clinicians to objectively and precisely monitor RGCs, as well as their axons and dendrites [25,26]. SS-OCT allows for a wider area in a single image, providing better imaging of the outermost temporal boundary of RNFL defects and brings the utility of SS-OCT wide-field RNFL mapping for early identification of glaucoma. Improved imaging and quantitative assessment of the lamina cribrosa (LC) structural alterations brought on by glaucomatous damage can also be provided by SS-OCT [24].

OCT angiography (OCTA) is a new method that allows for noninvasive and detailed imaging of the small blood vessels in the retina, choroid, and optic disc area. It also offers measurements of the amount of blood vessels in each layer, known as vascular density. Previous research has shown a relation between glaucoma and the flow of blood in the eyes, as well as the disparity between diastolic blood pressure and intraocular pressure (IOP). This discrepancy is linked to a higher occurrence of glaucoma [27–36].

3.2.1. Segmented Inner Retinal Layer Thickness

Numerous studies have indicated the potential utility of circumpapillary retinal nerve fiber layer (cpRNFL) measurements in the early detection of glaucoma [37]. Nonetheless, it is crucial to note that the depth of cpRNFL can be affected by individual variations in optic nerve head (ONH) structure, such as an oval-shaped and obliquely rotated ONH and peripapillary atrophy, which are commonly observed in individuals with high levels of myopia. However, when there is no concomitant disease, macular parameters are superior in producing more consonant pictures with less variance in structure between people [38]. Kim EK et al. reported that the RNFL, ganglion cell layer (GCL), and inner plexiform layer (IPL) changed as glaucoma progressed, which demonstrates that in individuals with glaucoma, the RGC experiences many dendritic (IPL) and soma (GCL) alterations and RGC axon damage induces rapid pathological alterations in RGC dendrites [4,39]. Slightly in advance of axonal thinning or soma shrinking, morphological alterations in RGC dendrites might be seen in pre-perimetric and early glaucoma [40]. These findings indicate that the measurement of IPL thickness might be a biomarker to detect impairment of RGC function in early glaucoma. Considering the structure–function correlation in segmented layers, Kim's study observed that IPL and GCIPL thickness have a stronger relationship than RNFL and GCL. And the confidence interval of IPL thickness over the disease progression is narrow. Therefore, measuring IPL thickness along with other segmented inner retinal layer thicknesses may be useful for the early diagnosis and monitoring of glaucoma [4]. Kouros et al. observed that global RNFL thickness had better performance in early glaucoma detection than GCIPL thickness, but sector GCIPL thickness measurements (inferotempereal and minimum GCIPL) had similar performance in sector RNFL thickness (inferior) [41]. Also, an asymmetry finding on the GCIPL thickness maps, the hemifield difference across the horizontal raphe, demonstrated a good early glaucoma detection ability for the GCIPL Hemifield Test [42,43].

3.2.2. Vessel Density, Flow Index, and Foveal Avascular Zone Parameters

The mobility of red blood cells inside blood arteries is the primary source of the signal fluctuation that OCTA detects between images [34]. The formation of a three-dimensional representation of the kinetic contrast resulting from the flow of blood is achieved through the acquisition of many photographs within a brief timeframe, which allows for the viewing and partial measurement of microvascular perfusion. One thing that should be brought to everyone's attention is the fact that every OCT device that is now on the market detects, represents, and analyzes OCTA signals and microvascular perfusion using a distinct algorithm [35]. Consequently, the results from various OCTA devices might not be directly comparable. However, most of the results can be applied to practical instruments currently on the market [44].

In the OCTA optic disc scan, pre-perimetric glaucomatous eyes was found to have a significant reduction in vessel density in the entire disc area, temporal region of the disc, and in the peripapillary area. And the flow index of these areas showed a considerable decrease compared to healthy individuals [45–47]. In the patients with unilateral perimetric glaucoma, the peripapillary and inferotemporal capillary beds were significantly decreased compared to the unaffected eye and in healthy individuals [48–51]. Kumar et al. reported that superior and temporal sectors of the OCTA images showed more vessel density decrease in glaucoma eyes then healthy eyes [52]. And the asymmetry of vascular density in bilateral eyes, measured by 4.5 $\times$ 4.5 mm disc-centered whole-image optic nerve head scans, distinguished healthy people from those who may have glaucoma [53]. The majority of research found a strong connection between the amount of vascular density loss and the severity of glaucoma. Hence, OCTA can identify decreases in blood flow in the ONH before any visible impairment to the visual field occurs. This indicates that OCTA could be valuable for early identification of glaucoma and assessing the risk of glaucoma development.

In the macular OCTA scans, the vessel density decrease is more noticeable in the inferior macular region and superficial vascular plexus layer (internal limiting membrane to inner plexiform layer)—which is now the most often employed OCTA parameter—than in the deep retinal layer because of the projection artifacts from the superficial plexus, and the wider field of the 6 $\times$ 6 mm scans centered on the fovea has a higher sensitivity in identifying changes in glaucoma in patients than the 3 $\times$ 3 mm scans [29,54–58]. A study using macular whole image vessel density found that a 0.11 μm/year faster decreasing rate of RNFL was associated with every 1% loss of macular vessel density [59]. Several studies also found a significant decrease of vessel density and flow density in deep retinal vascular plexus and the whole retina, and the diagnostic ability of glaucoma of the vessel density in the GCIPL might be better than in the superficial vascular plexus [49,60–65]. However, still some studies found that macular vessel density performed no better than OCT GCC thickness in distinguishing early glaucoma from healthy eyes [66–69]. Choi et al. reported that foveal avascular zone (FAZ)-related parameters (perimeter and circularity index) had a diagnostic value for discriminating glaucoma from healthy subjects. The circularity index would decrease once the FAZ did not have a purely circular shape owing to the progression of deterioration of the capillary network in the parafoveal region. The FAZ perimeter was higher and the circularity index was lower in the POAG eyes. Compared with GCIPL and RNFL thickness, the FAZ-related parameters have similar performance in distinguishing normal and glaucoma eyes [60].

3.2.3. Bruch's Membrane Opening–Minimum Rim Width (BMO-MRW) and Minimum Rim Area (MRA)

The clinically identified optic disc margin for the neuroretinal rim assessment has no solid anatomic foundation for two reasons: due to the invisible extensions of the Bruch's membrane (BM) within the disc margin from the image, and the optic nerve head's (ONH) rim tissue orientation not being traceable. The BM opening–minimum rim width (BMO-MRW) is a parameter that measures the length from the inner limiting membrane to its real anatomical outer border, BMO. The advantages of BMO-MRW include that it considers the expansions of BM that are clinically imperceptible but discovered by SD-OCT. Similar to current methods for measuring peripapillary retinal nerve fiber layer thickness, BMO-MRW measurement considers the varying path of axons across the location of measurement since it is made perpendicular to the axis of the neural tissue [70,71]. Chauhan et al. reported that compared to RNFL thickness, BMO-MRW produced better diagnostic results for glaucoma with current confocal scanning laser tomography (CSLT) or SD-OCT based ONH and RNFLT parameters, excluding the superiornasal quadrant, which exhibited a greater sensitivity to RNFL thickness [71–73]. Jonas et al. reported that RNFL thickness and BMO-MRW have comparable areas under the receiver operating characteristic curves (AUROCs) in distinguishing perimetric glaucoma eyes to normal eyes and both showed lower AUROCs in the pre-perimetric glaucoma group. If the specificity was fixed in 95% vs. 90%, RNFL thickness had a sensitivity of 84% vs. 84% and BMO-MRW had a sensitivity of 52% vs. 88% in distinguishing perimetric glaucoma to normal eyes. The BMO-MRW might be influenced by the retinal blood vessels since they may enter the ONH irregularly [74]. Moreover, when it comes to a larger disc, which might have a thinner BMO-MRW in general, a two-dimensional parameter, BMO–minimum rim area (MRA), might have a better diagnostic capability. Introduced by Gardiner et al., BMO-MRA was calculated using the total area of 48 trapeziums, each reaching the inner limiting membrane at an angle above the BMO plane from an identified BMO point [75]. As a result, when comparing different disc sizes, the BMO-MRA should be more beneficial than the BMO-MRW [76–78].

3.2.4. Lamina Cribrosa Morphology

The lamina cribrosa is a structure located deep within the eye, specifically within the optic nerve head. It is essentially a sieve-like structure made up of collagen fibers through which the retinal ganglion cell axons pass as they exit the eye to form the optic nerve. These axons transmit visual information from the retina to the brain and were thought to be vulnerable to the pressure gradient stress [79,80]. Over time, this pressure can lead to structural changes in the lamina cribrosa, such as thinning or deformation, which can impede the flow of nutrients to the optic nerve cells and cause damage to the nerve fibers themselves. Previous experimental studies suggested that the morphological changes of the lamina cribrosa precede the thinning of RNFL and defects of the visual field, which means the structural change of the lamina cribrosa could be found in the earliest stage of glaucoma [81,82]. Advanced image technologies including SS-OCT, enhanced depth imaging OCT (EDI-OCT), and adaptive optics -OCT, or -scanning laser ophthalmoscopy (SLO), improved the ability to evaluate the lamina cribrosa.

The lamina cribrosa thickness significantly influences the biomechanics of the optic nerve head (ONH), playing a crucial role in glaucomatous optic nerve change. Studies have shown that the mean laminar thickness was significantly thinner in glaucoma groups (215.41 ± 38.96 μm) than in the control groups (349.08 ± 23.34 μm). And the diagnostic value (as the area under the receiver operating characteristic curve) of the lamina cribrosa thickness for detecting POAG and NTG (0.941, 0.981) was slightly higher than the diagnostic performance of RNFL thickness measurement (0.928, 0.941) [83]. Besides the thinning of lamina cribrosa, posterior bowing, also posterior displacement of the laminar insertion, precedes the RNFL thinning in glaucoma patients. Another parameter which describes the morphology, the lamina cribrosa curvature index (LCCI), may help in distinguishing the glaucomatous optic neuropathy from the normal group and other neuropathies. It is measured by dividing the lamina cribrosa curve depth (LCCD) by the width of the anterior LC surface line and multiplying by 100 (introduced by Seung et al.) [84]. Jeong et al. reported that the greater the LCCI, the faster the RNFL loss rate [79]. The normal lamina cribrosa has a curve, that is, only when the posterior bowing surpasses a certain threshold will the optic nerve axons get injured. Seung et al. suggested the threshold of LCCI around 9.51 though it may differ among individuals and requires further refinement in a future investigation of greater magnitude.

3.3. *Magnetic Resonance Imaging (MRI)*

As a neurodegenerative disease, glaucoma causes damage not only to the retinal ganglion cells but also their dendrites and axons, and involves damage along the visual pathways to the brain, such as the optic tract, lateral geniculate nucleus (LGN), optic radiation, and visual cortex [85–90]. Recent studies have focused on the MRI utility of assessing the glaucomatous injuries within the brain, including atrophy and degeneration of the visual cortex and visual pathway, and the diffusion tensor imaging (DTI)-derived parameter, fractional anisotropy (FA) [91,92].

3.3.1. Morphometry

Anatomical magnetic resonance imaging (MRI) offers comprehensive details on the morphological characteristics of different brain areas, often pertaining to size and shape. With the advent of MRI scanners with field strengths of 3 Tesla or more, researchers can now produce images of exceptional quality that clearly distinguish different brain tissues and allow them to examine the relationships between different brain structures and biological, psychological, and clinical parameters. Morphometry is the quantitative measurement of a structure's dimensions and forms [93].

In a series of studies investigating the effects of glaucoma on the brain, several key findings were observed. Using voxel-based techniques, Bogorodzki et al. revealed that individuals with a loss of vision in one eye only due to advanced open-angle glaucoma exhibited a noticeable reduction in the thickness of the visual cortex compared to a normal age-matched group [94]. Another study using high-precision magnetic resonance imaging revealed a reduction in grey matter volume in patients with advanced glaucoma in a number of brain regions, including the lingual, calcarine, postcentral gyrus, inferior frontal, superior frontal gyrus, and Rolandic operculum, and also in the right cuneus, right inferior occipital gyrus, right supramarginal gyrus, and left paracentral lobule [95]. The findings collectively suggest that glaucoma can lead to structural changes in the brain, particularly in regions associated with vision processing. These changes may vary depending on the stage of the disease. Additionally, the cortical thickness of the visual cortex may serve as a potential diagnostic marker for glaucoma, especially when considering age-related changes in cortical thickness. Rodolfo et al. revealed that in an early glaucoma patient, a thinning cortex was majorly found in the primary visual cortex in MRI and the RNFL and GCL/IPL complex also showed morphological defects on OCT while the visual field exam still remained normal [96]. Early detection and monitoring of these brain changes through techniques like MRI could aid in the diagnosis and management of glaucoma.

3.3.2. Fractional Anisotropy (FA) Values and Mean Diffusivity (MD) of DTI

Postmortem examinations have shown the presence of glaucomatous neuronal degeneration in all regions of the central visual pathways, resulting in significant visual field impairments in both eyes. The quantitative measurement of anterior visual pathway compression may be achieved by the utilization of diffusion tensor imaging (DTI), which employs fractional anisotropy (FA) and mean diffusivity (MD). DTI measures the diffusion of water molecules in tissues, particularly in the brain's white matter tracts. It provides information about the microstructural organization and integrity of white matter fibers by analyzing the directionality and magnitude of water diffusion [97]. FA is a scalar value derived from the diffusion tensor, representing the degree of anisotropy within a voxel [98]. High FA values indicate highly directional diffusion, typically found in intact white matter tracts, while low FA values suggest disrupted or disorganized tissue structure. A drop in FA and an increase in MD may suggest the presence of structural impairment in the optic nerve axon among individuals diagnosed with glaucoma [99].

Prior research has demonstrated that individuals with glaucoma have notably elevated MD and reduced FA in relation to the optic nerve and optic radiation. These findings are consistent with the severity of glaucoma, as well as the morphological alterations observed in the optic nerve head and retinal nerve fiber layer [100–103]. The MD values exhibited a greater magnitude at the proximal location of the optic nerve head in comparison to the distal location. In contrast, a reduction in FA was seen solely in relation to the stage of the patient, regardless of the location of the optic nerve. Furthermore, in the early stage of glaucoma, there was a noticeable rise in comprehensive diffusivities at the proximal location. Conversely, at the distal location, a decrease was observed in the diffusivity that was the highest, whereas there was a rise in the diffusivities that were intermediate and the smallest. The results indicate that DTI, which has a high sensitivity for FA and a high specificity for MD, might be a useful additional diagnostic technique for evaluating structural changes in retinal ganglion cells and optic nerves in glaucoma [96,104].

4. Conclusions

Glaucoma may not even have any symptoms in the early stages and does not cause much restriction in daily life because the preservation of central vision comes at the expense of peripheral vision, which is more affected. It is only in the late stages, when significant and irreversible loss of vision has occurred causing weakened spatial perception and difficulties in certain daily activities, that it may be noted and diagnosed. Therefore, early diagnosis should be taken promptly.

The structural changes include the shortening scleral spur length, decreasing GCL/IPL thickness, BMO-MRW/MRA, decreasing vessel density/flow density, FAZ parameters, alteration of lamina cribrosa morphology, and the neurodegeneration noted from MRI. Relying merely on a single biomarker may not adequately assess glaucomatous changes, but combining multiple biomarkers and functional tests increases the sensitivity and specificity of early glaucoma diagnosis. Further investigation is warranted to examine the diagnostic and prognostic significance of these biomarkers combined with others, including perimetry and electrophysiological tests.

Author Contributions: Conceptualization, Y.-C.T. and D.-W.L.; validation, D.-W.L.; resources, D.-W.L.; writing—original draft preparation, Y.-C.T., T.-H.T. and H.-P.L.; writing—review and editing, Y.-H.C. and D.-W.L.; visualization, Y.-C.T., T.-H.T. and H.-P.L.; supervision, Y.-H.C. and D.-W.L. All authors have read and agreed to the published version of the manuscript.

Funding: This research received no external funding.

Conflicts of Interest: The authors declare no conflicts of interest.

References

1. Allison, K.; Patel, D.; Alabi, O. Epidemiology of Glaucoma: The Past, Present, and Predictions for the Future. *Cureus* **2020**, *12*, e11686. [CrossRef] [PubMed]
2. Al-Nosairy, K.O.; Hoffmann, M.B.; Bach, M. Non-invasive electrophysiology in glaucoma, structure and function-a review. *Eye* **2021**, *35*, 2374–2385. [CrossRef] [PubMed]
3. Mwanza, J.C.; Lee, G.; Budenz, D.L.; Warren, J.L.; Wall, M.; Artes, P.H.; Callan, T.M.; Flanagan, J.G. Validation of the UNC OCT Index for the Diagnosis of Early Glaucoma. *Transl. Vis. Sci. Technol.* **2018**, *7*, 16. [CrossRef] [PubMed]
4. Kim, E.K.; Park, H.L.; Park, C.K. Segmented inner plexiform layer thickness as a potential biomarker to evaluate open-angle glaucoma: Dendritic degeneration of retinal ganglion cell. *PLoS ONE* **2017**, *12*, e0182404. [CrossRef] [PubMed]
5. Fernández-Vega Cueto, A.; Álvarez, L.; García, M.; Álvarez-Barrios, A.; Artime, E.; Fernández-Vega Cueto, L.; Coca-Prados, M.; González-Iglesias, H. Candidate Glaucoma Biomarkers: From Proteins to Metabolites, and the Pitfalls to Clinical Applications. *Biology* **2021**, *10*, 763. [CrossRef]
6. Beykin, G.; Norcia, A.M.; Srinivasan, V.J.; Dubra, A.; Goldberg, J.L. Discovery and clinical translation of novel glaucoma biomarkers. *Prog. Retin. Eye Res.* **2021**, *80*, 100875. [CrossRef] [PubMed]
7. Von Thun Und Hohenstein-Blaul, N.; Kunst, S.; Pfeiffer, N.; Grus, F.H. Biomarkers for glaucoma: From the lab to the clinic. *Eye* **2017**, *31*, 225–231. [CrossRef]
8. Stein, J.D.; Khawaja, A.P.; Weizer, J.S. Glaucoma in Adults-Screening, Diagnosis, and Management: A Review. *JAMA* **2021**, *325*, 164–174. [CrossRef]
9. Goldmann, H.; Schmidt, T. Applanation tonometry. *Ophthalmologica* **1957**, *134*, 221–242. [CrossRef]
10. Lu, S.H.; Chong, I.T.; Leung, S.Y.Y.; Lam, D.C.C. Characterization of Corneal Biomechanical Properties and Determination of Natural Intraocular Pressure Using CID-GAT. *Transl. Vis. Sci. Technol.* **2019**, *8*, 10. [CrossRef]
11. Wagner, I.V.; Stewart, M.W.; Dorairaj, S.K. Updates on the Diagnosis and Management of Glaucoma. *Mayo Clin. Proc. Innov. Qual. Outcomes* **2022**, *6*, 618–635. [CrossRef]

12. Sathyan, P.; Shilpa, S.; Anitha, A. Optical Coherence Tomography in Glaucoma. *J. Curr. Glaucoma Pract.* **2012**, *6*, 1–5. [CrossRef] [PubMed]
13. Broadway, D.C. Visual field testing for glaucoma—A practical guide. *Community Eye Health* **2012**, *25*, 66–70. [PubMed]
14. Harasymowycz, P.; Birt, C.; Gooi, P.; Heckler, L.; Hutnik, C.; Jinapriya, D.; Shuba, L.; Yan, D.; Day, R. Medical Management of Glaucoma in the 21st Century from a Canadian Perspective. *J. Ophthalmol.* **2016**, *2016*, 6509809. [CrossRef] [PubMed]
15. Davis, B.M.; Crawley, L.; Pahlitzsch, M.; Javaid, F.; Cordeiro, M.F. Glaucoma: The retina and beyond. *Acta Neuropathol.* **2016**, *132*, 807–826. [CrossRef]
16. Mäepea, O.; Bill, A. The pressures in the episcleral veins, Schlemm's canal and the trabecular meshwork in monkeys: Effects of changes in intraocular pressure. *Exp. Eye Res.* **1989**, *49*, 645–663. [CrossRef] [PubMed]
17. Moses, R.A.; Grodzki, W.J., Jr. The scleral spur and scleral roll. *Investig. Ophthalmol. Vis. Sci.* **1977**, *16*, 925–931.
18. Rohen, J.W.; Lütjen, E.; Bárány, E. The relation between the ciliary muscle and the trabecular meshwork and its importance for the effect of miotics on aqueous outflow resistance. *Albrecht Graefes Arch. Klin. Exp. Ophthalmol.* **1967**, *172*, 23–47. [CrossRef] [PubMed]
19. Swain, D.L.; Ho, J.; Lai, J.; Gong, H. Shorter Scleral Spur in Eyes with Primary Open-Angle Glaucoma. *Investig. Ophthalmol. Vis. Sci.* **2015**, *56*, 1638–1648. [CrossRef]
20. Li, M.; Luo, Z.; Yan, X.; Zhang, H. Diagnostic power of scleral spur length in primary open-angle glaucoma. *Graefe's Arch. Clin. Exp. Ophthalmol.* **2020**, *258*, 1253–1260. [CrossRef]
21. Schuman, J.S.; Hee, M.R.; Arya, A.V.; Pedut-Kloizman, T.; Puliafito, C.A.; Fujimoto, J.G.; Swanson, E.A. Optical coherence tomography: A new tool for glaucoma diagnosis. *Curr. Opin. Ophthalmol.* **1995**, *6*, 89–95. [CrossRef]
22. Jaffe, G.J.; Caprioli, J. Optical coherence tomography to detect and manage retinal disease and glaucoma. *Am. J. Ophthalmol.* **2004**, *137*, 156–169. [CrossRef] [PubMed]
23. Ang, M.; Baskaran, M.; Werkmeister, R.M.; Chua, J.; Schmidl, D.; Aranha Dos Santos, V.; Garhöfer, G.; Mehta, J.S.; Schmetterer, L. Anterior segment optical coherence tomography. *Prog. Retin. Eye Res.* **2018**, *66*, 132–156. [CrossRef] [PubMed]
24. Shiga, Y.; Nishida, T.; Jeoung, J.W.; Di Polo, A.; Fortune, B. Optical Coherence Tomography and Optical Coherence Tomography Angiography: Essential Tools for Detecting Glaucoma and Disease Progression. *Front. Ophthalmol.* **2023**, *3*, 1217125. [CrossRef]
25. Kim, K.E.; Park, K.H. Update on the Prevalence, Etiology, Diagnosis, and Monitoring of Normal-Tension Glaucoma. *Asia Pac. J. Ophthalmol.* **2016**, *5*, 23–31. [CrossRef] [PubMed]
26. Mahmoudinezhad, G.; Mohammadzadeh, V.; Martinyan, J.; Edalati, K.; Zhou, B.; Yalzadeh, D.; Amini, N.; Caprioli, J.; Nouri-Mahdavi, K. Comparison of Ganglion Cell Layer and Ganglion Cell/Inner Plexiform Layer Measures for Detection of Early Glaucoma. *Ophthalmol. Glaucoma* **2023**, *6*, 58–67. [CrossRef] [PubMed]
27. Spaide, R.F.; Fujimoto, J.G.; Waheed, N.K.; Sadda, S.R.; Staurenghi, G. Optical coherence tomography angiography. *Prog. Retin. Eye Res.* **2018**, *64*, 1–55. [CrossRef] [PubMed]
28. Liu, L.; Jia, Y.; Takusagawa, H.L.; Pechauer, A.D.; Edmunds, B.; Lombardi, L.; Davis, E.; Morrison, J.C.; Huang, D. Optical Coherence Tomography Angiography of the Peripapillary Retina in Glaucoma. *JAMA Ophthalmol.* **2015**, *133*, 1045–1052. [CrossRef] [PubMed]
29. Takusagawa, H.L.; Liu, L.; Ma, K.N.; Jia, Y.; Gao, S.S.; Zhang, M.; Edmunds, B.; Parikh, M.; Tehrani, S.; Morrison, J.C.; et al. Projection-Resolved Optical Coherence Tomography Angiography of Macular Retinal Circulation in Glaucoma. *Ophthalmology* **2017**, *124*, 1589–1599. [CrossRef]
30. Bonomi, L.; Marchini, G.; Marraffa, M.; Bernardi, P.; Morbio, R.; Varotto, A. Vascular risk factors for primary open angle glaucoma: The Egna-Neumarkt Study. *Ophthalmology* **2000**, *107*, 1287–1293. [CrossRef]
31. Leske, M.C.; Wu, S.-Y.; Nemesure, B.; Hennis, A.; Group, B.E.S. Incident Open-Angle Glaucoma and Blood Pressure. *Arch. Ophthalmol.* **2002**, *120*, 954–959. [CrossRef]
32. Tielsch, J.M.; Katz, J.; Sommer, A.; Quigley, H.A.; Javitt, J.C. Hypertension, Perfusion Pressure, and Primary Open-angle Glaucoma: A Population-Based Assessment. *Arch. Ophthalmol.* **1995**, *113*, 216–221. [CrossRef] [PubMed]
33. Memarzadeh, F.; Ying-Lai, M.; Chung, J.; Azen, S.P.; Varma, R.; Group, L.A.L.E.S. Blood Pressure, Perfusion Pressure, and Open-Angle Glaucoma: The Los Angeles Latino Eye Study. *Investig. Ophthalmol. Vis. Sci.* **2010**, *51*, 2872–2877. [CrossRef] [PubMed]
34. Zheng, Y.; Wong, T.Y.; Mitchell, P.; Friedman, D.S.; He, M.; Aung, T. Distribution of Ocular Perfusion Pressure and Its Relationship with Open-Angle Glaucoma: The Singapore Malay Eye Study. *Investig. Ophthalmol. Vis. Sci.* **2010**, *51*, 3399–3404. [CrossRef] [PubMed]
35. Leske, M.C.; Heijl, A.; Hyman, L.; Bengtsson, B.; Dong, L.; Yang, Z. Predictors of Long-term Progression in the Early Manifest Glaucoma Trial. *Ophthalmology* **2007**, *114*, 1965–1972. [CrossRef] [PubMed]
36. Leske, M.C.; Wu, S.-Y.; Hennis, A.; Honkanen, R.; Nemesure, B. Risk Factors for Incident Open-angle Glaucoma: The Barbados Eye Studies. *Ophthalmology* **2008**, *115*, 85–93. [CrossRef] [PubMed]
37. Kuang, T.M.; Zhang, C.; Zangwill, L.M.; Weinreb, R.N.; Medeiros, F.A. Estimating Lead Time Gained by Optical Coherence Tomography in Detecting Glaucoma before Development of Visual Field Defects. *Ophthalmology* **2015**, *122*, 2002–2009. [CrossRef] [PubMed]

38. Cheng, L.; Wang, M.; Deng, J.; Lv, M.; Jiang, W.; Xiong, S.; Sun, S.; Zhu, J.; Zou, H.; He, X.; et al. Macular Ganglion Cell-Inner Plexiform Layer, Ganglion Cell Complex, and Outer Retinal Layer Thicknesses in a Large Cohort of Chinese Children. *Investig. Ophthalmol. Vis. Sci.* **2019**, *60*, 4792–4802. [CrossRef] [PubMed]
39. Della Santina, L.; Inman, D.M.; Lupien, C.B.; Horner, P.J.; Wong, R.O. Differential progression of structural and functional alterations in distinct retinal ganglion cell types in a mouse model of glaucoma. *J. Neurosci.* **2013**, *33*, 17444–17457. [CrossRef]
40. El-Danaf, R.N.; Huberman, A.D. Characteristic patterns of dendritic remodeling in early-stage glaucoma: Evidence from genetically identified retinal ganglion cell types. *J. Neurosci.* **2015**, *35*, 2329–2343. [CrossRef]
41. Nouri-Mahdavi, K.; Nowroozizadeh, S.; Nassiri, N.; Cirineo, N.; Knipping, S.; Giaconi, J.; Caprioli, J. Macular Ganglion Cell/Inner Plexiform Layer Measurements by Spectral Domain Optical Coherence Tomography for Detection of Early Glaucoma and Comparison to Retinal Nerve Fiber Layer Measurements. *Am. J. Ophthalmol.* **2013**, *156*, 1297–1307.e1292. [CrossRef]
42. Kim, Y.K.; Yoo, B.W.; Kim, H.C.; Park, K.H. Automated Detection of Hemifield Difference across Horizontal Raphe on Ganglion Cell--Inner Plexiform Layer Thickness Map. *Ophthalmology* **2015**, *122*, 2252–2260. [CrossRef] [PubMed]
43. Lee, W.J.; Na, K.I.; Kim, Y.K.; Jeoung, J.W.; Park, K.H. Diagnostic Ability of Wide-field Retinal Nerve Fiber Layer Maps Using Swept-Source Optical Coherence Tomography for Detection of Preperimetric and Early Perimetric Glaucoma. *J. Glaucoma* **2017**, *26*, 577–585. [CrossRef] [PubMed]
44. WuDunn, D.; Takusagawa, H.L.; Sit, A.J.; Rosdahl, J.A.; Radhakrishnan, S.; Hoguet, A.; Han, Y.; Chen, T.C. OCT Angiography for the Diagnosis of Glaucoma: A Report by the American Academy of Ophthalmology. *Ophthalmology* **2021**, *128*, 1222–1235. [CrossRef] [PubMed]
45. Jia, Y.; Morrison, J.C.; Tokayer, J.; Tan, O.; Lombardi, L.; Baumann, B.; Lu, C.D.; Choi, W.; Fujimoto, J.G.; Huang, D. Quantitative OCT angiography of optic nerve head blood flow. *Biomed. Opt. Express* **2012**, *3*, 3127–3137. [CrossRef] [PubMed]
46. Jia, Y.; Wei, E.; Wang, X.; Zhang, X.; Morrison, J.C.; Parikh, M.; Lombardi, L.H.; Gattey, D.M.; Armour, R.L.; Edmunds, B.; et al. Optical coherence tomography angiography of optic disc perfusion in glaucoma. *Ophthalmology* **2014**, *121*, 1322–1332. [CrossRef] [PubMed]
47. Lévêque, P.M.; Zéboulon, P.; Brasnu, E.; Baudouin, C.; Labbé, A. Optic Disc Vascularization in Glaucoma: Value of Spectral-Domain Optical Coherence Tomography Angiography. *J. Ophthalmol.* **2016**, *2016*, 6956717. [CrossRef] [PubMed]
48. Kim, S.B.; Lee, E.J.; Han, J.C.; Kee, C. Comparison of peripapillary vessel density between preperimetric and perimetric glaucoma evaluated by OCT-angiography. *PLoS ONE* **2017**, *12*, e0184297. [CrossRef] [PubMed]
49. Lu, P.; Xiao, H.; Liang, C.; Xu, Y.; Ye, D.; Huang, J. Quantitative Analysis of Microvasculature in Macular and Peripapillary Regions in Early Primary Open-Angle Glaucoma. *Curr. Eye Res.* **2020**, *45*, 629–635. [CrossRef]
50. Mansoori, T.; Sivaswamy, J.; Gamalapati, J.S.; Balakrishna, N. Radial Peripapillary Capillary Density Measurement Using Optical Coherence Tomography Angiography in Early Glaucoma. *J. Glaucoma* **2017**, *26*, 438–443. [CrossRef]
51. Akil, H.; Huang, A.S.; Francis, B.A.; Sadda, S.R.; Chopra, V. Retinal vessel density from optical coherence tomography angiography to differentiate early glaucoma, pre-perimetric glaucoma and normal eyes. *PLoS ONE* **2017**, *12*, e0170476. [CrossRef] [PubMed]
52. Kumar, R.S.; Anegondi, N.; Chandapura, R.S.; Sudhakaran, S.; Kadambi, S.V.; Rao, H.L.; Aung, T.; Sinha Roy, A. Discriminant Function of Optical Coherence Tomography Angiography to Determine Disease Severity in Glaucoma. *Investig. Ophthalmol. Vis. Sci.* **2016**, *57*, 6079–6088. [CrossRef] [PubMed]
53. Hou, H.; Moghimi, S.; Zangwill, L.M.; Shoji, T.; Ghahari, E.; Manalastas, P.I.C.; Penteado, R.C.; Weinreb, R.N. Inter-eye Asymmetry of Optical Coherence Tomography Angiography Vessel Density in Bilateral Glaucoma, Glaucoma Suspect, and Healthy Eyes. *Am. J. Ophthalmol.* **2018**, *190*, 69–77. [CrossRef] [PubMed]
54. Suh, M.H.; Zangwill, L.M.; Manalastas, P.I.; Belghith, A.; Yarmohammadi, A.; Medeiros, F.A.; Diniz-Filho, A.; Saunders, L.J.; Weinreb, R.N. Deep Retinal Layer Microvasculature Dropout Detected by the Optical Coherence Tomography Angiography in Glaucoma. *Ophthalmology* **2016**, *123*, 2509–2518. [CrossRef] [PubMed]
55. Penteado, R.C.; Bowd, C.; Proudfoot, J.A.; Moghimi, S.; Manalastas, P.I.C.; Ghahari, E.; Hou, H.; Shoji, T.; Zangwill, L.M.; Weinreb, R.N. Diagnostic Ability of Optical Coherence Tomography Angiography Macula Vessel Density for the Diagnosis of Glaucoma Using Difference Scan Sizes. *J. Glaucoma* **2020**, *29*, 245–251. [CrossRef] [PubMed]
56. Richter, G.M.; Madi, I.; Chu, Z.; Burkemper, B.; Chang, R.; Zaman, A.; Sylvester, B.; Reznik, A.; Kashani, A.; Wang, R.K.; et al. Structural and Functional Associations of Macular Microcirculation in the Ganglion Cell-Inner Plexiform Layer in Glaucoma Using Optical Coherence Tomography Angiography. *J. Glaucoma* **2018**, *27*, 281–290. [CrossRef] [PubMed]
57. Kurysheva, N.I.; Maslova, E.V.; Zolnikova, I.V.; Fomin, A.V.; Lagutin, M.B. A comparative study of structural, functional and circulatory parameters in glaucoma diagnostics. *PLoS ONE* **2018**, *13*, e0201599. [CrossRef] [PubMed]
58. Mansoori, T.; Gamalapati, J.; Sivaswamy, J.; Balakrishna, N. Optical coherence tomography angiography measured capillary density in the normal and glaucoma eyes. *Saudi J. Ophthalmol.* **2018**, *32*, 295–302. [CrossRef]
59. Moghimi, S.; Zangwill, L.M.; Penteado, R.C.; Hasenstab, K.; Ghahari, E.; Hou, H.; Christopher, M.; Yarmohammadi, A.; Manalastas, P.I.C.; Shoji, T.; et al. Macular and Optic Nerve Head Vessel Density and Progressive Retinal Nerve Fiber Layer Loss in Glaucoma. *Ophthalmology* **2018**, *125*, 1720–1728. [CrossRef]
60. Choi, J.; Kwon, J.; Shin, J.W.; Lee, J.; Lee, S.; Kook, M.S. Quantitative optical coherence tomography angiography of macular vascular structure and foveal avascular zone in glaucoma. *PLoS ONE* **2017**, *12*, e0184948. [CrossRef]
61. Chao, S.C.; Yang, S.J.; Chen, H.C.; Sun, C.C.; Liu, C.H.; Lee, C.Y. Early Macular Angiography among Patients with Glaucoma, Ocular Hypertension, and Normal Subjects. *J. Ophthalmol.* **2019**, *2019*, 7419470. [CrossRef] [PubMed]

62. Milani, P.; Urbini, L.E.; Bulone, E.; Nava, U.; Visintin, D.; Cremonesi, G.; Scotti, L.; Bergamini, F. The Macular Choriocapillaris Flow in Glaucoma and Within-Day Fluctuations: An Optical Coherence Tomography Angiography Study. *Investig. Ophthalmol. Vis. Sci.* **2021**, *62*, 22. [CrossRef] [PubMed]
63. Lommatzsch, C.; Rothaus, K.; Koch, J.M.; Heinz, C.; Grisanti, S. OCTA vessel density changes in the macular zone in glaucomatous eyes. *Graefes Arch. Clin. Exp. Ophthalmol.* **2018**, *256*, 1499–1508. [CrossRef] [PubMed]
64. Kromer, R.; Glusa, P.; Framme, C.; Pielen, A.; Junker, B. Optical coherence tomography angiography analysis of macular flow density in glaucoma. *Acta Ophthalmol.* **2019**, *97*, e199–e206. [CrossRef] [PubMed]
65. Shin, J.; Kwon, J.M.; Park, S.H.; Seo, J.H.; Jung, J.H. Diagnostic Ability of Macular Vessel Density in the Ganglion Cell-Inner Plexiform Layer on Optical Coherence Tomographic Angiography for Glaucoma. *Transl. Vis. Sci. Technol.* **2019**, *8*, 12. [CrossRef] [PubMed]
66. Hou, H.; Moghimi, S.; Zangwill, L.M.; Shoji, T.; Ghahari, E.; Penteado, R.C.; Akagi, T.; Manalastas, P.I.C.; Weinreb, R.N. Macula Vessel Density and Thickness in Early Primary Open-Angle Glaucoma. *Am. J. Ophthalmol.* **2019**, *199*, 120–132. [CrossRef] [PubMed]
67. Chung, J.K.; Hwang, Y.H.; Wi, J.M.; Kim, M.; Jung, J.J. Glaucoma Diagnostic Ability of the Optical Coherence Tomography Angiography Vessel Density Parameters. *Curr. Eye Res.* **2017**, *42*, 1458–1467. [CrossRef] [PubMed]
68. Kwon, J.; Choi, J.; Shin, J.W.; Lee, J.; Kook, M.S. Glaucoma Diagnostic Capabilities of Foveal Avascular Zone Parameters Using Optical Coherence Tomography Angiography According to Visual Field Defect Location. *J. Glaucoma* **2017**, *26*, 1120–1129. [CrossRef] [PubMed]
69. Triolo, G.; Rabiolo, A.; Shemonski, N.D.; Fard, A.; Di Matteo, F.; Sacconi, R.; Bettin, P.; Magazzeni, S.; Querques, G.; Vazquez, L.E.; et al. Optical Coherence Tomography Angiography Macular and Peripapillary Vessel Perfusion Density in Healthy Subjects, Glaucoma Suspects, and Glaucoma Patients. *Investig. Ophthalmol. Vis. Sci.* **2017**, *58*, 5713–5722. [CrossRef]
70. Reis, A.S.; O'Leary, N.; Yang, H.; Sharpe, G.P.; Nicolela, M.T.; Burgoyne, C.F.; Chauhan, B.C. Influence of clinically invisible, but optical coherence tomography detected, optic disc margin anatomy on neuroretinal rim evaluation. *Investig. Ophthalmol. Vis. Sci.* **2012**, *53*, 1852–1860. [CrossRef]
71. Chauhan, B.C.; O'Leary, N.; AlMobarak, F.A.; Reis, A.S.C.; Yang, H.; Sharpe, G.P.; Hutchison, D.M.; Nicolela, M.T.; Burgoyne, C.F. Enhanced detection of open-angle glaucoma with an anatomically accurate optical coherence tomography-derived neuroretinal rim parameter. *Ophthalmology* **2013**, *120*, 535–543. [CrossRef] [PubMed]
72. Lopes, F.S.S.; Matsubara, I.; Almeida, I.; Gracitelli, C.P.B.; Dorairaj, S.K.; Vessani, R.M.; Paranhos, A., Jr.; Prata, T.S. Using Enhanced Depth Imaging Optical Coherence Tomography-Derived Parameters to Discriminate between Eyes with and without Glaucoma: A Cross-Sectional Comparative Study. *Ophthalmic Res.* **2021**, *64*, 108–115. [CrossRef] [PubMed]
73. Bartlett, R.L.; Frost, B.E.; Mortlock, K.E.; Fergusson, J.R.; White, N.; Morgan, J.E.; North, R.V.; Albon, J. Quantifying biomarkers of axonal degeneration in early glaucoma to find the disc at risk. *Sci. Rep.* **2022**, *12*, 9366. [CrossRef]
74. Gmeiner, J.M.D.; Schrems, W.A.; Mardin, C.Y.; Laemmer, R.; Kruse, F.E.; Schrems-Hoesl, L.M. Comparison of Bruch's Membrane Opening Minimum Rim Width and Peripapillary Retinal Nerve Fiber Layer Thickness in Early Glaucoma Assessment. *Investig. Ophthalmol. Vis. Sci.* **2016**, *57*, OCT575–OCT584. [CrossRef] [PubMed]
75. Gardiner, S.K.; Ren, R.; Yang, H.; Fortune, B.; Burgoyne, C.F.; Demirel, S. A method to estimate the amount of neuroretinal rim tissue in glaucoma: Comparison with current methods for measuring rim area. *Am. J. Ophthalmol.* **2014**, *157*, 540–549.e2. [CrossRef]
76. Enders, P.; Adler, W.; Kiessling, D.; Weber, V.; Schaub, F.; Hermann, M.M.; Dietlein, T.; Cursiefen, C.; Heindl, L.M. Evaluation of two-dimensional Bruch's membrane opening minimum rim area for glaucoma diagnostics in a large patient cohort. *Acta Ophthalmol.* **2019**, *97*, 60–67. [CrossRef] [PubMed]
77. Enders, P.; Adler, W.; Schaub, F.; Hermann, M.M.; Dietlein, T.; Cursiefen, C.; Heindl, L.M. Novel Bruch's Membrane Opening Minimum Rim Area Equalizes Disc Size Dependency and Offers High Diagnostic Power for Glaucoma. *Investig. Ophthalmol. Vis. Sci.* **2016**, *57*, 6596–6603. [CrossRef] [PubMed]
78. Li, R.; Wang, X.; Wei, Y.; Fang, Y.; Tian, T.; Kang, L.; Li, M.; Cai, Y.; Pan, Y. Diagnostic capability of different morphological parameters for primary open-angle glaucoma in the Chinese population. *BMC Ophthalmol.* **2021**, *21*, 151. [CrossRef] [PubMed]
79. Kim, J.A.; Kim, T.W.; Weinreb, R.N.; Lee, E.J.; Girard, M.J.A.; Mari, J.M. Lamina Cribrosa Morphology Predicts Progressive Retinal Nerve Fiber Layer Loss in Eyes with Suspected Glaucoma. *Sci. Rep.* **2018**, *8*, 738. [CrossRef]
80. Abe, R.Y.; Gracitelli, C.P.; Diniz-Filho, A.; Tatham, A.J.; Medeiros, F.A. Lamina Cribrosa in Glaucoma: Diagnosis and Monitoring. *Curr. Ophthalmol. Rep.* **2015**, *3*, 74–84. [CrossRef]
81. Bellezza, A.J.; Rintalan, C.J.; Thompson, H.W.; Downs, J.C.; Hart, R.T.; Burgoyne, C.F. Deformation of the lamina cribrosa and anterior scleral canal wall in early experimental glaucoma. *Investig. Ophthalmol. Vis. Sci.* **2003**, *44*, 623–637. [CrossRef] [PubMed]
82. Strouthidis, N.G.; Fortune, B.; Yang, H.; Sigal, I.A.; Burgoyne, C.F. Longitudinal change detected by spectral domain optical coherence tomography in the optic nerve head and peripapillary retina in experimental glaucoma. *Investig. Ophthalmol. Vis. Sci.* **2011**, *52*, 1206–1219. [CrossRef] [PubMed]
83. Park, H.Y.; Park, C.K. Diagnostic capability of lamina cribrosa thickness by enhanced depth imaging and factors affecting thickness in patients with glaucoma. *Ophthalmology* **2013**, *120*, 745–752. [CrossRef] [PubMed]
84. Lee, S.H.; Kim, T.W.; Lee, E.J.; Girard, M.J.; Mari, J.M. Diagnostic Power of Lamina Cribrosa Depth and Curvature in Glaucoma. *Investig. Ophthalmol. Vis. Sci.* **2017**, *58*, 755–762. [CrossRef] [PubMed]

85. Zhou, W.; Muir, E.R.; Chalfin, S.; Nagi, K.S.; Duong, T.Q. MRI Study of the Posterior Visual Pathways in Primary Open Angle Glaucoma. *J. Glaucoma* **2017**, *26*, 173–181. [CrossRef]
86. Schmidt, M.A.; Knott, M.; Heidemann, R.; Michelson, G.; Kober, T.; Dörfler, A.; Engelhorn, T. Investigation of lateral geniculate nucleus volume and diffusion tensor imaging in patients with normal tension glaucoma using 7 tesla magnetic resonance imaging. *PLoS ONE* **2018**, *13*, e0198830. [CrossRef]
87. Wang, J.; Zhang, Y.; Meng, X.; Liu, G. Application of diffusion tensor imaging technology in glaucoma diagnosis. *Front. Neurosci.* **2023**, *17*, 1125638. [CrossRef] [PubMed]
88. Song, X.Y.; Puyang, Z.; Chen, A.H.; Zhao, J.; Li, X.J.; Chen, Y.Y.; Tang, W.J.; Zhang, Y.Y. Diffusion Tensor Imaging Detects Microstructural Differences of Visual Pathway in Patients with Primary Open-Angle Glaucoma and Ocular Hypertension. *Front. Hum. Neurosci.* **2018**, *12*, 426. [CrossRef] [PubMed]
89. Crish, S.D.; Sappington, R.M.; Inman, D.M.; Horner, P.J.; Calkins, D.J. Distal axonopathy with structural persistence in glaucomatous neurodegeneration. *Proc. Natl. Acad. Sci. USA* **2010**, *107*, 5196–5201. [CrossRef]
90. Yücel, Y.H.; Zhang, Q.; Weinreb, R.N.; Kaufman, P.L.; Gupta, N. Effects of retinal ganglion cell loss on magno-, parvo-, koniocellular pathways in the lateral geniculate nucleus and visual cortex in glaucoma. *Prog. Retin. Eye Res.* **2003**, *22*, 465–481. [CrossRef]
91. Li, M.; Ke, M.; Song, Y.; Mu, K.; Zhang, H.; Chen, Z. Diagnostic utility of central damage determination in glaucoma by magnetic resonance imaging: An observational study. *Exp. Ther. Med.* **2019**, *17*, 1891–1895. [CrossRef] [PubMed]
92. Colbert, M.K.; Ho, L.C.; van der Merwe, Y.; Yang, X.; McLellan, G.J.; Hurley, S.A.; Field, A.S.; Yun, H.; Du, Y.; Conner, I.P.; et al. Diffusion Tensor Imaging of Visual Pathway Abnormalities in Five Glaucoma Animal Models. *Investig. Ophthalmol. Vis. Sci.* **2021**, *62*, 21. [CrossRef] [PubMed]
93. Bansal, R.; Gerber, A.J.; Peterson, B.S. Brain morphometry using anatomical magnetic resonance imaging. *J. Am. Acad. Child. Adolesc. Psychiatry* **2008**, *47*, 619–621. [CrossRef] [PubMed]
94. Bogorodzki, P.; Piątkowska-Janko, E.; Szaflik, J.; Szaflik, J.P.; Gacek, M.; Grieb, P. Mapping cortical thickness of the patients with unilateral end-stage open angle glaucoma on planar cerebral cortex maps. *PLoS ONE* **2014**, *9*, e93682. [CrossRef] [PubMed]
95. Chen, W.W.; Wang, N.; Cai, S.; Fang, Z.; Yu, M.; Wu, Q.; Tang, L.; Guo, B.; Feng, Y.; Jonas, J.B.; et al. Structural brain abnormalities in patients with primary open-angle glaucoma: A study with 3T MR imaging. *Investig. Ophthalmol. Vis. Sci.* **2013**, *54*, 545–554. [CrossRef] [PubMed]
96. Mastropasqua, R.; Agnifili, L.; Mattei, P.A.; Caulo, M.; Fasanella, V.; Navarra, R.; Mastropasqua, L.; Marchini, G. Advanced Morphological and Functional Magnetic Resonance Techniques in Glaucoma. *BioMed Res. Int.* **2015**, *2015*, 160454. [CrossRef] [PubMed]
97. Graham, K.L.; Johnson, P.J.; Barry, E.F.; Pérez Orrico, M.; Soligo, D.J.; Lawlor, M.; White, A. Diffusion tensor imaging of the visual pathway in dogs with primary angle-closure glaucoma. *Vet. Ophthalmol.* **2021**, *24* (Suppl. S1), 63–74. [CrossRef]
98. Li, Y.; Zhang, W. Quantitative evaluation of diffusion tensor imaging for clinical management of glioma. *Neurosurg. Rev.* **2020**, *43*, 881–891. [CrossRef]
99. Li, K.; Lu, C.; Huang, Y.; Yuan, L.; Zeng, D.; Wu, K. Alteration of fractional anisotropy and mean diffusivity in glaucoma: Novel results of a meta-analysis of diffusion tensor imaging studies. *PLoS ONE* **2014**, *9*, e97445. [CrossRef]
100. Fiedorowicz, M.; Dyda, W.; Rejdak, R.; Grieb, P. Magnetic resonance in studies of glaucoma. *Med. Sci. Monit.* **2011**, *17*, Ra227–Ra232. [CrossRef]
101. Michelson, G.; Wärntges, S.; Engelhorn, T.; El-Rafei, A.; Hornegger, J.; Dörfler, A. Integrity/demyelination of the optic radiation, morphology of the papilla, and contrast sensitivity in glaucoma patients. *Klin. Monbl Augenheilkd.* **2012**, *229*, 143–148. [CrossRef] [PubMed]
102. Nucci, C.; Mancino, R.; Martucci, A.; Bolacchi, F.; Manenti, G.; Cedrone, C.; Culasso, F.; Floris, R.; Cerulli, L.; Garaci, F.G. 3-T Diffusion tensor imaging of the optic nerve in subjects with glaucoma: Correlation with GDx-VCC, HRT-III and Stratus optical coherence tomography findings. *Br. J. Ophthalmol.* **2012**, *96*, 976–980. [CrossRef] [PubMed]
103. Garaci, F.G.; Bolacchi, F.; Cerulli, A.; Melis, M.; Spanò, A.; Cedrone, C.; Floris, R.; Simonetti, G.; Nucci, C. Optic nerve and optic radiation neurodegeneration in patients with glaucoma: In vivo analysis with 3-T diffusion-tensor MR imaging. *Radiology* **2009**, *252*, 496–501. [CrossRef] [PubMed]
104. Bolacchi, F.; Garaci, F.G.; Martucci, A.; Meschini, A.; Fornari, M.; Marziali, S.; Mancino, R.; Squillaci, E.; Floris, R.; Cerulli, L.; et al. Differences between proximal versus distal intraorbital optic nerve diffusion tensor magnetic resonance imaging properties in glaucoma patients. *Investig. Ophthalmol. Vis. Sci.* **2012**, *53*, 4191–4196. [CrossRef] [PubMed]

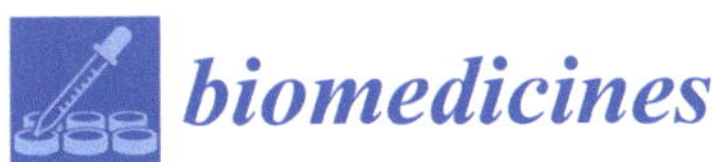

MDPI

Review

Nicotinamide: Bright Potential in Glaucoma Management

Silvia Babighian [1], Irene Gattazzo [1], Maria Sole Zanella [1], Alessandro Galan [1], Fabiana D'Esposito [2,3], Mutali Musa [4,5], Caterina Gagliano [6,7], Lucia Lapenna [8] and Marco Zeppieri [9,*]

1 Department of Ophthalmology, Ospedale Sant'Antonio, Azienda Ospedaliera, 35127 Padova, Italy; silvia.babighian@aopd.veneto.it (S.B.)
2 Imperial College Ophthalmic Research Group (ICORG) Unit, Imperial College, 153-173 Marylebone Rd, London NW15QH, UK
3 Department of Neurosciences, Reproductive Sciences and Dentistry, University of Naples Federico II, Via Pansini 5, 80131 Napoli, Italy
4 Department of Optometry, University of Benin, Benin City 300238, Nigeria
5 Africa Eye Laser Centre, Km 7, Benin 300105, Nigeria
6 Department of Medicine and Surgery, University of Enna "Kore", Piazza dell'Università, 94100 Enna, Italy
7 Eye Clinic Catania University San Marco Hospital, Viale Carlo Azeglio Ciampi, 95121 Catania, Italy
8 U.O.C Oculistica, Ospedale "DI Venere", 70012 Bari, Italy
9 Department of Ophthalmology, University Hospital of Udine, 33100 Udine, Italy
* Correspondence: markzeppieri@hotmail.com; Tel.: +39-0432-552743

Abstract: Background: Glaucoma is a major cause of incurable ocular morbidity and poses significant challenges in its management due to the limited treatment options and potential adverse effects. Nicotinamide, a naturally occurring diet-rich nutrient, has emerged as a promising therapeutic agent for glaucoma, offering neuroprotective effects and the potential modulation of intraocular pressure (IOP) regulation pathways. This comprehensive review sought to analyze the current literature on nicotinamide in glaucoma management, exploring its mechanisms of action, efficacy, and safety profile. Methods: A systematic search of the PubMed database was conducted to identify relevant records on the therapeutic actions of nicotinamide in ocular hypertension and glaucoma. Publications evaluating nicotinamide's effects on retinal ganglion cells (RGCs), optic nerve function, IOP regulation, and neuroinflammatory pathways were included. Results: The literature review revealed the preclinical evidence supporting nicotinamide's neuroprotective effects on RGCs, the preservation of optic nerve integrity, and the modulation of glaucoma-associated neuroinflammation. Additionally, nicotinamide may exert IOP-lowering effects through its influence on ocular blood flow and aqueous humor dynamics. Conclusions: Nicotinamide holds promise as a novel therapeutic approach in glaucoma management, offering potential neuroprotective and IOP-lowering effects. The authors recommend more research to determine the nicotinamide efficacy, safe dosing parameters, and any long-term safety concerns in glaucoma patients.

Keywords: nicotinamide; glaucoma; intraocular pressure

Citation: Babighian, S.; Gattazzo, I.; Zanella, M.S.; Galan, A.; D'Esposito, F.; Musa, M.; Gagliano, C.; Lapenna, L.; Zeppieri, M. Nicotinamide: Bright Potential in Glaucoma Management. *Biomedicines* **2024**, *12*, 1655. https://doi.org/10.3390/biomedicines12081655

Academic Editor: Da-Wen Lu

Received: 21 June 2024
Revised: 22 July 2024
Accepted: 22 July 2024
Published: 25 July 2024

1. Introduction

Glaucomas are a diverse group of conditions that cause irreversible vision loss and affect over 70 million people all over the world [1]. The hallmark of glaucoma is a gradual destruction of retinal ganglion cells (RGCs) and optic nerve injury, with abnormal intraocular pressure (IOP) being the primary cause [2]. As a result, glaucoma management requires the administration of hypotensive pharmacological agents to reduce IOP or surgery [3].

Glaucoma presents as either open-angle, or closed-angle. Primary open-angle glaucoma presents with an anterior chamber (AC) angle which is open/deep, suggesting that the aqueous humor outflow is not impeded. In closed-angle glaucoma, the AC is narrow, or even closed, suggesting that the aqueous humor outflow is actively impeded [1]. Glaucoma can be classified as either primary or secondary, depending on whether it develops independently (primary) or as a consequence of another disease process. Given that glaucoma often presents without noticeable symptoms in its initial stages, approximately 10–50% of those affected are typically diagnosed only at advanced stages of the disease. Consequently, a search for an effective therapeutic approach to glaucoma remains a top priority [4]. Currently, any vision loss caused by glaucoma cannot be retrieved by any known means. Therefore, early detection and effective treatment are crucial. Due to the emergence of better healthcare options to society, people are generally expected to live longer, and this will come with a higher incidence and prevalence of glaucoma, highlighting the need for improved detection methods and quality care to prevent unnecessary blindness [5].

The first line of management for glaucoma is prostaglandin analogues, closely followed by beta-blockers, alpha-agonists, etc. [4]. All these therapies are currently aimed at reducing intraocular pressure, but do little in terms of protecting the neural tissue potentially damaged by the disease [4].

Nowadays, the goal of glaucoma research is to find intraocular-pressure-independent techniques to reducing the likelihood and severity of glaucomatous optic nerve damage. Recent advances in trial design and technology developments that allow for the early detection of pathogenic alterations have revived interest in neuroprotection research. This increased interest is fueled by a clearer knowledge of the processes behind RGC degeneration and breakthroughs in basic research targeted at finding possible treatment targets [5].

While a definitive consensus on the precise cause of glaucomatous optic neuropathy remains elusive, the cellular mechanisms leading to RGC death encompass the exposure to neurotoxic substances like nitric oxide (NO) and glutamate, as well as the deprivation of internal trophic factors, impairment of cellular self-repair processes, and intracellular destructive pathways [6].

The rationale behind the treatment lies in restoring the balance between cellular death and survival signals, thereby preserving visual function. Consequently, numerous ongoing trials are investigating the potential benefits of neuroprotective agents including Memantine, Brimonidine, nerve growth factor (NGF), and Nicotinamide [7]. Despite the limited clinical validation confirming its therapeutic properties in glaucoma management, Nicotinamide (Vitamin B3) is already advocated as an adjunct treatment for this disease especially in sufferers experiencing the progression of visual field loss despite adequate intraocular pressure control [8,9].

Nicotinamide is a water-soluble nutrient which is largely obtained by consuming nutrient-rich foods such as poultry and fish [7]. Its chemical structure is shown below in Figure 1.

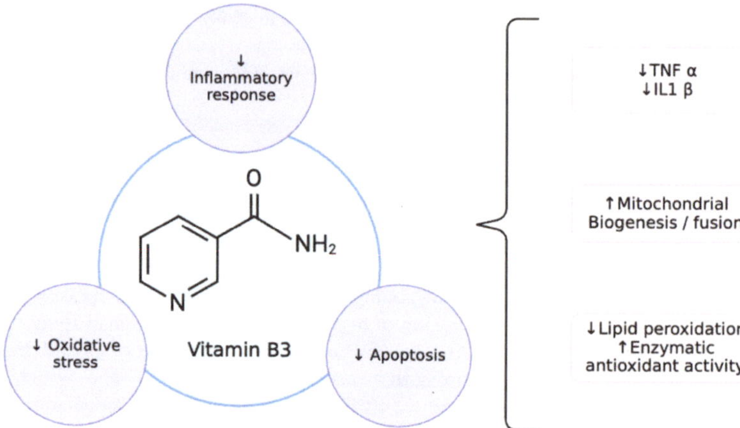

Figure 1. NAD structure and mechanisms of action. Up arrow = increase, downward arrow = decrease.

2. Materials and Methods

For this review, an electronic search was carried out using PubMed and Medline databases for all published articles up to 20 May 2024. The comprehensive literature analysis included articles published between 2000 and 2024, utilizing a combination of the following terms: nicotinamide, glaucoma, intraocular pressure, nicotinamide riboside, and neuroprotection. A total of five results were returned. Relevant cross-references from the selected articles were also included in the review. Records which were not in English language or out of scope as related to this manuscript were excluded. Moreover, records without complete research data and those with errata were excluded. The literature search was performed by three authors (I.G., M.Z., and S.B.). Any disagreements were resolved through open discussion with senior authors.

3. Nicotinamide: Mechanisms of Action

Nicotinamide (NAM) is a substance that is water-soluble. It is part of the niacin and/or vitamin B3 complex, together with nicotinic acid (NA) and nicotinamide riboside (NR). It acts as a precursor to nicotinamide adenine dinucleotide (NAD+), and is crucial for essential cellular activities [10]. These substances are precursors in the food for the production of the beneficial molecules nicotinamide adenine dinucleotide without (NAD) and with phosphate (NADP). Nicotinamide is an essential part of the glycolysis pathway. It helps in the production of NAD+ which is necessary for generating ATP and controlling cellular energy levels as well as several metabolic activities [11].

There are three types of vitamin B3, of which the most commonly encountered as a component of human diet are NAM and NA. Upon intestinal absorption in the human body, NA is converted into NAM [12]. A lesser proportion of NAM is retained in the liver, as the majority is either removed as urine or utilized in the production of critical substances such as NAD [13–15]. NAM is acquired through dietary sources, predominantly found in eggs, beef, fish, and mushrooms, with lesser quantities present in vegetables. Additionally, nicotinamide is derived from dietary tryptophan. Tryptophan is an essential amino acid [16].

The properties attributed to NAM are manifold, encompassing anti-inflammatory, neuroprotective, and antioxidant effects. Concerning its anti-inflammatory properties, it has photoprotective properties on the skin, reducing hyperpigmentation, wrinkles, ultraviolet-exposure-related immunosuppression, and sebum synthesis [12]. Consequently, it finds application in dermatology for the treatment of conditions such as pemphigoid, acne, skin cancer, and atopic dermatitis [17], as well as in rheumatology as an antipsoriatic agent [18].

Nicotinamide's neuroprotective impact is due to its role in neuronal formation, survival, and function in the central nervous system. Its function in the production of NAD emphasizes its critical position for cells prone to diminishing NAD amounts, notably neuronal cells [13], which have been shown to decline with age [19]. As a result, nicotinamide is expected to be of critical importance in neuronal development and neuroprotection, contributing to both neuronal death and neuroprotective activity. Numerous studies emphasize its role in neurological diseases and neurodegenerative illnesses [20].

Furthermore, NAM has antioxidant capabilities that maintain membrane integrity, and prevent cellular damage, phagocytosis, programmed cell death, and the development of venous thrombosis [21]. Furthermore, it appears to be implicated as a treatment factor in three major neurodegenerative conditions. These are namely Alzheimer's, Parkinson's, and Huntington's diseases [14,22], and it has exhibited protective properties in multiple investigative models of neurodegenerative conditions [23,24].

4. Potential Mechanisms through Which Nicotinamide May Exert Its Effects in Glaucoma Management

Although raised IOP appears to be the primary cause of glaucoma, which might hinder axonal transmission among the neuronal tissue that make up the second cranial nerve [25,26], other variables might also exacerbate RGC mortality, either independently or in concert with increased IOP [27].

Impaired blood flow autoregulation leading to local hypoxia [1], glutamatergic system overstimulation [28,29], abnormal immunological responses [30], oxidative stress [31,32], and mitochondrial dysfunction [33–36] are some of the causes that may be linked to RGC depletion.

Among these variables, oxidative damage and mitochondrial dysfunction are strong reasons to investigate the possible utility of NAM and its riboside in treating glaucoma, considering their anti-oxidative qualities and capacity to modulate mitochondrial activity [9,16,37]. Zeng has explored the possible impacts and processes of NR on a fibrosis and oxidative stress model using cells from the human trabecular meshwork (HTM). The study found that NR pretreatment boosted the survival and proliferation of HTM cells, protecting them against oxidative stress and fibrosis [38].

Camalleri et al. observed that dietary supplementation with antioxidant compounds, including a combination of forskolin, homotaurine, and spearmint extract, with selected B vitamins, resulted in the restoration of impaired retinal parameters assessed through electrophysiological examinations. Consequently, the authors suggested possible neuroprotection alternatives independent of IOP, proposing that dietary supplementation might attenuate inflammatory processes initiated by glial cell activation, thereby safeguarding RGCs [39].

In glaucoma, the elevated mutation rate observed in mitochondrial DNA has proven the presence of a mitochondrial dysfunction [40,41]. Furthermore, the activity of the mitochondrial respiratory complex I seems to be reduced by 18% in the lymphoblasts of primary open-angle glaucoma sufferers when compared to a non-POAG group ($p = 0.032$), resulting in comparable reductions in ATP production in both groups [42]. The redox imbalance in glaucoma is worsened due to the astrocyte and RGC mitochondrial malfunction in [43], that hampers the sustenance of the increased energy request due to metabolic stress in cases of higher IOP [1].

Moreover, there is an age-related increase in NAD consumption, resulting in diminished NAD availability across various tissues. Notably, this reduction in NAD levels is particularly pronounced in individuals with glaucoma [14,44,45].

A reduction in NAD levels increases the likelihood of mitochondrial malfunction, making RGCs more vulnerable to extrinsic influences such a high IOP [14,45–47]. Notably, individuals with POAG had a 30% lower plasma level of NAM, a precursor of NAD, compared to age- and gender-matched controls [48,49]. However, systemic NR administration causes a considerable rise in NAD bioavailability in numerous tissues, inclusive of components of the central nervous system [24,50]. It, therefore, makes sense that dietary supplementation with either NAM or NR, aiming at increasing the NAD bioavailability, might offer a viable therapeutic strategy in the treatment of glaucoma [33,51].

5. Studies on the Use of NAM and NR in Glaucoma

There have been many animal studies looking at the potential of NAM as a neuroprotective agent in glaucoma. Williams et al. compared mitochondrial abnormalities and lower NAD+ concentrations in DBA/2J mice, a glaucoma-like rodent model, to controls [52]. They next showed that the supplementation of exogenous nicotinamide (at a level comparable to 2.5 g daily in a 60 kg human) may restore the function of RGCs in elderly mice prone to glaucoma mice, resulting in a tenfold reduction in the chance of developing glaucoma [47,52].

Chou et al. studied D2 mice utilizing flickering-light-pattern electroretinography (F-PERG) to determine the effect of nicotinamide supplementation (equivalent dosage of 2 g per day) on RGC function. The adaption of F-PERG declined with age and was significantly poorer in untreated D2 mice ($p < 0.01$). Furthermore, they found that, utilizing immunohistochemical methods, the treated group had a higher RGC density than the control group [53].

Zhang et al. administered mice with nicotinamide riboside or phosphate-buffered saline (PBS) daily for five days to see how NR treatment affected NAD levels in RGCs. In comparison to the PBS-injected control group, NR treatment almost quadrupled NAD levels in the retina ($p < 0.01$) [54].

Tribble et al. conducted another investigation on mice with ocular hypertension and found that nicotinamide therapy was effective. They demonstrated that nicotinamide may increase mitochondrial activity and have a neuroprotective impact on defective RGCs. Using a retinal explant model, they also investigated the protective benefits of nicotinamide (NAM) against an acute, axon-specific damage. Retinas dissected and cultivated in solutions diluted with two doses (100 mM or 500 mM) of NAD showed the reduced loss of retinal RGCs and less shrinkage of cell nuclei as compared to retinal explants cultured ex vivo without NAM supplementation [9].

Yu et al. examined RGC alterations in rat models of chronic ocular hypertension. After providing NADPH and N-acetylcysteine (NAC), they detected decreased glutathione (GSH) production, apoptosis, axonal damage, and peroxidation in RGCs. Furthermore, electrophysiological function increased while Müller cell gliosis was decreased [55].

Boodram evaluated the impact of dietary nicotinamide supplementation on axonal microtubule degradation, which seems to play an important part in the development of glaucoma. They discovered that administering 550 mg per day in a mouse model of glaucoma protected the volume of retinal nerve fibers [56]. Kim et al. assessed a direct administration approach using NAM extracellular vesicles (EVs) in mice glaucoma models. A quantitative study of dendritic integrity demonstrated NAM's ability to protect RGCs [57].

6. Clinical Evidence on the Use of NAM or NR in Glaucoma

Hui et al. carried out a randomized, double-blind, case–control investigative study on 57 POAG patients, separated into two categories. One set of mice received NAM at 1.5 g/day for 6 weeks, then half the starting dose for the remaining 6 weeks, whereas another set group received a placebo for 3 months. After 12 weeks, the groups changed treatments. Assessments, including comprehensive eye examinations, visual field tests, and electroretinography, were performed at the beginning and every six weeks [8].

Out of the 49 participants who took part in the study, those who received NAM showed improved electroretinographic characteristics associated with the inner retina ($p = 0.02$). Slight changes in automated perimetry were observed. In the group that took 3 g/day of NAM, there was a greater improvement in the mean deviation (MD) of $\geq$1 dB from the baseline compared to the placebo group (27% vs. 16%, $p = 0.02$). Patients who took a high dose of NAM had fewer decreases in MD of $\geq$1 dB when compared to the placebo group (4% vs. 12%, $p = 0.02$). However, after 12 weeks, no significant difference was observed in the average MD between the placebo and treatment groups ($p = 0.53$). NAM supplementation did not have any effect on the intraocular pressure (IOP), mean arterial pressure, visual acuity, or retinal nerve fiber layer thickness. However, this research was limited by an inadequate follow-up period, different forms of glaucoma in the participants, and incomplete ocular pressure data during the study [8].

Moraes et al. conducted a double-masked experiment on POAG, assessing the effects of NAM- and pyruvate (PYR)-fortified diets. Thirty-two participants with moderate POAG were placed into two groups: one group received up to 3000 mg/day of dietary NAM and PYR for 6 weeks, while the second group received a placebo for the same time period. Participants were subjected to four visual field tests spanning two weeks at the beginning and conclusion of the research, with two extra tests administered four weeks in and one week after supplementation finished.

The treatment group had a significantly average improvement on the total deviation plot ($p = 0.005$), and a threefold higher probability of improving the thresholds of the tested points ($p = 0.02$), notwithstanding the initial sensitivity, and higher rates of improvements in the pattern standard deviation (PSD). However, there were no significant changes in the visual field indices, mean deviation, ocular coherence tomography, nor MoCA scores.

The findings revealed that the locations exhibiting improvement initially had an intermediate sensitivity, indicating that supplementing may be improving the function of the defective RGCs. Despite the apparent functional gains, the study's brief length precludes the extrapolation to long-term effects, and no information on IOP behavior in either group was found [58].

Leung et al. performed a randomized clinical study at the Chinese University of Hong Kong to assess the outcome of 300 mg of NR augmentation on 125 POAG patients who were randomly allocated to receive either NR or a placebo over 24 months. Ocular examinations of the retinal nerve fiber layer (RNFL) and visual field (VF) tests are planned at the beginning of the research, after one month, four months, and then every two months until the 24-month period is completed. The major aim is to establish if NR may delay the pace of RNFL thinning over 24 months by evaluating the VF progression and OCT parameters [59].

Thus far, four important ongoing clinical studies deserve to be noted.

Garthway-Heath et al. are carrying out a random-sampled, placebo-controlled, multicenter, phase 3 trial at the University College of London, to measure the reduction in average visual field sensitivity over 27 months in POAG sufferers administered an increasing dose of NAM (from 1.5 g per day for 6 weeks, then rising to 3.0 g daily) compared to those receiving placebo tablets, as well as to assess the safety of NAM and its effects on mitochondrial activity (NCT05405868) [60].

Another prospective, randomized, placebo-controlled, double-masked trial led by Jennie Nyman at Umea University, Sweden and the Australian Centre for Eye Research (NCT05275738) aims to assess the VF progression indices, with the participants to be administered 3.0 g/day of NAM or a placebo over a two-year period [61].

Furthermore, Kolomeyer is conducting another work of clinical research that intends to assess the changes in vision and visual function after six months of therapy. POAG subjects are being administered GlaucoCetin containing NAM, while a control group receives a placebo. The trial will also evaluate improvements in quality of life, electrophysiological responsiveness, and contrast sensitivity (NCT04784234 [62]).

Finally, Columbia University is conducting an interventional, randomized clinical trial to investigate changes in the central visual field, RNFL, and RGC layer using optical coherence tomography in 188 OAG patients that will be taking pyruvate and nicotinamide versus placebo for a total of 20 months (NCT05695027) [63].

7. Safety Profile

Nicotinamide is considered a dietary supplement rather than a drug formulation. The oral administration of this substance results in efficient absorption and distribution throughout the body's tissues. It undergoes hepatic metabolism and renal excretion. The recommended daily nicotinamide intake is about 15 mg, and the occurrence of negative effects is uncommon, even at the high levels used in pharmacological treatments. Even when these negative effects occur, they are generally mild and may include gastrointestinal discomfort [58], headache, nausea, tinnitus [8], and vertigo. These complaints were reported to resolve spontaneously after stopping NAM administration [64]. Only one serious adverse event of drug-induced liver injury (DILI) has been reported related to the use of NAM. A 73-year-old woman who was participating in the NCT05695027 trial, dosing over the first 3 weeks, with 1 g/day of nicotinamide and 3 g/day of calcium pyruvate in the first week, 2 g/day of each component in the second week, and 3 g/day for each element in the third week, experienced severe acute transaminitis within 5 weeks of treatment. However, the DILI appeared to be idiosyncratic and not related to the pharmacological properties of the drug [65]. Concerns have been raised about its safety in long-term use due to a hypothesis of increased cell proliferation and tumorigenesis following the erased intracellular NAD. Maric et al. has reported a higher prevalence of neoplastic growths in the mammary glands of murine models treated with NR, but the study lacked statistical analysis, and the dose used (400 mg/kg) was extremely high compared to typical human doses [66].

On the opposite hand, NAD may actually prevent cancer, as it is a substrate for the DNA-repair enzyme PARP-1, which prevents cancer-promoting mutations [67]. Additionally, NAD supplementation has been shown to improve the effectiveness of tumor immunotherapy [68]. A human study found that nicotinamide boosted the metabolism and survival of natural killer cells, aiding in remission in non-Hodgkin lymphoma patients [69]. Moreover, no increased tumor incidence has been reported among subjects taking high doses of nicotinamide for dermatological disorders or cancer prevention, nor in diabetic patients on high doses for prolonged periods [70,71]. Glaucoma management needs to be personalized and tailored to the severity of the disease and the individual needs of the patients to ensure a proper quality of life. It is imperative that patients undergo pertinent testing, examinations, differential diagnosis, and treatment to provide the best clinical outcomes and treatments for each patient [72–74].

While generally well-tolerated, nicotinamide can pose risks for certain individuals. People with pre-existing liver disease or a history of jaundice should exercise caution due to the potential worsening of liver function. Similarly, those with diabetes may experience blood sugar fluctuations, so monitoring blood sugar levels is crucial [75]. Nicotinamide might also interact with medications that affect blood clotting or how the body breaks down certain drugs, so it is important to consult a doctor before taking it alongside other medications.

8. NAD Fortification and Supplementation in the Body

Multiple compounds have been reported to increase NAD levels in the body. Van der Muelen et al. [76] carried out a study on bifidobacterial metabolism. They reported that sugar consumption and subsequent succinic acid production resulted in the production of NAD+. Apigenin has also been shown to upregulate NAD dehydrogenase quinone [77], and increase the activation factor of NAD [77]. Resveratrol is another compound, and it has been reported to show synergistic activities with other compounds, promoting the production of NAD+, thereby prolonging good health [78]. Nicotinamide is, however, a drug of choice because of its ability to augment the activity of other NAD+-promoting compounds [77]. Glaucomatous damage results from increased pressure intraocularly and can begin at any point in the disease progression [79]. Hence, NAM supplementation/intake is advised at all times.

9. Review Summary

A summary of the sampled publications used in this paper is shown in Table 1 below.

Table 1. Summary of sampled studies.

Author	Type of Study	Study Sample	Methods	Conclusion
Hui et al. [8]	In vivo	57 glaucoma patients	Change in inner retinal function	Nicotinamide supplementation can improve inner retinal function.
Tribble et al. [9]	In vivo	Murine models	Optical coherence tomography of the outer RGC layer	A nicotinamide-enriched diet significantly reduced RGC loss compared to normal diet.
Chou et al. [53]	In vivo	10 DBA/2J mice	Electroretinogram (PERG) of RGC function	NAM-fed D2 showed increased RGC density (2.4×), and larger RGC soma size (2×) when compared to controls
Zhang et al. [54]	In vivo	Murine models	PERG of RGC function	Mice treated with NAM precursors showed significantly preserved RGC function.

Table 1. *Cont.*

Author	Type of Study	Study Sample	Methods	Conclusion
Nzoughet et al. [48]	In vitro	34 POAG patients	Liquid chromatography and mass spectrometry was used to assess NAM levels in blood plasma compared to controls.	Plasma NAM levels were significantly lower in the glaucoma cohort when compared with controls.
Williams et al. [47]	In vitro	Murine models	Metabolites of age- and glaucoma-compromised RGCs were studied (outer retina).	NAD and NAD+ levels were found to be reduced, suggesting they play a role in keeping RGCs healthy.
Zeng et al. [38]	In vitro	Human trabecular meshwork cells (HTM)	Hoechst staining and MTT assays were used to assess HTM viability.	NAM had a protective effect on oxidative stress, prolonging HTM viability.
Sasaki et al. [37]	In vitro	Mouse models	Axonal degeneration in extracted dorsal root ganglia (DRG) from rat embryos	NAM synthesized from different precursors slowed the rate of axonal degeneration.
Tribble et al. [9]	In vitro	Murine models	Observed nuclear shrinkage in cultured RGC axons	NAM fortification resulted in less RGC axon loss and shrinkage.

10. Limitations to This Study

Nicotinamide is a novel therapy for glaucoma management. Hence, the literature on its efficacy and comparative use is relatively scarce. The authors suggest that this review should spur further research on this nutrient. Moreover, while this review correctly describes the usefulness of Nicotinamide as a drug, as shown in its safety profile above, there still needs to be concern about the clinically safe dosing and treatment regimen.

Another limitation encountered in the course of this review was the relative paucity of data evidenced by the low number of records returned by the search criteria. The authors attempted to widen the search net but the records returned were not relevant to this study.

11. Conclusions

The quest for new treatments to enhance glaucoma management is ongoing. Studies have indicated that NAM and nicotinamide riboside (NR) support mitochondrial health and may shield RGCs from stressors like increased IOP. These protective effects have been confirmed in various experimental models of axonal injury. Short-term NAM supplementation has improved retinal function and visual field sensitivity in clinical settings. NR is currently being evaluated in glaucoma patients, though no results have been published yet. While these compounds generally have a good safety record, their long-term effects are still unclear. Additionally, there is no definitive pharmacokinetic study that establishes the bioavailability of NMN when administered orally or topically. As a result, the bioavailability of NMN remains uncertain and could potentially limit its effectiveness and use.

Author Contributions: Conceptualization, S.B., I.G., M.S.Z., A.G., F.D., M.M., C.G., L.L. and M.Z.; methodology, S.B., I.G., M.S.Z., A.G., C.G., L.L. and M.Z.; software, S.B., I.G., M.S.Z., A.G., F.D. and M.Z.; validation, S.B., I.G., M.S.Z., A.G., F.D., M.M., C.G., L.L. and M.Z.; formal analysis, S.B., I.G., A.G., F.D., C.G. and M.Z.; investigation, S.B., I.G., M.S.Z., A.G., F.D., M.M., C.G. and M.Z.; resources, S.B., A.G., C.G. and L.L.; data curation, S.B., I.G., M.S.Z., A.G., F.D., M.M., C.G., L.L. and M.Z.; writing—original draft preparation, S.B., I.G., M.S.Z., A.G. and M.Z.; writing—review and editing, S.B., I.G., M.S.Z., A.G., F.D., M.M., C.G., L.L. and M.Z.; visualization, S.B., I.G., M.S.Z., A.G., F.D., M.M., C.G., L.L. and M.Z.; supervision, A.G., C.G., L.L. and M.Z.; project administration, S.B., A.G., M.M., C.G. and M.Z. All authors have read and agreed to the published version of the manuscript.

Funding: This research received no external funding.

Institutional Review Board Statement: Not applicable.

Informed Consent Statement: Not applicable.

Data Availability Statement: Data sharing is not applicable.

Acknowledgments: The authors thank Francesca Gattazzo for proofreading the manuscript.

Conflicts of Interest: The authors declare no conflicts of interest.

References

1. Weinreb, R.N.; Aung, T.; Medeiros, F.A. The pathophysiology and treatment of glaucoma: A review. *J. Am. Med. Assoc.* **2014**, *311*, 1901–1911. [CrossRef] [PubMed]
2. Adornetto, A.; Rombolà, L.; Morrone, L.A.; Nucci, C.; Corasaniti, M.T.; Bagetta, G.; Russo, R. Natural Products: Evidence for Neuroprotection to Be Exploited in Glaucoma. *Nutrients* **2020**, *12*, 3158. [CrossRef] [PubMed]
3. Esporcatte, B.L.; Tavares, I.M. Normal-tension glaucoma: An update. *Arq. Bras. Oftalmol.* **2016**, *79*, 270–276. [CrossRef] [PubMed]
4. Dietze, J.; Blair, K.; Zeppieri, M.; Havens, S.J. Glaucoma. In *StatPearls*; StatPearls Publishing: Treasure Island, FL, USA, 2024. [PubMed]
5. Jayaram, H.; Kolko, M.; Friedman, D.S.; Gazzard, G. Glaucoma: Now and beyond. *Lancet* **2023**, *402*, 1788–1801. [CrossRef] [PubMed]
6. Schwartz, M.; Yoles, E. Neuroprotection: A new treatment modality for glaucoma? *Curr. Opin. Ophthalmol.* **2000**, *11*, 107–111. [CrossRef] [PubMed]
7. Musa, M.; Zeppieri, M.; Atuanya, G.N.; Enaholo, E.S.; Topah, E.K.; Ojo, O.M.; Salati, C. Nutritional Factors: Benefits in Glaucoma and Ophthalmologic Pathologies. *Life* **2023**, *13*, 1120. [CrossRef] [PubMed] [PubMed Central]
8. Hui, F.; Tang, J.; Williams, P.A.; McGuinness, M.B.; Hadoux, X.; Casson, R.J.; Coote, M.; Trounce, I.A.; Martin, K.R.; van Wijngaarden, P.; et al. Improvement in inner retinal function in glaucoma with nicotinamide (vitamin B3) supplementation: A crossover randomized clinical trial. *Clin. Exp. Ophthalmol.* **2020**, *48*, 903–914. [CrossRef] [PubMed]
9. Tribble, J.R.; Otmani, A.; Sun, S.; Ellis, S.A.; Cimaglia, G.; Vohra, R.; Jöe, M.; Lardner, E.; Venkataraman, A.P.; Domínguez-Vicent, A.; et al. Nicotinamide provides neuroprotection in glaucoma by protecting against mitochondrial and metabolic dysfunction. *Redox Biol.* **2021**, *43*, 101988. [CrossRef] [PubMed]
10. Rennie, G.; Chen, A.C.; Dhillon, H.; Vardy, J.; Damian, D.L. Nicotinamide and neurocognitive function. *Nutr. Neurosci.* **2015**, *18*, 193–200. [CrossRef] [PubMed]
11. Petriti, B.; Williams, P.A.; Lascaratos, G.; Chau, K.Y.; Garway-Heath, D.F. Neuroprotection in Glaucoma: NAD(+)/NADH Redox State as a Potential Biomarker and Therapeutic Target. *Cells* **2021**, *10*, 1402. [CrossRef] [PubMed]
12. Rolfe, H.M. A review of nicotinamide: Treatment of skin diseases and potential side effects. *J. Cosmet. Dermatol.* **2014**, *13*, 324–328. [CrossRef] [PubMed]
13. Fricker, R.A.; Green, E.L.; Jenkins, S.I.; Griffin, S.M. The Influence of Nicotinamide on Health and Disease in the Central Nervous System. *Int. J. Tryptophan Res.* **2018**, *11*, 1178646918776658. [CrossRef] [PubMed]
14. Williams, A.; Ramsden, D. Nicotinamide: A double edged sword. *Park. Relat. Disord.* **2005**, *11*, 413–420. [CrossRef] [PubMed]
15. Institute of Medicine (US) Standing Committee on the Scientific. Evaluation of Dietary Reference Intakes and its Panel on Folate, Other B Vitamins, and Choline. Dietary Reference Intakes for Thiamin, Riboflavin, Niacin, Vitamin B6, Folate, Vitamin B12, Pantothenic Acid, Biotin, and Choline. In *The National Academies Collection: Reports Funded by National Institutes of Health*; National Academies Press (US): Washington, DC, USA, 1998. Available online: http://www.ncbi.nlm.nih.gov/books/NBK114310/ (accessed on 2 May 2024).
16. Bogan, K.L.; Brenner, C. Nicotinic acid, nicotinamide, and nicotinamide riboside: A molecular evaluation of NAD+ precursor vitamins in human nutrition. *Annu. Rev. Nutr.* **2008**, *28*, 115–130. [CrossRef] [PubMed]
17. Forbat, E.; Al-Niaimi, F.; Ali, F.R. Use of nicotinamide in dermatology. *Clin. Exp. Dermatol.* **2017**, *42*, 137–144. [CrossRef] [PubMed]
18. Namazi, M.R. Nicotinamide: A potential addition to the anti-psoriatic weaponry. *FASEB J.* **2003**, *17*, 1377–1379. [CrossRef] [PubMed]
19. Gomes, A.P.; Price, N.L.; Ling, A.J.; Moslehi, J.J.; Montgomery, M.K.; Rajman, L.; White, J.P.; Teodoro, J.S.; Wrann, C.D.; Hubbard, B.P.; et al. Declining NAD(+) induces a pseudohypoxic state disrupting nuclear-mitochondrial communication during aging. *Cell* **2013**, *155*, 1624–1638. [CrossRef] [PubMed]
20. Gasperi, V.; Sibilano, M.; Savini, I.; Catani, M.V. Niacin in the Central Nervous System: An Update of Biological Aspects and Clinical Applications. *Int. J. Mol. Sci.* **2019**, *20*, 974. [CrossRef] [PubMed]
21. Maiese, K.; Chong, Z.Z. Nicotinamide: Necessary nutrient emerges as a novel cytoprotectant for the brain. *Trends Pharmacol. Sci.* **2003**, *24*, 228–232. [CrossRef] [PubMed]
22. Beal, M.F.; Henshaw, D.R.; Jenkins, B.G.; Rosen, B.R.; Schulz, J.B. Coenzyme Q10 and nicotinamide block striatal lesions produced by the mitochondrial toxin malonate. *Ann. Neurol.* **1994**, *36*, 882–888. [CrossRef] [PubMed]

23. Vaur, P.; Brugg, B.; Mericskay, M.; Li, Z.; Schmidt, M.S.; Vivien, D.; Orset, C.; Jacotot, E.; Brenner, C.; Duplus, E. Nicotinamide riboside, a form of vitamin B(3), protects against excitotoxicity-induced axonal degeneration. *FASEB J.* **2017**, *31*, 5440–5452. [CrossRef] [PubMed]
24. Gong, B.; Pan, Y.; Vempati, P.; Zhao, W.; Knable, L.; Ho, L.; Wang, J.; Sastre, M.; Ono, K.; Sauve, A.A.; et al. Nicotinamide riboside restores cognition through an upregulation of proliferator-activated receptor-γ coactivator 1α regulated β-secretase 1 degradation and mitochondrial gene expression in Alzheimer's mouse models. *Neurobiol. Aging* **2013**, *34*, 1581–1588. [CrossRef] [PubMed]
25. Fechtner, R.D.; Weinreb, R.N. Mechanisms of optic nerve damage in primary open angle glaucoma. *Surv. Ophthalmol.* **1994**, *39*, 23–42. [CrossRef] [PubMed]
26. Quigley, H.A.; McKinnon, S.J.; Zack, D.J.; Pease, M.E.; Kerrigan-Baumrind, L.A.; Kerrigan, D.F.; Mitchell, R.S. Retrograde axonal transport of BDNF in retinal ganglion cells is blocked by acute IOP elevation in rats. *Investig. Ophthalmol. Vis. Sci.* **2000**, *41*, 3460–3466.
27. Weinreb, R.N.; Khaw, P.T. Primary open-angle glaucoma. *Lancet* **2004**, *363*, 1711–1720. [CrossRef] [PubMed]
28. Yoles, E.; Schwartz, M. Elevation of intraocular glutamate levels in rats with partial lesion of the optic nerve. *Arch. Ophthalmol.* **1998**, *116*, 906–910. [CrossRef] [PubMed]
29. Dreyer, E.B.; Zurakowski, D.; Schumer, R.A.; Podos, S.M.; Lipton, S.A. Elevated glutamate levels in the vitreous body of humans and monkeys with glaucoma. *Arch. Ophthalmol.* **1996**, *114*, 299–305. [CrossRef] [PubMed]
30. Tezel, G.; Edward, D.P.; Wax, M.B. Serum autoantibodies to optic nerve head glycosaminoglycans in patients with glaucoma. *Arch. Ophthalmol.* **1999**, *117*, 917–924. [CrossRef] [PubMed]
31. Liu, B.; Neufeld, A.H. Nitric oxide synthase-2 in human optic nerve head astrocytes induced by elevated pressure in vitro. *Arch. Ophthalmol. Chic. Ill 1960* **2001**, *119*, 240–245.
32. Nita, M.; Grzybowski, A. The Role of the Reactive Oxygen Species and Oxidative Stress in the Pathomechanism of the Age-Related Ocular Diseases and Other Pathologies of the Anterior and Posterior Eye Segments in Adults. *Oxid. Med. Cell Longev.* **2016**, *2016*, 3164734. [CrossRef] [PubMed]
33. Liebmann, J.M.; Cioffi, G.A. Nicking Glaucoma with Nicotinamide? *N. Engl. J. Med.* **2017**, *376*, 2079–2081. [CrossRef] [PubMed]
34. Lopez Sanchez, M.I.; Crowston, J.G.; Mackey, D.A.; Trounce, I.A. Emerging Mitochondrial Therapeutic Targets in Optic Neuropathies. *Pharmacol. Ther.* **2016**, *165*, 132–152. [CrossRef] [PubMed]
35. Osborne, N.N.; Álvarez, C.N.; del Olmo Aguado, S. Targeting mitochondrial dysfunction as in aging and glaucoma. *Drug Discov. Today* **2014**, *19*, 1613–1622. [CrossRef] [PubMed]
36. Lee, S.; Van Bergen, N.J.; Kong, G.Y.; Chrysostomou, V.; Waugh, H.S.; O'Neill, E.C.; Crowston, J.G.; Trounce, I.A. Mitochondrial dysfunction in glaucoma and emerging bioenergetic therapies. *Exp. Eye Res.* **2011**, *93*, 204–212. [CrossRef] [PubMed]
37. Sasaki, Y.; Araki, T.; Milbrandt, J. Stimulation of nicotinamide adenine dinucleotide biosynthetic pathways delays axonal degeneration after axotomy. *J. Neurosci.* **2006**, *26*, 8484–8491. [CrossRef] [PubMed]
38. Zeng, Y.; Lin, Y.; Yang, J.; Wang, X.; Zhu, Y.; Zhou, B. The Role and Mechanism of Nicotinamide Riboside in Oxidative Damage and a Fibrosis Model of Trabecular Meshwork Cells. *Transl. Vis. Sci. Technol.* **2024**, *13*, 24. [CrossRef] [PubMed]
39. Cammalleri, M.; Dal Monte, M.; Amato, R.; Bagnoli, P.; Rusciano, D. A Dietary Combination of Forskolin with Homotaurine, Spearmint and B Vitamins Protects Injured Retinal Ganglion Cells in a Rodent Model of Hypertensive Glaucoma. *Nutrients* **2020**, *12*, 1189. [CrossRef] [PubMed]
40. Banerjee, D.; Banerjee, A.; Mookherjee, S.; Vishal, M.; Mukhopadhyay, A.; Sen, A.; Basu, A.; Ray, K. Mitochondrial genome analysis of primary open angle glaucoma patients. *PLoS ONE* **2013**, *8*, e70760. [CrossRef] [PubMed]
41. Abu-Amero, K.K.; Morales, J.; Bosley, T.M. Mitochondrial abnormalities in patients with primary open-angle glaucoma. *Investig. Ophthalmol. Vis. Sci.* **2006**, *47*, 2533–2541. [CrossRef] [PubMed]
42. Van Bergen, N.J.; Crowston, J.G.; Craig, J.E.; Burdon, K.P.; Kearns, L.S.; Sharma, S.; Hewitt, A.W.; Mackey, D.A.; Trounce, I.A. Measurement of Systemic Mitochondrial Function in Advanced Primary Open-Angle Glaucoma and Leber Hereditary Optic Neuropathy. *PLoS ONE* **2015**, *10*, e0140919. [CrossRef] [PubMed]
43. Ju, W.K.; Kim, K.Y.; Lindsey, J.D.; Angert, M.; Duong-Polk, K.X.; Scott, R.T.; Kim, J.J.; Kukhmazov, I.; Ellisman, M.H.; Perkins, G.A.; et al. Intraocular pressure elevation induces mitochondrial fission and triggers OPA1 release in glaucomatous optic nerve. *Investig. Ophthalmol. Vis. Sci.* **2008**, *49*, 4903–4911. [CrossRef] [PubMed]
44. Katsyuba, E.; Romani, M.; Hofer, D.; Auwerx, J. NAD(+) homeostasis in health and disease. *Nat. Metab.* **2020**, *2*, 9–31. [CrossRef] [PubMed]
45. Cimaglia, G.; Votruba, M.; Morgan, J.E.; André, H.; Williams, P.A. Potential Therapeutic Benefit of NAD(+) Supplementation for Glaucoma and Age-Related Macular Degeneration. *Nutrients* **2020**, *12*, 2871. [CrossRef] [PubMed]
46. Pietris, J. The Role of NAD(+) and Nicotinamide (Vitamin B3) in Glaucoma: A Literature Review. *J. Nutr. Sci. Vitaminol.* **2022**, *68*, 151–154. [CrossRef] [PubMed]
47. Williams, P.A.; Harder, J.M.; Foxworth, N.E.; Cochran, K.E.; Philip, V.M.; Porciatti, V.; Smithies, O.; John, S.W. Vitamin B(3) modulates mitochondrial vulnerability and prevents glaucoma in aged mice. *Science* **2017**, *355*, 756–760. [CrossRef] [PubMed]
48. Kouassi Nzoughet, J.; Chao de la Barca, J.M.; Guehlouz, K.; Leruez, S.; Coulbault, L.; Allouche, S.; Bocca, C.; Muller, J.; Amati-Bonneau, P.; Gohier, P.; et al. Nicotinamide Deficiency in Primary Open-Angle Glaucoma. *Investig. Ophthalmol. Vis. Sci.* **2019**, *60*, 2509–2514. [CrossRef] [PubMed]

49. Wang, J.; He, Z. NAD and axon degeneration: From the Wlds gene to neurochemistry. *Cell Adh Migr.* **2009**, *3*, 77–87. [CrossRef] [PubMed]
50. Schöndorf, D.C.; Ivanyuk, D.; Baden, P.; Sanchez-Martinez, A.; De Cicco, S.; Yu, C.; Giunta, I.; Schwarz, L.K.; Di Napoli, G.; Panagiotakopoulou, V.; et al. The NAD+ Precursor Nicotinamide Riboside Rescues Mitochondrial Defects and Neuronal Loss in iPSC and Fly Models of Parkinson's Disease. *Cell Rep.* **2018**, *23*, 2976–2988. [CrossRef] [PubMed]
51. Williams, P.A.; Harder, J.M.; John, S.W.M. Glaucoma as a Metabolic Optic Neuropathy: Making the Case for Nicotinamide Treatment in Glaucoma. *J. Glaucoma* **2017**, *26*, 1161–1168. [CrossRef] [PubMed]
52. Williams, P.A.; Harder, J.M.; Cardozo, B.H.; Foxworth, N.E.; John, S.W.M. Nicotinamide treatment robustly protects from inherited mouse glaucoma. *Commun. Integr. Biol.* **2018**, *11*, e1356956. [CrossRef] [PubMed]
53. Chou, T.H.; Romano, G.L.; Amato, R.; Porciatti, V. Nicotinamide-Rich Diet in DBA/2J Mice Preserves Retinal Ganglion Cell Metabolic Function as Assessed by PERG Adaptation to Flicker. *Nutrients* **2020**, *12*, 1910. [CrossRef] [PubMed]
54. Zhang, X.; Zhang, N.; Chrenek, M.A.; Girardot, P.E.; Wang, J.; Sellers, J.T.; Geisert, E.E.; Brenner, C.; Nickerson, J.M.; Boatright, J.H.; et al. Systemic Treatment with Nicotinamide Riboside Is Protective in Two Mouse Models of Retinal Ganglion Cell Damage. *Pharmaceutics* **2021**, *13*, 893. [CrossRef] [PubMed]
55. Yu, N.; Wu, X.; Zhang, C.; Qin, Q.; Gu, Y.; Ke, W.; Liu, X.; Zhang, Q.; Liu, Z.; Chen, M.; et al. NADPH and NAC synergistically inhibits chronic ocular hypertension-induced neurodegeneration and neuroinflammation through regulating p38/MAPK pathway and peroxidation. *Biomed. Pharmacother.* **2024**, *175*, 116711. [CrossRef] [PubMed]
56. Boodram, V.; Lim, H. Protective effects of nicotinamide in a mouse model of glaucoma DBA/2 studied by second-harmonic generation microscopy. *bioRxiv* **2024**. [CrossRef] [PubMed]
57. Kim, M.; Kim, J.Y.; Rhim, W.K.; Cimaglia, G.; Want, A.; Morgan, J.E.; Williams, P.A.; Park, C.G.; Han, D.K.; Rho, S. Extracellular vesicle encapsulated nicotinamide delivered via a trans-scleral route provides retinal ganglion cell neuroprotection. *Acta Neuropathol. Commun.* **2024**, *12*, 65. [CrossRef] [PubMed]
58. De Moraes, C.G.; John, S.W.M.; Williams, P.A.; Blumberg, D.M.; Cioffi, G.A.; Liebmann, J.M. Nicotinamide and Pyruvate for Neuroenhancement in Open-Angle Glaucoma: A Phase 2 Randomized Clinical Trial. *JAMA Ophthalmol.* **2022**, *140*, 11–18. [CrossRef] [PubMed]
59. Leung, C.K.S.; Ren, S.T.; Chan, P.P.M.; Wan, K.H.N.; Kam, A.K.W.; Lai, G.W.K.; Chiu, V.S.M.; Ko, M.W.L.; Yiu, C.K.F.; Yu, M.C.Y. Correction to: Nicotinamide riboside as a neuroprotective therapy for glaucoma: Study protocol for a randomized, double-blind, placebo-control trial. *Trials* **2022**, *23*, 134. [CrossRef] [PubMed]
60. University College, London. A Phase III, Double-Masked, Randomised, Placebo-Controlled Trial Investigating the Safety and Efficacy of Nicotinamide (NAM) to Slow Visual Field Loss in Adults with Open-Angle Glaucoma. clinicaltrials.gov; Report No.: NCT05405868. May 2024. Available online: https://clinicaltrials.gov/study/NCT05405868 (accessed on 2 May 2024).
61. Umeå University. The Glaucoma Nicotinamide Trial—A Prospective, Randomized, Placebo-Controlled, Double-Masked Trial. clinicaltrials.gov; Report No.: NCT05275738. July 2023. Available online: https://clinicaltrials.gov/study/NCT05275738 (accessed on 2 May 2024).
62. Kolomeyer, N.N. A Prospective Randomized Controlled Trial of GlaucoCetin vs Placebo in Glaucoma Patients with Visual Field Loss. clinicaltrials.gov; Report No.: NCT04784234. June 2022. Available online: https://clinicaltrials.gov/study/NCT04784234 (accessed on 2 May 2024).
63. Shukla, A.G. Nicotinamide and Pyruvate for Open Angle Glaucoma: A Randomized Clinical Study. clinicaltrials.gov; Report No.: NCT05695027. July 2023. Available online: https://clinicaltrials.gov/study/NCT05695027 (accessed on 2 May 2024).
64. Hwang, E.S.; Song, S.B. Possible Adverse Effects of High-Dose Nicotinamide: Mechanisms and Safety Assessment. *Biomolecules* **2020**, *10*, 687. [CrossRef] [PubMed]
65. Garg Shukla, A.; Cioffi, G.A.; Liebmann, J.M. Drug-Induced Liver Injury During a Glaucoma Neuroprotection Clinical Trial. *J. Glaucoma* **2024**. [CrossRef] [PubMed]
66. Maric, T.; Bazhin, A.; Khodakivskyi, P.; Mikhaylov, G.; Solodnikova, E.; Yevtodiyenko, A.; Giordano Attianese, G.M.P.; Coukos, G.; Irving, M.; Joffraud, M.; et al. A bioluminescent-based probe for in vivo non-invasive monitoring of nicotinamide riboside uptake reveals a link between metastasis and NAD(+) metabolism. *Biosens. Bioelectron.* **2023**, *220*, 114826. [CrossRef] [PubMed]
67. Miwa, M.; Masutani, M. PolyADP-ribosylation and cancer. *Cancer Sci.* **2007**, *98*, 1528–1535. [CrossRef] [PubMed]
68. Morandi, F.; Horenstein, A.L.; Malavasi, F. The Key Role of NAD(+) in Anti-Tumor Immune Response: An Update. *Front. Immunol.* **2021**, *12*, 658263. [CrossRef] [PubMed]
69. Cichocki, F.; Zhang, B.; Wu, C.Y.; Chiu, E.; Day, A.; O'Connor, R.S.; Yackoubov, D.; Simantov, R.; McKenna, D.H.; Cao, Q.; et al. Nicotinamide enhances natural killer cell function and yields remissions in patients with non-Hodgkin lymphoma. *Sci. Transl. Med.* **2023**, *15*, eade3341. [CrossRef] [PubMed]
70. Madaan, P.; Sikka, P.; Malik, D.S. Cosmeceutical Aptitudes of Niacinamide: A Review. *Recent Adv. Anti-Infect. Drug Discov.* **2021**, *16*, 196–208. [CrossRef] [PubMed]
71. Knip, M.; Douek, I.F.; Moore, W.P.; Gillmor, H.A.; McLean, A.E.; Bingley, P.J.; Gale, E.A. European Nicotinamide Diabetes Intervention Trial Group. Safety of high-dose nicotinamide: A review. *Diabetologia* **2000**, *43*, 1337–1345. [CrossRef] [PubMed]
72. Salvetat, M.L.; Zeppieri, M.; Tosoni, C.; Brusini, P.; Medscape. Baseline factors predicting the risk of conversion from ocular hypertension to primary open-angle glaucoma during a 10-year follow-up. *Eye* **2016**, *30*, 784–795. [CrossRef] [PubMed]

73. Della Mea, G.; Bacchetti, S.; Zeppieri, M.; Brusini, P.; Cutuli, D.; Gigli, G.L. Nerve fibre layer analysis with GDx with a variable corneal compensator in patients with multiple sclerosis. *Ophthalmologica* **2007**, *221*, 186–189. [CrossRef] [PubMed]
74. Salvetat, M.L.; Zeppieri, M.; Tosoni, C.; Parisi, L.; Brusini, P. Non-conventional perimetric methods in the detection of early glaucomatous functional damage. *Eye* **2010**, *24*, 835–842. [CrossRef] [PubMed]
75. Curry, A.M.; Rymarchyk, S.; Herrington, N.B.; Donu, D.; Kellogg, G.E.; Cen, Y. Nicotinamide riboside activates SIRT5 deacetylation. *FEBS J.* **2023**, *290*, 4762–4776. [CrossRef] [PubMed] [PubMed Central]
76. Van der Meulen, R.; Adriany, T.; Verbrugghe, K.; De Vuyst, L. Kinetic analysis of bifidobacterial metabolism reveals a minor role for succinic acid in the regeneration of NAD+ through its growth-associated production. *Appl. Environ. Microbiol.* **2006**, *72*, 5204–5210. [CrossRef] [PubMed] [PubMed Central]
77. Zhou, N.; Tian, Y.; Liu, W.; Tu, B.; Xu, W.; Gu, T.; Zou, K.; Lu, L. Protective Effects of Resveratrol and Apigenin Dietary Supplementation on Serum Antioxidative Parameters and mRNAs Expression in the Small Intestines of Diquat-Challenged Pullets. *Front. Vet. Sci.* **2022**, *9*, 850769. [CrossRef] [PubMed] [PubMed Central]
78. Sharma, A.; Chabloz, S.; Lapides, R.A.; Roider, E.; Ewald, C.Y. Potential Synergistic Supplementation of NAD+ Promoting Compounds as a Strategy for Increasing Healthspan. *Nutrients* **2023**, *15*, 445. [CrossRef] [PubMed] [PubMed Central]
79. Yanez, M.; Jhanji, M.; Murphy, K.; Gower, R.M.; Sajish, M.; Jabbarzadeh, E. Nicotinamide Augments the Anti-Inflammatory Properties of Resveratrol through PARP1 Activation. *Sci. Rep.* **2019**, *9*, 10219. [CrossRef] [PubMed] [PubMed Central]

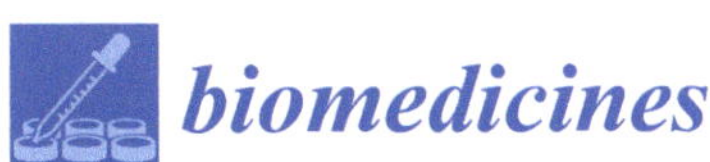

MDPI

Article

Endocyclophotocoagulation Combined with Phacoemulsification in Glaucoma Treatment: Five-Year Results

Bartłomiej Bolek [1,2,*], Adam Wylęgała [3], Małgorzata Rebkowska-Juraszek [2] and Edward Wylęgała [1,2]

1 Chair and Clinical Department of Ophthalmology, School of Medicine in Zabrze, Medical University of Silesia in Katowice, 40-760 Katowice, Poland
2 Clinical Department of Ophthalmology, District Railway Hospital, 40-760 Katowice, Poland
3 Health Promotion and Obesity Management, Pathophysiology Department, Medical University of Silesia in Katowice, 40-752 Katowice, Poland
* Correspondence: bartlomiej.bolek@sum.edu.pl; Tel.: +48-32-605-35-92

Abstract: Background: this study aimed to assess the effectiveness and safety of phaco-endocyclophotocoagulation (phaco-ECP) in patients with glaucoma over five consecutive years. Methods: Thirty-eight patients (38 eyes) with primary and secondary glaucoma were enrolled to undergo phaco-ECP (Endo Optiks URAM E2, Beaver-Visitec International, Waltham, MA, USA). The primary outcome measures were intraocular pressure (IOP) reduction, success rates, glaucoma medication use, and visual acuity after phaco-ECP. An IOP reduction of 20% compared to the baseline value without re-intervention was considered a successful treatment. Complete success was defined as a cessation of antiglaucoma medications. Secondary outcome measures included intraoperative and postoperative complications. Measurements were performed preoperatively and in the first week and 1, 3, 6, 12, 18, 24, 30, 36, 42, 48, 54, and 60 months postoperatively. Results: The mean ± SD values of IOP preoperatively, at 12, 24, 36, 48, and 60 months postoperatively were 22.6 ± 6.7 mmHg, 15.9 ± 3.9 mmHg ($p < 0.001$), 15.9 ± 2.9 mmHg ($p < 0.001$), 15.6 ± 2.7 mmHg ($p < 0.001$), 15.5 ± 3.8 mmHg ($p < 0.001$), and 15.2 ± 2.6 mmHg ($p < 0.001$), respectively. The mean IOP at the last follow-up was reduced by 32.7%. The decrease in the number of antiglaucoma medications was statistically significant at each follow-up visit compared to the baseline. The qualified success rate was 40.6%. All patients at the 60-month follow-up visit required the use of antiglaucoma medications—none of the patients achieved complete success. During the follow-up period, nine patients (28.3%) that required retreatment due to nonachievement of the target IOP were considered failures. Six patients (15.8%) were lost from the follow-up. A total of 23 patients were evaluated 60 months after their phaco-ECP. Complications directly associated with the procedure, such as corneal edema (25.6%), IOP spikes (20.5%), IOL dislocation (2.6%), and uveitis (12.8%), were observed in our patients. Hypotony was not observed in any of our patients. Conclusions: The phaco-ECP procedure was effective, well-tolerated, and safe for reducing IOP in glaucoma patients with cataracts over a long-term follow-up. Randomized, larger-scale studies are required to validate the results obtained.

Keywords: cyclodestruction; glaucoma; endocyclophotocoagulation; transscleral cyclophotocoagulation; cataract

Citation: Bolek, B.; Wylęgała, A.; Rebkowska-Juraszek, M.; Wylęgała, E. Endocyclophotocoagulation Combined with Phacoemulsification in Glaucoma Treatment: Five-Year Results. *Biomedicines* **2024**, *12*, 186. https://doi.org/10.3390/biomedicines12010186

Academic Editor: Da-Wen Lu

Received: 5 December 2023
Revised: 29 December 2023
Accepted: 10 January 2024
Published: 15 January 2024

1. Introduction

Cyclodestructive techniques are used to treat moderate and severe manifestations of glaucoma [1–3]. These methods induce a decrease in intraocular pressure (IOP) by attenuating the production of aqueous humor through partial damage to the non-pigmented epithelium of the ciliary body. In comparison to the commonly used transscleral diode laser cyclodestruction (TSCPC), endocyclophotocoagulation (ECP) for glaucoma treatment allows for direct visualization of the ciliary processes, precise laser application, and has demonstrated superior safety and selectivity over TSCPC [4–6]. More recently, to enhance the safety profile of existing cyclophotocoagulation methods, two innovative approaches have been introduced: micropulse cyclophotocoagulation and ultrasound cycloplasty. In the former, each laser pulse is divided into extremely short-duration phases, thereby minimizing heat accumulation and reducing the disruption of the non-pigmented epithelium and adjacent tissues [2,7–10]. In the latter, high-intensity focused ultrasound technology is utilized, and energy is delivered via a specially designed probe. This technique enables precise focusing of ultrasound energy at the desired depth, minimizing uncontrolled absorption and thereby reducing damage to adjacent tissues [11–13]. In juxtaposition to the transscleral methodology, ECP enables the precise titration of diode laser therapy targeting the ciliary body through direct visualization via endoscopy. This ability to directly observe the target tissue represents the foremost benefit of this method. Nonetheless, it is an invasive procedure typically indicated for patients with glaucoma who are concurrently undergoing cataract surgery [14,15].

To date, only one study with a follow-up period exceeding 36 months has assessed the effectiveness of endoscopic cyclophotocoagulation (ECP) or its combination with phacoemulsification (phaco-ECP). This study aims to assess the effectiveness and safety of the phaco-ECP treatment in glaucoma patients over a consecutive 60-month follow-up period. The primary outcome measures included post-procedure intraocular pressure (IOP) reduction, success rates, glaucoma medication usage, and visual acuity. Secondary outcome measures encompassed any procedure-related complications or postoperative adverse events. The extended period between surgery and the last follow-up visit enables a more precise determination of the effectiveness of the procedure and the need for reintervention, which is crucial in glaucoma management for the preservation of visual acuity.

2. Materials and Methods

This was a non-randomized, prospective, single-arm, single-center, follow-up clinical study. It received approval from the institutional review board of the Medical University of Silesia (KNW-0022-KB1-131-16) and followed the tenets of the Declaration of Helsinki. Patients were recruited between November 2016 and September 2018. All enrolled patients provided written informed consent prior to participating in the study.

Inclusion criteria for the study encompassed adult patients ($\geq$18 years) with uncontrolled glaucoma (IOP > 21 mmHg, despite the maximum tolerated doses of antiglaucoma medications) or intolerance to glaucoma medications despite well-controlled IOP. Exclusion criteria included pregnant women, ocular and non-ocular disorders that can significantly affect the visual field other than glaucoma or cataract, and patients less than 18 years of age. Comprehensive ophthalmic examinations were conducted, which involved measurements of IOP using the standard Goldmann applanation tonometer (GAT), an assessment of the number of antiglaucoma medications, a and determination of best-corrected logMAR visual acuity. These examinations were performed preoperatively and at 1 day, 1 week, 1, 3, 6, 12, 18, 24, 30, 36, 42, 48, 54, and 60 months postoperatively. The IOP measurements adhered to the guidelines set forth by the World Glaucoma Association for the design and reporting of glaucoma surgical trials [16]. Visual field tests were performed using a Humphrey Visual Field Analyzer III (Carl Zeiss Meditec, Dublin, CA, USA) set for a full threshold 24-2 testing strategy preoperatively and at 12, 24, 36, 48, and 60 months postoperatively. To measure VF loss the mean deviation (MD) parameter was used. Glaucoma stages of patients in the study group were based on the MD (early glaucomatous loss—MD $\leq$ 6 dB; moderate glaucomatous loss—6 dB > MD $\leq$ 12 dB; advanced glaucomatous loss—MD > 12 dB) [17]. The study considered a treatment successful (qualified success) if there was a 20% reduction in IOP and the IOP remained below 21 mmHg during the 60-month period of follow-up visits compared to the baseline value without requiring additional surgical intervention [16]. Complete success was defined as a cessation of antiglaucoma medications. Failure was defined as the IOP not being reduced by at least 20% from the baseline and above 21 mmHg (over two consecutive visits), and/or the necessity for further glaucoma surgical intervention. In cases where IOP was not sufficiently lowered during follow-up and the number of antiglaucoma medications was reduced compared to the baseline, additional medications were added. If needed, further glaucoma surgery was performed based on the patient's clinical conditions.

Standard phacoemulsification surgery was performed, with intraocular lens implantation in the capsular bag. An ECP (Endo Optiks URAM E2, Beaver-Visitec International, Waltham, MA, USA) probe was carefully introduced into the sulcus, and diode laser treatment was applied between 270 and 360 degrees, continuing until whitening and shrinkage of the ciliary processes were observed. The power was initially set at 250 mW and was then adjusted based on the observed effect.

All surgical procedures were executed by one unchanging surgeon (E.W.). Postoperative management involved a reassessment of intraocular pressure (IOP), with adjustments made to the preoperative antiglaucoma medication regimen based on these readings. Subsequent to surgery, patients were administered topical ofloxacin (five times a day for two weeks) and dexamethasone (five times a day for two weeks, followed by three times a day for two weeks). Statistical analyses were carried out using Statistica Software version 13 (TIBCO Software Inc., Palo Alto, CA, USA). Group comparisons for specific parameters were conducted using either the Wilcoxon signed-rank test or a paired t-test, contingent upon the data distribution. Kaplan–Meier survival curves were employed to evaluate the qualified and complete success of the treatment over time. The results of IOP are visually represented through a scatter plot, illustrating preoperative IOP on the x-axis versus 60-month postoperative IOP on the y-axis. A p-value of ≤ 0.05 was deemed statistically significant.

3. Results

Thirty-eight patients (38 eyes) diagnosed with primary and secondary glaucoma were included in this study of phaco-ECP. Detailed patient characteristics can be found in Table 1. The glaucoma stages of the patients enrolled in the study, based on their VF, are presented in Table 2. Preoperatively, sixteen of our patients had early glaucomatous loss, thirteen of our patients had moderate glaucomatous loss, and 9 of our patients had advanced glaucomatous loss. Throughout the follow-up period, nine eyes (28.3%) required re-treatment due to not achieving the target IOP and were categorized as failures. Among these, three eyes (7.9%) underwent TSCPC surgery approximately 23 months later, two patients (5.3%) received UCP treatment around 30 months post procedure, one patient (2.6%) underwent trabeculectomy 18 months after the initial intervention, and microshunt implantation was performed in two patients (5.3%) approximately 42 months later. Additionally, one patient (2.6%) had non-penetrating deep sclerectomy 24 months following the phaco-ECP. Six patients (15.8%) were lost to the follow-up during the study period. Of these, three patients died from causes unrelated to glaucoma, while three patients discontinued their participation in the study visits due to reasons of a medical or non-medical nature that were unrelated to glaucoma. As a result, a total of 23 patients were included in the evaluation at the 60-month follow-up following their phaco-ECP.

The mean $\pm$ SD values of IOP preoperatively at 1 day, 1 week, 1, 3, 6, 12, 18, 24, 30, 36, 42, 48, 54, and 60 months postoperatively are presented in Table 3. A statistically significant reduction in IOP was observed at each follow-up timepoint compared to the baseline. The mean IOP at the last follow-up showed a reduction of 32.7% (Table 3). The qualified success rate was 40.6% (13 out of 32 eyes). Among the patients who did not achieve qualified success, nine eyes required additional surgical interventions. Furthermore, ten patients did not meet the minimum IOP reduction success criterion. At the 60-month follow-up, all patients still required antiglaucoma medications, and none achieved complete success. Visual representations of the data are provided as the Kaplan–Meier survival curves (Figures 1 and 2) and a scatter plot (Figure 3). It is important to note that patients lost to the follow-up were excluded from the analysis of success rates.

Table 1. Demographic characteristics. Demographic data, type of glaucoma, and history of prior glaucoma surgeries of patients enrolled in the study.

Demographic Characteristics		
Age (years)		
Mean ± SD Range	78.03 ± 9.13 52.00–98.00	
	No. (%)	
Gender		
Female	24	(63.2)
Male	14	(36.8)
Type of glaucoma:		
Primary open-angle glaucoma	26	(68.4)
Secondary open-angle glaucoma		
Post-penetrating keratoplasty glaucoma	1	(2.6)
Exfoliative	3	(7.9)
Pigmentary	0	(0.0)
Uveitic glaucoma	1	(2.6)
Neovascular glaucoma	1	(2.6)
Other	3	(7.9)
Primary angle-closure glaucoma	3	(7.9)
Secondary angle-closure glaucoma	0	(0.0)
Aniridic glaucoma	0	(0.0)
Prior glaucoma surgeries:		
Trabeculectomy Deep sclerectomy Surgery (tube/stents) Transscleral cyclophotocoagulation Ultrasound Cyclo Plasty	4 1 0 0 0	

SD—standard deviation, MD—mean deviation.

Table 2. Glaucoma staging of patients enrolled in the study.

Glaucoma Staging		
	No. (%)	
Early glaucomatous loss MD ≤ 6 dB	16	(42.1)
Moderate glaucomatous loss 6 dB > MD ≤ 12 dB	13	(34.2)
Advanced glaucomatous loss MD > 12 dB	9	(23.7)

The mean ± SD values of the number of antiglaucoma medications taken preoperatively and 1 day, 1 week, 1, 3, 6, 12, 18, 24, 30, 36, 42, 48, 54, and 60 months postoperatively are presented in Table 3. A statistically significant reduction in the number of antiglaucoma medications was observed at each follow-up timepoint compared to the baseline. Before undergoing phaco-ECP, three patients required systemic carbonic anhydrase administration. During the 60-month follow-up, thirteen eyes maintained the same number of antiglaucoma medications as at baseline. Conversely, other patients showed a reduction in their number of antiglaucoma medications at the last follow-up compared to baseline. None of the patients experienced an increase in the number of antiglaucoma medications compared to their preoperative regimen during the last visit. In a few cases, systemic carbonic anhydrase was added during follow-up just before surgical re-intervention to lower intraocular pressure, and these cases were considered treatment failures. None of the eyes required systemic carbonic anhydrase at the 60-month follow-up.

Table 3. Intraocular pressure and number of hypotensive medications taken after phaco-ECP—60-month follow-up.

	Mean IOP ± SD	*p*-Value	Number of Hypotensive Medications ± SD	*p*-Value	% IOP Reduction	No. Patients
Preop	22.6 ± 6.7		3.4 ± 0.9		-	38
1 day	18.4 ± 5.0	0.009	1.4 ± 1.4	<0.001	18.6	38
1 week	18.4 ± 7.3	0.007	1.6 ± 1.2	<0.001	18.5	38
1 month	16.4 ± 5.5	<0.001	1.9 ± 1.1	<0.001	27.3	38
3 months	16.8 ± 6.1	0.003	1.7 ± 0.9	<0.001	25.4	38
6 months	15.6 ± 3.7	<0.001	2.0 ± 1.2	<0.001	31.0	38
12 months	15.9 ± 3.9	<0.001	2.2 ± 1.1	<0.001	29.5	38
18 months	16.9 ± 5.0	<0.001	2.5 ± 1.2	<0.001	24.9	36
24 months	15.9 ± 2.9	<0.001	2.6 ± 1.2	0.001	29.4	35
30 months	16.6 ± 4.1	0.001	2.6 ± 1.3	0.005	26.4	33
36 months	15.6 ± 2.7	<0.001	2.6 ± 1.3	0.005	30.7	31
42 months	15.9 ± 4.5	0.006	2.3 ± 1.3	0.001	29.7	27
48 months	15.5 ± 3.8	0.001	2.1 ± 1.3	0.002	31.3	25
54 months	15.5 ± 2.8	<0.001	2.8 ± 0.9	0.013	31.4	23
60 months	15.2 ± 2.6	<0.001	2.7 ± 1.1	0.009	32.7	23

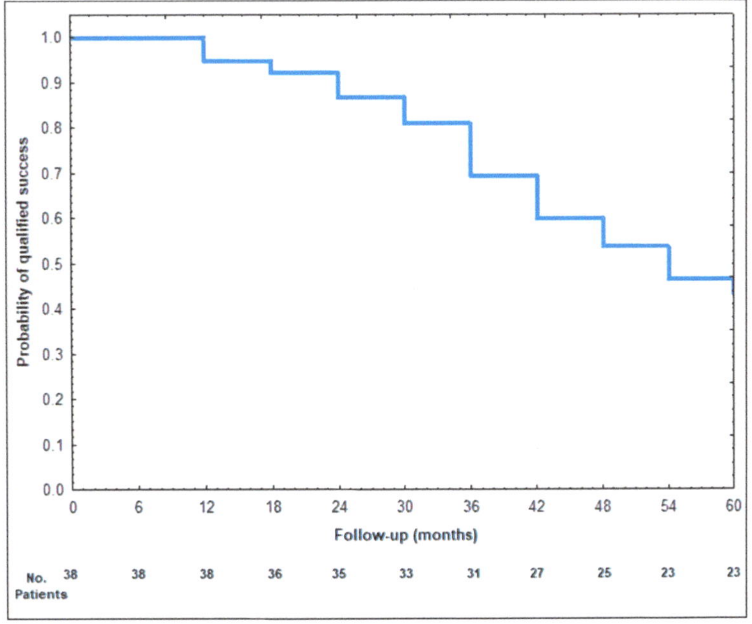

Figure 1. Kaplan–Meier survival curve of qualified success after phaco-ECP—60-month follow-up.

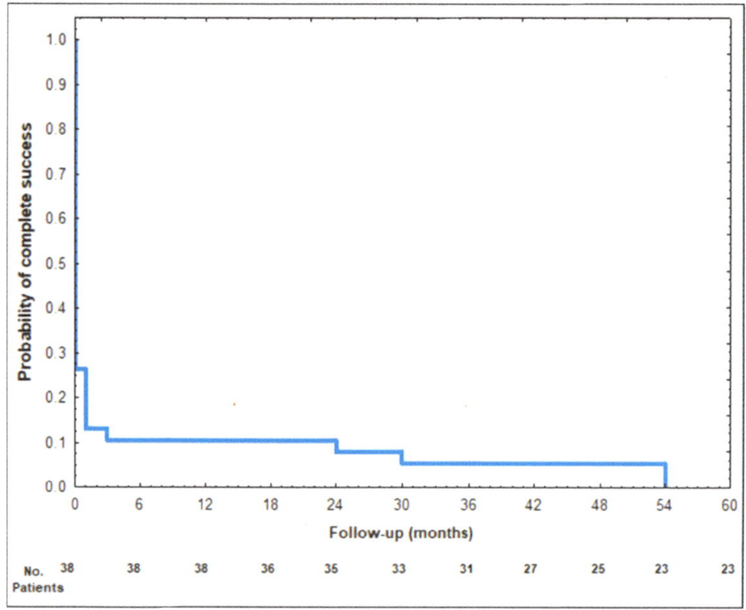

Figure 2. Kaplan–Meier survival curve of complete success after phaco-ECP—60-month follow-up.

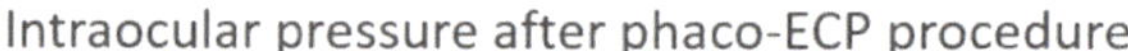

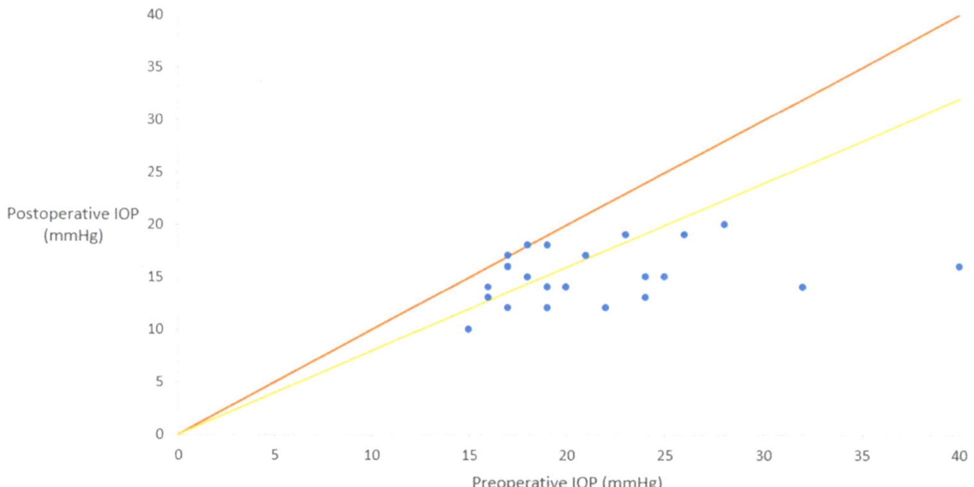

Figure 3. Scatter plot of preoperative IOP (*x*-axis) versus 60-month postoperative IOP (*y*-axis). Each point represents one eye showing the preoperative IOP and the postoperative IOP. Orange line indicates no change. Yellow diagonal line represents 20% IOP reduction. phaco-ECP—phaco-endocyclophotocoagulation, IOP—intraocular pressure.

The best-corrected logMAR visual acuities ± SD values preoperatively and 1 day, 1 week, 1, 3, 6, 12, 18, 24, 30, 36, 42, 48, 54, and 60 months postoperatively are presented in Table 3. There were statistically differences in this parameter at each significant follow-up timepoint compared to the baseline.

The VF mean deviation ± SD values preoperatively and 12, 24, 36, 48, and 60 months postoperatively were −9.07 ± 7.50 dB, −9.59 ± 10.26 dB (p = 0.215), −9.44 ± 8.71 dB (p = 0.255), −10.26 ± 9.41 dB (p = 0.483), −9.21 ± 8.01 dB (p = 0.937), and −9.46 ± 10.03 dB (p = 0.191), respectively.

Table 4 lists the postoperative complications encountered during the study. Corneal edema was observed in ten patients (26.3%), which resolved over time without corneal decompensation. An IOP spike occurred in eight patients (21.1%). In one patient (2.6%), there was an IOL dislocation (subluxation) 36 months post-procedure. Three patients (7.9%) developed macular edema, while four patients (10.5%) experienced the development of an epiretinal membrane approximately 46 months after the phaco-ECP procedure. One patient (2.6%) encountered a full-thickness macular hole 12 months after the initial procedure. Anterior uveitis was observed in five patients (13.2%) immediately after the procedure. Five patients (13.2%) required Nd:YAG capsulotomy due to a secondary cataract approximately 24 months after the procedure. Notably, no other significant intraoperative or postoperative complications were observed.

Table 4. Intraoperative and postoperative complications after phaco-ECP—60-month follow-up.

Complications		
	No. (%)	
Epithelial defects	0/38	(0.0)
Corneal edema	10/38	(26.3)
Corneal decompensation	0/38	(0.0)
IOP spike	8/38	(21.1)
IOL dislocation	1/38	(2.6)
Hypotony, choroid detachment	0/38	(0.0)
Macular edema	3/38	(7.9)
Macular hole	1/38	(2.6)
Epiretinal membrane	4/38	(10.5)
Retinal detachment	1/38	(2.6)
Phthisis bulbi	0/38	(0.0)
Uveitis	5/38	(13.2)

phaco-ECP—phaco-endocyclophotocoagulation, IOP—intraocular pressure, IOL—intraocular lens.

4. Discussion

To summarize, this is one of the longest long-term prospective single-center studies of glaucoma patients who have undergone phaco-ECP. At the final follow-up, the mean intraocular pressure (IOP) demonstrated a reduction exceedingly greater than a quarter. The qualified success rate was observed to be reasonable. The incidence of adverse events aligns with the findings reported in prior publications [15,18–21].

Lowering intraocular pressure (IOP) continues to be the principal and evidence-based strategy in the therapeutic management of glaucoma [22,23]. This can be achieved through various strategies, including pharmacological and surgical interventions aimed at reducing aqueous humor production and improving outflow. Within these approaches, inducing targeted damage to the non-pigmented epithelium of the ciliary body using methods like laser photocoagulation, cryotherapy, or ultrasound energy has been commonly practiced. Among these interventions, transscleral cyclophotocoagulation (TSCPC) stands out as the most prevalent and efficacious technique. The mechanism of action of TSCPC involves the destruction of the pigmented ciliary body epithelium, leading to indirect destruction of the non-pigmented cells and an increase in uveoscleral outflow [24,25]. This method is primarily used in severe cases of refractory glaucoma when prior pharmacological or surgical interventions, such as filtration or seton procedures, have proven ineffective [26].

Cyclodestruction techniques, including TSCPC, come with two major limitations in glaucoma treatment. Firstly, there is a lack of selectivity for the target tissue, which may lead to potential damage to adjacent structures. Secondly, predicting the therapeutic effect in relation to the applied dosage can be challenging. Additionally, TSCPC entails the risk of complications such as pain, conjunctival burn, scleral thinning, and uveitis [24,27–29]. While rare, more serious complications include hypotension, choroidal detachment, choroiditis, retinal detachment, and, extremely rarely, phthisis bulbi [7].

To address these challenges and enhance the safety profile of existing cyclophotocoagulation methods, two innovative approaches have emerged: micropulse cyclophotocoagulation and ultrasound cycloplasty, briefly mentioned in the introduction. In contrast to the transscleral methodology, endoscopic cyclophotocoagulation (ECP) enables the precise modulation of diode laser therapy, targeting the ciliary body by directly visualizing the tissue via endoscopy. The ability to directly observe the target tissue is the primary advantage of this method and has been proven to possess superior safety and selectivity over TSCPC [4–6]. Nonetheless, it is an invasive procedure typically indicated for patients with moderate glaucoma who are concurrently undergoing cataract surgery [14,15].

It is imperative to acknowledge that this procedure is not devoid of side effects. The most frequently observed complications include IOP spikes, heightened inflammation (in comparison to phacoemulsification without ECP), and the potential for intraocular lens dislocation [30,31]. In our study, corneal edema was noted in ten patients (26.3%), which spontaneously resolved over time without corneal decompensation or the need for corneal grafting. IOP spikes manifested in eight patients (21.1%), successfully managed with topical IOP-lowering medications, negating the necessity for further intervention. In one patient (2.6%), IOL dislocation (subluxation) was observed 36 months post-procedure, resulting in a decline in visual acuity. However, surgical intervention was not pursued, as the patient chose not to undergo the procedure. Hypotony was not observed in any of our patients. Macular edema occurred in three patients (7.9%) one month after the procedure and resolved within two months through pharmacotherapy, involving topical nonsteroidal anti-inflammatory drugs and oral carbonic anhydrase inhibitors. Epiretinal membranes were detected approximately 46 months after the initial procedure in four of our patients (10.5%), but surgical intervention was not required during the study follow-up due to the minimal progression of the condition. One patient (2.6%) developed a full-thickness macular hole 12 months after the initial procedure, necessitating subsequent vitrectomy surgery. Uveitis occurred in five of our patients (13.2%) approximately one month after the procedure. In four cases, it was minor and resolved after treatment with the topical steroid dexamethasone, without further complications. One patient developed fibrinous anterior uveitis with posterior synechiae formation, requiring intensive treatment with systemic prednisone therapy and subconjunctival steroid injections, which yielded positive results. No other significant intraoperative or postoperative complications were observed. The incidence of major complications in our study is comparable to the results published to date [15,18–21].

It is widely known that glaucoma is a progressive disease, and surgical interventions often need to be repeated periodically to maintain proper glaucoma control. Longer observation periods yield more data regarding the effectiveness of the procedure. Therefore, a crucial question in glaucoma management is how long a given procedure will suffice for maintaining proper glaucoma control. Moreover, there is a commonly held opinion that the ciliary body can regenerate after cyclodestruction, potentially leading to an increase in IOP and decreasing the long-term efficacy of the procedure, with the necessity of reperforming that procedure. In analyzing the limited literature on ciliary body regeneration, which is primarily based on animal studies, it remains challenging to definitively prove this opinion. A few studies have shown some epithelial regeneration in pars plicata [27] and the reperfusion of the ciliary processes [5,28], particularly in favor of ECP [5]. However, authors consistently conclude that the capillary network regeneration of the ciliary processes is mostly incomplete, and the regenerated epithelium is always disorganized, with a lack of a well-developed pigment epithelial layer, which may result in limited functionality concerning secretory function [27].

Many studies on ECP exhibit limited follow-up data, with our search identifying only one available study reporting 60-month outcomes and four studies presenting data with a 36months follow-up period. Other studies related to phaco-ECP have shorter follow-up durations. Oberfeld et al. [20] reported a 12% success rate at 60 months after phaco-ECP, with an 18% reduction in intraocular pressure (IOP) among the 9 patients who remained in the study out of the initial 78 enrolled. After 36 months, the same authors reported 27 patients still in the study, with a 25% reduction in IOP and a 34% success rate. Other studies with 36 months of follow-up showed a 25% reduction in IOP and a 40% success rate [18], a 26% reduction in IOP and a 45% success rate [19], or a 13% reduction in IOP with a 70% success rate [15,21]. Similarly, studies with a 24-month follow-up period reported IOP reductions ranging from 30% to 40% [32,33].

In our study, a decrease in IOP and the number of antiglaucoma medications was statistically significant at each follow-up time point. The mean IOP at the 60-month follow-up was reduced by 32.7%, with a qualified success rate of 40%. These results exceed those of the only available 5-year study conducted by Oberfeld et al. [20]. We attribute this difference to the extent of the ciliary process treatment, which in their study covered 90–360 degrees, whereas in our study it spanned 270–360 degrees. Other studies mentioned above, although with shorter follow-up durations, have reported higher success rates and IOP reductions, like our findings at the 36-month post-procedure mark, where the success rate of our study reached 60%.

It is crucial to recognize the limitations associated with assessing intraocular pressure (IOP), particularly the presence of regression to the mean, an inherent challenge in non-randomized studies such as this one. To minimize the influence of IOP measurement variability, we conducted multiple assessments in accordance with the recommendations of the World Glaucoma Association [16]. While this approach helps mitigate the impact of regression to the mean, it remains a factor that warrants consideration when interpreting the results. Throughout the follow-up period, no significant changes in visual acuity were observed. While there was no statistically significant loss in the visual field (VF) at each follow-up time point within the study group, individual patient analyses revealed that a minority experienced substantial VF deterioration, typically necessitating re-treatment. Regarding different glaucoma subtypes, whether patients were treatment-naïve or had previously undergone surgical interventions, we did not identify any significant differences in outcomes following phaco-ECP.

It is noteworthy that phaco-ECP, due to its similar approach and low complication rate, should be compared to other glaucoma surgeries commonly performed in conjunction with phacoemulsification, such as an iStent injection, Hydrus Microstent implantation (HMS), or trabecular excision using a Kahook Dual Blade (KDB) as part of Microinvasive Glaucoma Surgery (MIGS). At the time of writing, publications directly comparing phaco-ECP to different combined procedures are limited. One publication that compared phaco-ECP with phaco-trabeculectomy showed similar IOP reductions at 24 months post operation [34]. With a shorter one-year follow-up period, Moghimi et al. [35] conducted a comparison between phaco-ECP, phaco-trabeculectomy, and phaco-viscocanalostomy, demonstrating the comparable effectiveness between the first two procedures and the superior effectiveness of the latter. Regarding trabeculectomy, it is noteworthy that common opinion and published clinical studies indicate a decreased success rate when it is combined with cataract surgery compared to when performed as a standalone procedure. This decrease is attributed to increased inflammation and bleb fibrosis [36,37]. In the aforementioned earlier study by Oberfeld et al. [20], notable for its extensive follow-up duration, a comparative analysis was conducted between phaco-ECP, phaco-KDB, and PEcK (combined phacoemulsification, ECP, and KDB). This study revealed similar results between the phaco-ECP and phaco-KDB groups but a greater reduction in the PEcK group [20]. Other published studies on ECP and MIGS compare combined phaco-ECP with or without other MIGS (KDB, iStent), presenting superior results in triple procedures [38,39]. Studies of MIGS procedures combined with cataract surgery in terms of extended observation, like our study with a 60-month follow-up, are limited and consist mainly of non-comparative studies or studies comparing phaco-MIGS to phaco alone. The Manchester iStent study even presented 7-year results, with a success rate of 46% of patients and a 20% IOP reduction after 60 months [40]. Arriola-Villalobos et al. reported outcomes from the same procedure, with a 16% decrease in IOP and a success rate of 40% among the 13 patients who completed 60 months of follow-up [41]. In contrast, while the two studies concerning iStent demonstrate a high success rate for that procedure, the HORIZON study, which focused on HMS procedures, presents quite the opposite results. After 5 years, there was a 6% reduction in IOP, and this was not statistically significant compared to phaco-alone procedures [42]. However, the authors found a reduced need for medication to achieve IOP control and a decreased need for incisional IOP-lowering procedures. The limited availability of studies with a 60-month follow-up period presents challenges in drawing definitive conclusions regarding the long-term effectiveness of these procedures and their comparison to phaco-ECP. More studies on MIGS, including phaco-ECP, with extended follow-up durations are undoubtedly necessary to provide a comprehensive assessment. This will help address the question of the most effective and safe treatment option for patients with uncontrolled glaucoma and concomitant cataract. It is important to note that comparing and analyzing the aforementioned studies is complicated due to variations in methodology, particularly in terms of defining a successful outcome.

The current study has several limitations, including its retrospective, noncomparative design and a moderate number of cases. Analyzing the results, these facts should be acknowledged and data validation is necessary from larger-scale studies. Nevertheless, it stands as one of the longest clinical studies and has the largest number of follow-up patients in the literature.

In conclusion, regarding ECP studies with a 60-month follow-up, only one study is available. Our study, conducted over the same follow-up period, demonstrates a reasonable success rate and IOP reduction, along with a favorable safety profile. By amalgamating this information from 60 months of follow-up data with our results after 36 months (where the success rate stands ranges from 40–70%) we can present a more comprehensive picture of the duration of ECP's effects, which is satisfactory, in our opinion. These findings support its suitability as a viable option for patients with uncontrolled glaucoma and cataract. For this type of patient, when the cataract is operable, a combined procedure is recommended. In terms of patients with controlled glaucoma and operable cataract, despite this not being the primary focus of the study, and based on our experience, ECP is also a viable option to reduce the number of medications. However, in such cases, it is advisable to avoid inducing hypotony. Therefore, the number of drops and preoperative IOP should not be excessively low (low or mid-teens), considering that we are reducing the IOP by 30% with this method. Using this information, clinicians can determine the suitability and duration of a particular procedure in the treatment of glaucoma for individual patients. This is invaluable for the preservation of vision in glaucoma patients.

5. Conclusions

The phaco-ECP procedure is effective, well-tolerated, and safe for reducing the IOP in glaucoma patients with cataracts over a long-term follow-up. Randomized, larger-scale studies are required to validate the results obtained.

Author Contributions: Conceptualization, B.B. and M.R.-J.; methodology, B.B. and M.R.-J.; formal analysis, A.W.; investigation, B.B. and M.R.-J.; resources, B.B. and M.R.-J.; data curation, B.B and A.W.; writing—original draft preparation, B.B.; writing—review and editing, B.B., A.W. and E.W.; visualization, B.B. and A.W.; supervision, E.W.; project administration, B.B. and A.W. All authors have read and agreed to the published version of the manuscript.

Funding: This research received no external funding. The APC was funded by the Medical University of Silesia in Katowice.

Institutional Review Board Statement: This study adhered to the principles outlined in the Declaration of Helsinki, and received approval from the Medical University of Silesia board (KNW-0022-KB1-131-16).

Informed Consent Statement: Informed consent was obtained from all subjects involved in the study.

Data Availability Statement: The datasets generated during and/or analyzed during the current study are available from the corresponding author upon reasonable request.

Conflicts of Interest: The authors declare no conflicts of interest.

Abbreviations

IOP	Intraocular Pressure
MD	Mean Deviation
SS-OCT	Swept-Source Optical Coherence Tomography
ECP	Endocyclophotocoagulation
phaco-ECP	Phaco-endocyclophotocoagulation
TSCPC	Transscleral Cyclophotocoagulation
μCPC	Transscleral Microcyclophotocoagulation
UCP	Ultrasound Ciliary Plasty
KDB	Kahook Dual Blade
MIGS	Microinvasive Glaucoma Surgery
HMS	Hydrus Microstent implantation

References

1. Souissi, S.; Le Mer, Y.; Metge, F.; Portmann, A.; Baudouin, C.; Labbé, A.; Hamard, P. An update on continuous-wave cyclophotocoagulation (CW-CPC) and micropulse transscleral laser treatment (MP-TLT) for adult and paediatric refractory glaucoma. *Acta Ophthalmol.* **2021**, *99*, E621–E653. [CrossRef] [PubMed]
2. Dastiridou, A.I.; Katsanos, A.; Denis, P.; Francis, B.A.; Mikropoulos, D.G.; Teus, M.A.; Konstas, A.-G. Cyclodestructive Procedures in Glaucoma: A Review of Current and Emerging Options. *Adv. Ther.* **2018**, *35*, 2103–2127. [CrossRef]
3. Michelessi, M.; Bicket, A.K.; Lindsley, K. Cyclodestructive procedures for non-refractory glaucoma. *Cochrane Database Syst Rev.* **2018**, *4*. [CrossRef] [PubMed]
4. Pantcheva, M.B.; Kahook, M.Y.; Schuman, J.S.; Noecker, R.J. Comparison of acute structural and histopathological changes in human autopsy eyes after endoscopic cyclophotocoagulation and trans-scleral cyclophotocoagulation. *Br. J. Ophthalmol.* **2007**, *91*, 248–252. [CrossRef]
5. Lin, S.C.; Chen, M.J.; Lin, M.S.; Howes, E.; Stamper, R.L. Vascular effects on ciliary tissue from endoscopic versus trans-scleral cyclophotocoagulation. *Br. J. Ophthalmol.* **2006**, *90*, 496–500. [CrossRef] [PubMed]
6. Pastor, S.A.; Singh, K.; Lee, D.A.; Juzych, M.S.; Lin, S.C.; Netland, P.A.; Nguyen, N.T. Cyclophotocoagulation A report by the american academy of ophthalmology. *Ophthalmology* **2001**, *108*, 2130–2138. [CrossRef]
7. Tan, A.M.; Chockalingam, M.; Aquino, M.C.; Lim, Z.I.; See, J.L.; Chew, P.T. Micropulse transscleral diode laser cyclophotocoagulation in the treatment of refractory glaucoma. *Clin. Exp. Ophthalmol.* **2010**, *38*, 266–272. [CrossRef] [PubMed]
8. Aquino, M.C.D.; Barton, K.; Tan, A.M.W.; Sng, C.; Li, X.; Loon, S.C.; Chew, P.T. Micropulse versus continuous wave transscleral diode cyclophotocoagulation in refractory glaucoma: A randomized exploratory study. *Clin. Exp. Ophthalmol.* **2015**, *43*, 40–46. [CrossRef]
9. Maslin, J.S.; Chen, P.P.; Sinard, J.; Nguyen, A.T.; Noecker, R. Histopathologic changes in cadaver eyes after MicroPulse and continuous wave transscleral cyclophotocoagulation. *Can. J. Ophthalmol.* **2020**, *55*, 330–335. [CrossRef]
10. Moussa, K.; Feinstein, M.; Pekmezci, M.; Lee, J.H.; Bloomer, M.; Oldenburg, C.; Sun, Z.; Lee, R.K.; Ying, G.-S.; Han, Y. Histologic changes following continuous wave and micropulse transscleral cyclophotocoagulation: A randomized comparative study. *Transl. Vis. Sci. Technol.* **2020**, *9*, 22. [CrossRef]
11. Aptel, F.; Charrel, T.; Palazzi, X.; Chapelon, J.-Y.; Denis, P.; Lafon, C. Histologic effects of a new device for High-Intensity focused Ultrasound Cyclocoagulation. *Investig. Opthalmol. Vis. Sci.* **2010**, *51*, 5092–5098. [CrossRef]
12. Charrel, T.; Aptel, F.; Birer, A.; Chavrier, F.; Romano, F.; Chapelon, J.-Y.; Denis, P.; Lafon, C. Development of a Miniaturized HIFU Device for Glaucoma Treatment with Conformal Coagulation of the Ciliary Bodies. *Ultrasound Med. Biol.* **2011**, *37*, 742–754. [CrossRef] [PubMed]

13. Aptel, F.; Lafon, C. Therapeutic applications of ultrasound in ophthalmology. *Int. J. Hyperth.* **2012**, *28*, 405–418. [CrossRef] [PubMed]
14. Berke, S.; Cohen, A.; Sturm, R.; Caronia, R.; Nelson, D. Endoscopic Cyclophotocoagulation (Ecp) and Phacoemulsification in the Treatment of Medically Controlled Primary Open-Angle Glaucoma. *J. Glaucoma* **2000**, *9*, 129. [CrossRef]
15. Siegel, M.J.; Boling, W.S.; Faridi, O.S.; Gupta, C.K.; Kim, C.; Boling, R.C.; Citron, M.E.; Siegel, M.J.; Siegel, L.I. Combined endoscopic cyclophotocoagulation and phacoemulsification versus phacoemulsification alone in the treatment of mild to moderate glaucoma. *Clin. Exp. Ophthalmol.* **2015**, *43*, 531–539. [CrossRef] [PubMed]
16. Shaarawy, T.M.; Sherwood, M.B.; Grehn, F. *Guidelines on Design and Reporting of Surgical Trials—World Glaucoma Association. WGA Guidelines on Design and Reporting of Glaucoma Surgical Trials*; Kugler Publications: Amsterdam, The Netherlands, 2009.
17. Augusto, A.-B.; Bagnasco, L.; Bagnis, A.; Breda, J.; Bonzano, C.; Brezhnev, A.; Bron, A.; Cutolo, C.; Cvenkel, B.; Gandolf, S.; et al. European Glaucoma Society Terminology and Guidelines for Glaucoma, 5th Edition. *Br. J. Ophthalmol.* **2021**, *105*, 1–169.
18. Smith, M.; Byles, D.; Lim, L.-A. Phacoemulsification and endocyclophotocoagulation in uncontrolled glaucoma: Three-year results. *J. Cataract. Refract. Surg.* **2018**, *44*, 1097–1102. [CrossRef]
19. Yap, T.E.; Zollet, P.; Husein, S.; Murad, M.M.M.; Ameen, S.; Crawley, L.; Bloom, P.A.; Ahmed, F. Endocyclophotocoagulation combined with phacoemulsification in surgically naive primary open-angle glaucoma: Three-year results. *Eye* **2022**, *36*, 1890–1895. [CrossRef]
20. Oberfeld, B.; Pahlaviani, F.G.; Hall, N.; Falah-Trzcinski, H.; Trzcinski, J.; Chang, T.; Valle, D.S.-D. Combined MIGS: Comparing Additive Effects of Phacoemulsification, Endocyclophotocoagulation, and Kahook Dual Blade. *Clin. Ophthalmol.* **2023**, *17*, 1647–1659. [CrossRef]
21. Francis, B.A.; Berke, S.J.; Dustin, L.; Noecker, R. Endoscopic cyclophotocoagulation combined with phacoemulsification versus phacoemulsification alone in medically controlled glaucoma. *J. Cataract. Refract. Surg.* **2014**, *40*, 1313–1321. [CrossRef]
22. Kass, M.A.; Heuer, D.K.; Higginbotham, E.J.; Johnson, C.A.; Keltner, J.L.; Miller, J.P.; Parrish, R.K.; Wilson, M.R.; Gordon, M.O. The Ocular Hypertension Treatment Study: A randomized trial determines that topical ocular hypotensive medication delays or prevents the onset of primary open-angle glaucoma. *Arch. Ophthalmol.* **2002**, *120*, 701–713. [CrossRef] [PubMed]
23. Heijl, A.; Leske, M.C.; Bengtsson, B.; Hyman, L.; Bengtsson, B.; Hussein, M. Early Manifest Glaucoma Trial Group. Reduction of intraocular pressure and glaucoma progression: Results from the Early Manifest Glaucoma Trial. *Arch. Ophthalmol.* **2002**, *120*, 1268–1279. [CrossRef] [PubMed]
24. Frezzotti, P.; Mittica, V.; Martone, G.; Motolese, I.; Lomurno, L.; Peruzzi, S.; Motolese, E. Longterm follow-up of diode laser transscleral cyclophotocoagulation in the treatment of refractory glaucoma. *Acta Ophthalmol.* **2010**, *88*, 150–155. [CrossRef] [PubMed]
25. Grueb, M.; Rohrbach, J.M.; Bartz-Schmidt, K.U.; Schlote, T. Transscleral diode laser cyclophotocoagulation as primary and secondary surgical treatment in primary open-angle and pseudoexfoliatve glaucoma. *Graefe's Arch. Clin. Exp. Ophthalmol.* **2006**, *244*, 1293–1299. [CrossRef] [PubMed]
26. Jankowska-Szmul, J.; Dobrowolski, D.; Wylegala, E. CO_2 laser-assisted sclerectomy surgery compared with trabeculectomy in primary open-angle glaucoma and exfoliative glaucoma. A 1-year follow-up. *Acta Ophthalmol.* **2018**, *96*, e582–e591. [CrossRef]
27. Vernon, S.A.; Koppens, J.M.; Menon, G.J.; Negi, A.K. Diode laser cycloablation in adult glaucoma: Long-term results of a standard protocol and review of current literature. *Clin. Exp. Ophthalmol.* **2006**, *34*, 411–420. [CrossRef]
28. Walland, M.J. Diode laser cyclophotocoagulation: Longer term follow up of a standardized treatment protocol. *Clin. Exp. Ophthalmol.* **2000**, *28*, 263–267. [CrossRef]
29. Pucci, V.; Tappainer, F.; Borin, S.; Bellucci, R. Long-Term follow-up after transscleral diode laser photocoagulation in refractory glaucoma. *Ophthalmologica* **2003**, *217*, 279–283. [CrossRef]
30. Noecker, R.J.; Kahook, M.Y.; Berke, S.J.M.; Nichamin, L.D.; Weston, J.-M.; Mackool, R.; Tyson, F.; Lima, F.; Kleinfeldt, N. Uncontrolled intraocular pressure after endoscopic cyclophotocoagulation. *J. Glaucoma* **2008**, *17*, 250–251. [CrossRef]
31. Noecker, R.J. *ECP Collaborative Study Group. Complications of Endoscopic Cyclophotocoagulation*; The ASCRS Symposium on Cataract, IOL and Refractive Surgery; ECP Collaborative Study Group: San Diego, CA, USA, 2007.
32. Lindfield, D.; Ritchie, R.W.; Griffiths, M.F. 'Phaco–ECP': Combined endoscopic cyclophotocoagulation and cataract surgery to augment medical control of glaucoma. *BMJ Open* **2012**, *2*, e000578. [CrossRef]
33. Izquierdo Villavicencio, J.C.; Gonzalez Mendez, A.L.; Ramirez Jimenez, I.; Baltodano, F.P.Q.; Segura, R.C.A.; Franco, L.S.; Ponte-Dávila, M.C. Clinical Results of Endocyclophotocoagulation in Patients with Cataract and Open-Angle Glaucoma at Oftalmosalud Eye Institute, Lima-Peru. *J. Clin. Exp. Ophthalmol.* **2018**, *9*, 1–5. [CrossRef]
34. Gayton, J.L.; Van Der Karr, M.; Sanders, V. Combined cataract and glaucoma surgery: Trabeculectomy versus endoscopic laser cycloablation. *J. Cataract. Refract. Surg.* **1999**, *25*, 1214–1219. [CrossRef] [PubMed]
35. Moghimi, S.; Hamzeh, N.; Mohammadi, M.; Khatibi, N.; Bowd, C.; Weinreb, R.N. Combined glaucoma and cataract surgery: Comparison of viscocanalostomy, endocyclophotocoagulation, and ab interno trabeculectomy. *J. Cataract. Refract. Surg.* **2018**, *44*, 557–565. [CrossRef] [PubMed]
36. Murthy, S.K.; Damji, K.F.; Pan, Y.; Hodge, W.G. Trabeculectomy and phacotrabeculectomy, with mitomycin-C, show similar two-year target IOP outcomes. *Can. J. Ophthalmol.* **2006**, *41*, 51–59. [CrossRef] [PubMed]
37. Cillino, S.; Di Pace, F.; Casuccio, A.; Calvaruso, L.; Morreale, D.; Vadalà, M.; Lodato, G. Deep Sclerectomy Versus Punch Trabeculectomy with or without Phacoemulsification. *J. Glaucoma* **2004**, *13*, 500–506. [CrossRef] [PubMed]

38. Izquierdo, J.C.; Agudelo, N.; Rubio, B.; Camargo, J.; Ruiz-Montenegro, K.; Gajardo, C.; Rincon, M. Combined Phacoemulsification and 360-Degree Endocyclophotocoagulation with and without a Kahook Dual Blade in Patients with Primary Open-Angle Glaucoma. *Clin. Ophthalmol.* **2021**, *15*, 11–17. [CrossRef]
39. Pantalon, A.D.; Barata, A.D.D.O.; Georgopoulos, M.; Ratnarajan, G. Outcomes of phacoemulsification combined with two iStent inject trabecular microbypass stents with or without endocyclophotocoagulation. *Br. J. Ophthalmol.* **2020**, *104*, 1378–1383. [CrossRef] [PubMed]
40. Ziaei, H.; Au, L. Manchester iStent study: Long-term 7-year outcomes. *Eye* **2021**, *35*, 2277–2282. [CrossRef]
41. Arriola-Villalobos, P.; Martínez-De-La-Casa, J.M.; Díaz-Valle, D.; Fernández-Pérez, C.; García-Sánchez, J.; García-Feijoó, J. Combined iStent trabecular micro-bypass stent implantation and phacoemulsification for coexistent open-angle glaucoma and cataract: A long-term study. *Br. J. Ophthalmol.* **2012**, *96*, 645–649. [CrossRef]
42. Ahmed, I.I.K.; De Francesco, T.; Rhee, D.; McCabe, C.; Flowers, B.; Gazzard, G.; Samuelson, T.W.; Singh, K.; HORIZON Investigators. Long-term Outcomes from the HORIZON Randomized Trial for a Schlemm's Canal Microstent in Combination Cataract and Glaucoma Surgery. *Ophthalmology* **2022**, *129*, 742–751. [CrossRef]

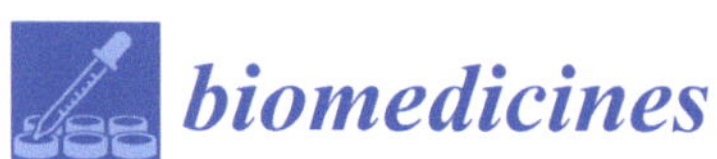

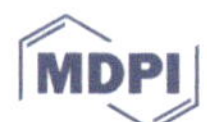

Article

Long-Term Clinical Outcomes of Ahmed Valve Implantation in Aniridic Glaucoma

Bartłomiej Bolek [1,2], Edward Wylęgała [1,2] and Dorota Tarnawska [2,3,*]

1 Chair and Clinical Department of Ophthalmology, School of Medicine in Zabrze, Medical University of Silesia in Katowice, 40-760 Katowice, Poland; bartlomiej.bolek@sum.edu.pl (B.B.)
2 Clinical Department of Ophthalmology, District Railway Hospital, 40-760 Katowice, Poland
3 Institute of Biomedical Engineering, Faculty of Science and Technology, University of Silesia in Katowice, 75 Pułku Piechoty 1A, 41-500 Chorzów, Poland
* Correspondence: dorota.tarnawska@us.edu.pl; Tel.: +48-32-349-7567

Abstract: Background: This study assessed the efficacy and safety of Ahmed valve implantation in patients with aniridic glaucoma for three consecutive years. Methods: Six adult patients (seven eyes) with Ahmed valve (AV) implants for aniridic glaucoma were enrolled in the study. The primary outcome measures were intraocular pressure reduction, glaucoma medication use, success rates, and visual acuity after AV implantation. A 30% reduction in IOP from baseline without the need for re-intervention was considered an effective treatment. The cessation of antiglaucoma medications was defined as complete success. Intraoperative and postoperative complications were included as secondary outcome measures. Measurements were performed preoperatively, at the first week, and 1, 3, 6, 12, 18, 24, 30, and 36 months postoperatively. Results: A total of seven eyes (6 patients) were evaluated 36 months after AV implantation. The mean ± SD values of IOP preoperatively at 1 day, 1 week, and 1, 3, 6, 12, 18, 24, 30, and 36 months postoperatively were 30.4 ± 4.0 mmHg, 14.6 ± 4.6 mmHg, 16.1 ± 4.6 mmHg, 20.7 ± 7.0 mmHg, 14.5 ± 2.7 mmHg, 16.5 ± 5.9 mmHg, 16.2 ± 4.0 mmHg, 16.3 ± 4.3 mmHg, 17.2 ± 10.1 mmHg, 17.6 ± 6.9 mmHg, and 18.2 ± 5.5 mmHg, respectively. At the last follow up, the mean IOP was reduced by 40.2%. The qualified success rate was 85.7%. One patient (one eye) at the last follow-up visit did not require antiglaucoma medications, resulting in a complete success rate of 14.3%. Intra- and postoperative mild or moderate subconjunctival bleeding was observed in all the patients. No other major/minor intraoperative or postoperative complications were noted. Conclusions: In long-term follow up, the AV implantation procedure is well-tolerated and relatively safe for reducing IOP in adult aniridia patients with glaucoma. These results should be validated through studies involving a larger patient cohort.

Keywords: Ahmed valve; aniridia; glaucoma; glaucoma drainage device; intraocular pressure

Citation: Bolek, B.; Wylęgała, E.; Tarnawska, D. Long-Term Clinical Outcomes of Ahmed Valve Implantation in Aniridic Glaucoma. *Biomedicines* **2023**, *11*, 2996. https://doi.org/10.3390/biomedicines11112996

Academic Editor: Da-Wen Lu

Received: 1 October 2023
Revised: 31 October 2023
Accepted: 3 November 2023
Published: 8 November 2023

1. Introduction

Aniridia is a profoundly visually impairing rare genetic disorder primarily caused by a heterozygous mutation in paired box 6 (PAX6) [1,2]. This condition leads to the underdevelopment or abnormal development of the iris, and is associated with various ocular abnormalities, including keratopathy, cataract, nystagmus, foveal hypoplasia, optic nerve hypoplasia, and glaucoma. Secondary glaucoma usually develops during the first two decades of life with prevalence from 6% to 75% [3–5], or even higher [6]. Rudimentary iris stroma extends forwards onto the trabecular meshwork, at first resembling anterior synechiae, followed by forming a sheet that results in eventual angle closure [3]. Other mechanisms implicated in the pathogenesis of glaucoma involve the absence of the Schlemm canal [7]. Various surgical techniques, including goniosurgery, trabeculotomy, trabeculectomy, the use of glaucoma drainage devices (GDD), and cyclodestructive procedures, have been employed to address this type of glaucoma, yielding variable degrees of success [8–16].

The purpose of this study was to evaluate the long-term outcomes and complication rates of Ahmed valve (AV) implantation in patients with glaucoma secondary to congenital aniridia. The primary outcome measures encompassed reductions in intraocular pressure (IOP), changes in the usage of glaucoma medications, success rates, and alterations in visual acuity following the AV implantation. Additionally, secondary outcome measures involved the evaluation of both intraoperative and postoperative complications.

2. Materials and Methods

This study was a retrospective, single-arm case series, conducted in a noncomparative manner at a single center. The study received approval from the institutional review board of the Medical University of Silesia (Approval number: KNW/0022/KB1/131/16) and adhered to the principles of the Declaration of Helsinki. Patients who underwent AV implantation procedure (model FP7, New World Medical, Rancho Cucamonga, CA, USA) for aniridic glaucoma operated upon between November 2008 and April 2019 were included in the study. All patients provided informed consent for the AV implantation procedure. The study enrolled participants who met the following inclusion criteria: congenital aniridia, adult patients (≥18 years), AV implantation due to uncontrolled aniridic glaucoma (IOP > 21 mmHg, despite maximum tolerated doses of antiglaucoma medications), intolerance to glaucoma medications despite well-controlled IOP, 36-month follow-up period. Exclusion criteria encompassed the following: pregnant women, patients aged <18 years. Patients with a history of other treatments/surgeries for glaucoma were not excluded from the study.

A retrospective review of medical and surgical records was performed to collect the following data: complete ophthalmic examination with IOP measurements, number of antiglaucoma medications, and best-corrected log MAR visual acuity recorded preoperatively and at 1 day, 1 week, and 1, 3, 6, 12, 18, 24, 30, and 36 months after surgery.

All follow-up time points and IOP measurements in our clinic are always made according to the World Glaucoma Association Guidelines on Design and Reporting of Glaucoma Surgical Trials—the average of three measurements obtained with the standard Goldmann applanation tonometer (GAT) [17]. Data also extracted were age, sex, concomitant ocular disorders, history of other intraocular surgeries, lens status, intraoperative complications, postoperative complications, and re-interventions.

Treatment was deemed successful (qualified success) if, during 36-month follow-up assessments, there was a 30% reduction in IOP compared to the baseline value, and this reduction was achieved without requiring surgical re-intervention. Increased IOP was counted as a failure if it occurred at two consecutive follow-up visits. IOP spikes to 3 months after AV implantation were not considered as a failure. Complete success was defined as cessation of antiglaucoma medications.

In cases where IOP was not adequately reduced during follow up, additional ocular hypotensive medications were added. In the event of failure to achieve IOP control with up to three topical medications, the planned intervention in the study group was to be transscleral cyclophotocoagulation (TSCPC).

AV implantation procedure was performed under peribulbar or general anesthesia. All the plates were implanted at the superior temporal quadrant of the eye. First, a traction suture was placed into the superior limbal cornea. A 10 mm conjunctival and a fornix-based opening were created in the superior temporal quadrant. The plate was placed in sub-Tenon space 8–9 mm from the limbus between the lateral and superior rectus muscles and sutured to the superficial sclera with 8-0 Prolene nonabsorbable sutures. Next, the tube was trimmed to extend 2–3 mm into the anterior chamber. A 23-gauge needle was used to penetrate sclera 2–3 mm posterior to the corneal limbus, directed parallel to the iris surface. The tube was inserted bevel up through the tunnel into the anterior chamber and secured to the sclera using one 10-0 nylon anchoring suture. The silicone tube near the limbus was then covered with a 5 × 6 mm full-thickness donor sclera graft, sutured with four 7-0 absorbable (polyglactin) sutures. The conjunctiva was closed using interrupted 10-0 nylon sutures. A subconjunctival steroid and antibiotic injection were performed. All the procedures were performed by two experienced surgeons (D.T. and E.W.).

In the first week after surgery, anti-glaucoma medication was withdrawn in all but one patient. At subsequent follow-up visits, they were added as needed, depending on IOP.

Postoperatively, patients were treated topically with dexamethasone (five times a day for two weeks and tapered over two months) and ofloxacin (five times a day for two weeks). Statistical analysis utilized Statistica Software version 13 (TIBCO Software Inc., Palo Alto, CA, USA). Datasets were compared based on data distribution, with the Wilcoxon signed-rank test or paired t-test applied for relevant parameters. Kaplan–Meier survival curves assessed treatment success over time, and IOP results were visualized using a scatter plot comparing preoperative IOP (x-axis) with 3-year postoperative IOP (y-axis). A significance level of $p \leq 0.05$ denoted statistical significance.

3. Results

Six adult patients (seven eyes) with aniridic glaucoma were enrolled for AV implantation. Patient characteristics are detailed in Table 1. None of the patients required reoperation throughout the follow-up period due to failure to achieve the target IOP. In the data collected, there were three follow-up time-points not available due to patient missed visits (case n6—day 1 visit; case n4—18-month visit; case n1—30-month visit). The mean ± SD values of IOP preoperatively at 1 day, 1 week, and 1, 3, 6, 12, 18, 24, 30, and 36 months postoperatively were 30.4 ± 4.0 mmHg, 14.6 ± 4.6 mmHg, 16.1 ± 4.6 mmHg, 20.7 ± 7.0 mmHg, 14.5 ± 2.7 mmHg, 16.5 ± 5.9 mmHg, 16.2 ± 4.0 mmHg, 16.3 ± 4.3 mmHg, 17.2 ± 10.1 mmHg, 17.6 ± 6.9 mmHg, and 18.2 ± 5.5 mmHg, respectively (Tables 1 and 2, Figure 1). The mean IOP at the final follow up exhibited a reduction of 40.2% (Table 2). The qualified success rate was 85,7% (six eyes). One patient (one eye) (at 30- and 36-month follow-up visit) did not achieve IOP reduction at two consecutive follow-up visits; this was considered a failure and qualified for TSCPC. However, the procedure was canceled because the patient had an intraocular pressure of 18 mmHg on the day of admission to the laser procedure. In further follow up, already beyond the three-year period of the study, the patient maintained an effectively lowered IOP, and at the 84-month visit 16 mm IOP was recorded with two antiglaucoma medications.

Table 1. Patient characteristics and intraocular pressure outcome. IOP—intraocular pressure; LE—lens extraction; LE + IOL—lens extraction with intraocular lens implantation; PKP—penetrating keratoplasty; TSCPC—transscleral cyclophotocoagulation; Trab—trabeculectomy.

Case	Age (Years)	Gender	Prior Surgeries	Lens Status	Preoperative IOP (mmHg)	Postoperative IOP 36 Months (mmHg)
1	53	M	LE, TSCPC	Aphakic	30	18
2	52	M	LE	Aphakic	30	19
3	37	F	LE + IOL, TSCPC, Trab	Pseudophakic	36	16
4	40	F	LE + IOL, Trab	Pseudophakic	27	14
5	48	F	LE + IOL, PKP	Pseudophakic	35	30
6	50	F	LE + IOL, PKP, Trab	Pseudophakic	30	17
7	40	F	LE + IOL, Trab	Pseudophakic	25	14

Table 2. Intraocular pressure and number of hypotensive medications after AV implantation.

	Mean IOP ± SD			Number of Hypotensive Medications ± SD			% IOP Reduction
Preop	30.4	±	4.0	4.0	±	1.0	-
1 day	14.6	±	4.6	0.2	±	0.4	52.0
1 week	16.1	±	4.6	0.1	±	0.4	46.9
1 month	20.7	±	7.0	0.3	±	0.5	32.1
3 months	14.5	±	2.7	0.8	±	0.8	52.3
6 months	16.5	±	5.9	0.8	±	0.8	45.8
12 months	16.2	±	4.0	1.3	±	0.5	46.9
18 months	16.3	±	4.3	1.5	±	1.3	46.6
24 months	17.2	±	10.1	1.8	±	1.1	43.5
30 months	17.6	±	6.9	1.4	±	0.9	42.2
36 months	18.2	±	5.5	1.3	±	0.6	40.2

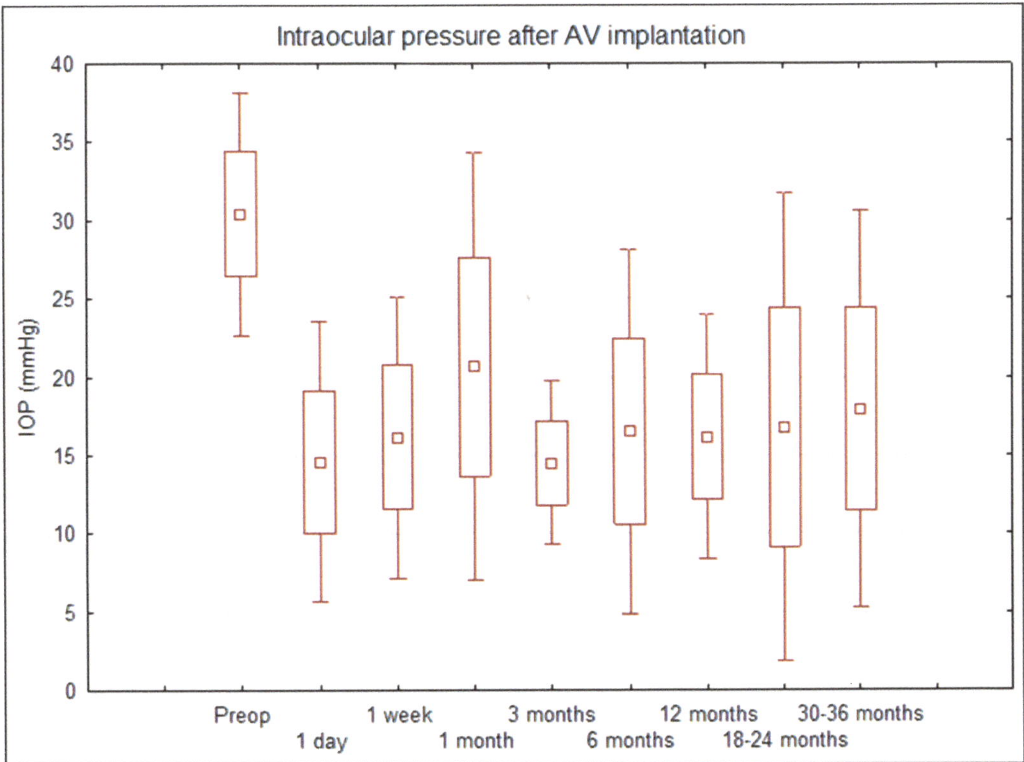

Figure 1. Intraocular pressure after AV implantation—36-month follow up. *AV—Ahmed valve; IOP—intraocular pressure.*

At the 36-month follow up, one patient (one eye) no longer needed antiglaucoma medications. The complete success rate was 14.3% (Figures 2 and 3—Kaplan-Meier survival curves, Figure 4—scatter plot).

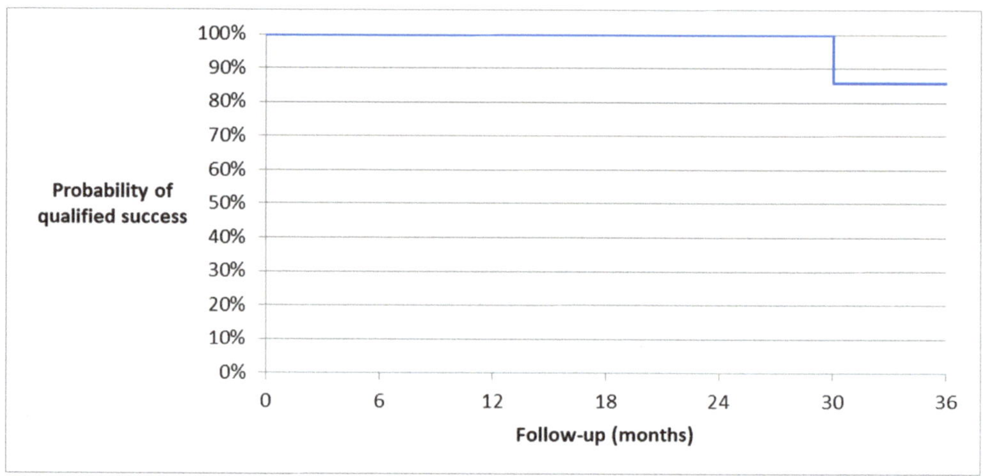

Figure 2. Kaplan–Meier survival curve of qualified success after AV implantation—36-month follow up.

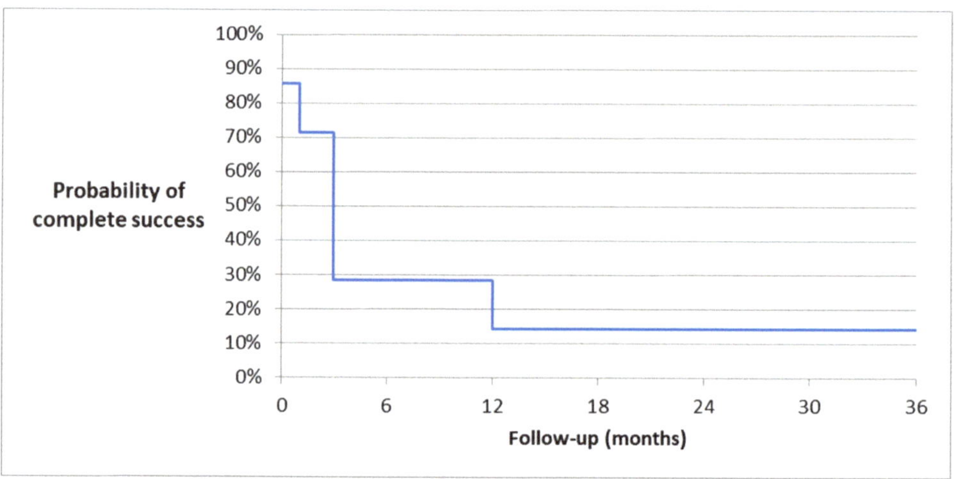

Figure 3. Kaplan–Meier survival curve of complete success after AV implantation—36-month follow up.

The mean ± SD values of the number of antiglaucoma medications preoperatively and at 1 day, 1 week, and 1, 3, 6, 12, 18, 24, 30, and 36 months postoperatively were 4.0 ± 1.0, 0.2 ± 0.4, 0.1 ± 0.4, 0.3 ± 0.5, 0.8 ± 0.8, 0.8 ± 0.8, 1.3 ± 0.5, 1.5 ± 1.3, 1.8 ± 1.1, 1.4 ± 0.9, and 1.3 ± 0.6, respectively (Table 2, Figure 5). Before AV implantation, two patients required systemic carbonic anhydrase therapy. However, none of the patients needed systemic carbonic anhydrase treatment at the 36-month follow-up visit. Five patients had reduced the number of antiglaucoma medications they were taking, and two had maintained the same number of medications at the last follow-up visit compared to the baseline. Importantly, none of the patients required more antiglaucoma medications compared to their preoperative regimen at the last visit. None of the patients required systemic carbonic anhydrase during the 36-month follow up.

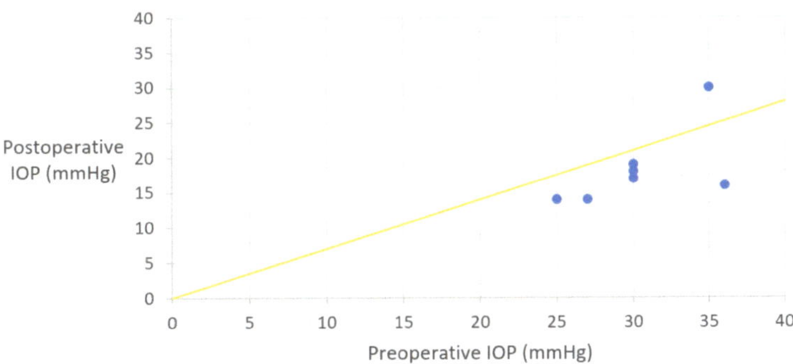

Figure 4. Scatter plot as preoperative IOP (*x*-axis) versus 3-year postoperative IOP (*y*-axis). Yellow slope diagonal line represents 30% IOP reduction. *AV—Ahmed valve, IOP—intraocular pressure.*

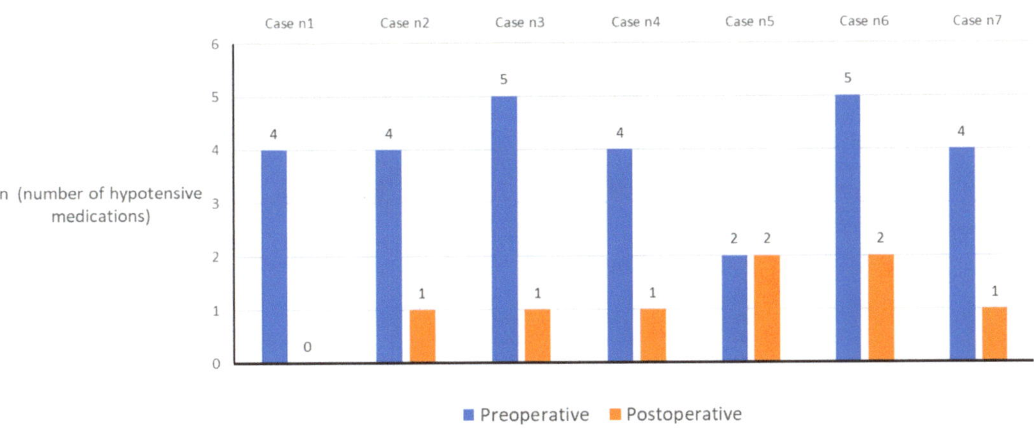

Figure 5. Number of antiglaucoma medications preoperative and postoperative at last follow up. *AV—Ahmed valve.*

The mean best-corrected log MAR visual acuity preoperatively at 1 day, 1 week, and 1, 3, 6, 12, 18, 24, 30, and 36 months postoperatively were 1.64 ± 0.32, 1.72 ± 0.23, 1.64 ± 0.35, 1.33 ± 0.23, 1.53 ± 0.37, 1.57 ± 0.30, 1.58 ± 0.35, 1.90 ± 0.76, 1.56 ± 0.15, 1.52 ± 0.22, and 1.53 ± 0.25, respectively.

Table 3 provides a comprehensive list of both intraoperative and postoperative complications. An IOP spike was observed in two patients (28.6%). Intra- and postoperative mild or moderate subconjunctival bleeding was observed in all the patients. No other major/minor intraoperative or postoperative complications occurred (Figure 6. Aniridia patient after AV implantation).

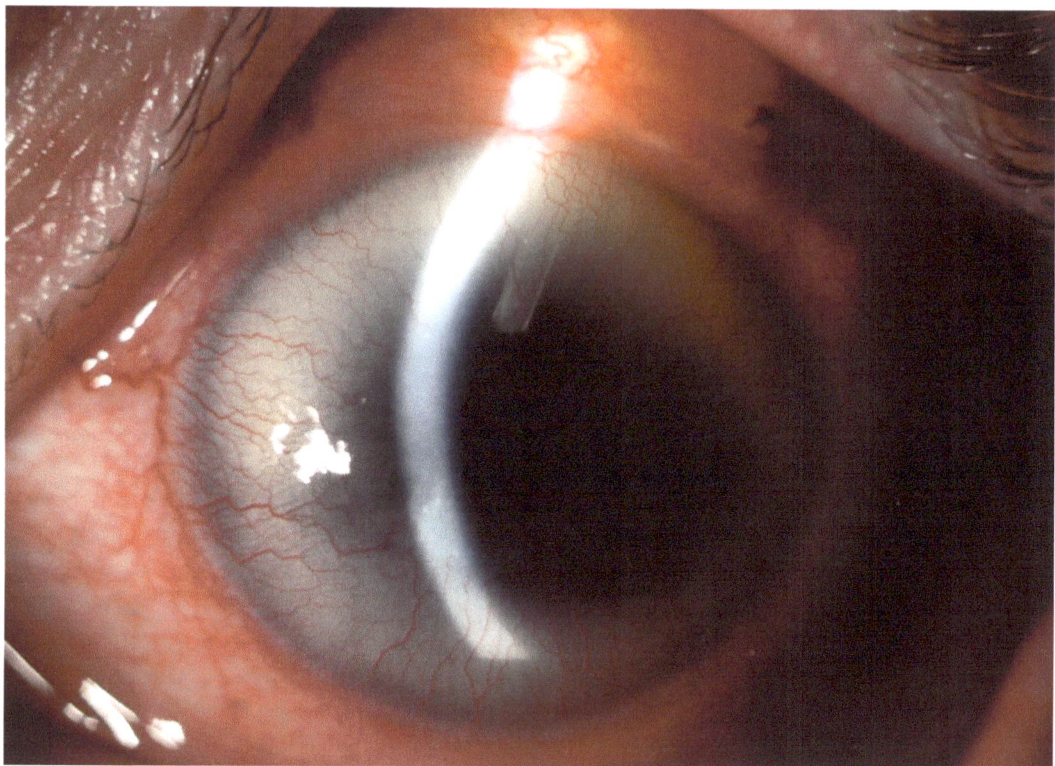

Figure 6. Left eye of the patient with aniridia and aphakia after Ahmed valve implantation. The valve tube in the anterior chamber is visible. Grade 2 aniridia-associated keratopathy can be noted.

Table 3. Intraoperative and postoperative complications after AV implantation.

Complications	No.	%
Intraoperative		
Scleral/iris perforation	0/7	0
Anterior chamber shallowing	0/7	0
Subconjunctival hemorrhage	7/7	100
Postoperative		
Early		
Conjunctival hyperemia	3/7	42.9
Subconjunctival hemorrhage	7/7	100
Epithelial defects	2/7	28.6
IOP spike	3/7	42.9
Hypotony, choroid detachment	0/7	0
Hyphema	0/7	0
Uveitis	0/7	0
Vitreous hemorrhage	0/7	0

Table 3. *Cont.*

Complications	No.	%
Late		
Tube exposure	0/7	0
Diplopia/strabismus	0/7	0
Hypotony, choroid detachment	0/7	0
Corneal decompensation	0/7	0
Retinal detachment	0/7	0
Phthisis bulbi	0/7	0

4. Discussion

Glaucoma secondary to aniridia is difficult to control with intraocular pressure-lowering medication. Frequently a surgical approach is needed, and few types of procedures are performed; however, the success rate is highly variable. Studies report the use of (1) aqueous drainage devices, (2) angle surgeries, especially before the angle closure is extensive, (3) filtering operations, and (4) cyclodestructive procedures.

Cyclocryotherapy and transscleral diode laser cyclophotocoagulation (TSCPC) are the two most common cyclodestructive methods described in the literature in aniridia-related glaucoma. The efficacy of the first method is mediocre/average, with a relatively high complication rate. Wallace and associates report that in six of nine procedures (performed in one or more sessions), IOP control was achieved; nonetheless, authors add that they would now prefer performing trabeculectomy or seton implantation before cyclocryotherapy [16]. Wiggins and associates evaluated different types of glaucoma surgeries in aniridia [7]. In the cyclocryotherapy group, 5 of 20 of the performed procedures were successful. The authors reported complications of this procedure, like phthisis bulbi and cataract. In their study, other glaucoma surgeries like trabeculotomy, trabeculectomy, and Molteno implant placement were performed, with a conclusion that the best results occurred after Molteno implants in aniridia patients, and authors advocate this method. Another study concerning cyclocryotherapy treatment reported that four (50%) of eight aniridic eyes had a "devastating complication developed, three of which represented phthisis and the fourth which represented a retinal detachment followed by phthisis" [18]. TSCPC is another type of cyclodestructive procedure which is used in patients with aniridia. The efficacy is similar to cyclocryotherapy; however, the complication rate is lower, with no literature reports of phthisis bulbi [14]. Three patients in our study had TSCPC before AV implantation. We did not observe any major complications postoperatively. However, due to worsening IOP control, these patients underwent AV implantation (an average of two years after TSCPC) and were enrolled in the study. The above-mentioned cyclodestrutive methods usually need to be repeated to achieve proper IOP control.

Therapeutic goniotomy is usually unsuccessful [10,19]. However, a few authors reported success of this procedure as a prophylactic before glaucoma develops [8,19]. Compared to goniotomy, better effectiveness in the treatment of aniridic glaucoma is achieved with trabeculotomy [10]. Adachi and associates reported that ten (83%) of twelve eyes obtained IOP control after the first or second trabeculotomy with a mean follow up of around ten years.

Trabeculectomy is a frequently performed procedure in aniridia, usually as a primary surgical approach. However, results in this type of glaucoma are unsatisfactory. In a previously cited paper, Wiggins and associates analyzed the efficacy of trabeculectomy with or without fluorouracil in aniridia patients [7]. The results were poor—out of fifteen procedures only one was successful. Similarly, in a different study, cited above, all five patients initially treated with trabeculectomy needed another glaucoma surgery in less than a one year follow up [9]. Durai and associates compared trabeculectomy to the Aurolab Aqueous Drainage Implant [11]. Again, the results of trabeculectomy were mediocre (the probability of failure at 2 years was 58.3%) and the efficacy of the Aurolab Aqueous Drainage Implant was definitely better (the probability of failure at two years was 11.1%). As mentioned in the description of patients' characteristics, three of our patients had trabeculectomy before AV implantation. In these few cases, the efficacy of this procedure lasted longer, with an average of five years until AV implantation.

Few studies report the usage of different types of GDD in aniridic glaucoma. In a study mentioned earlier conducted by Wiggins and associates, out of five eyes with Molteno implants, only one required reoperation during a mean of 28 months' follow up [7]. The same implant used by Molteno and associates allowed successful IOP control (defined as IOP < 20 mm Hg without medical treatment) in all three aniridia patients in a mean follow up of 5 years [13]. Billson and associates also reported reasonable IOP control with Molteno GDD over a three-year follow-up period in two patients [20]. In the study mentioned earlier conducted by Adachi and associates [9], the authors also implanted Molteno GDD with comparably good results—a success rate of 83% (five of six eyes had IOP < 21 mm Hg in the mean follow-up period of 10.4 years).

Only one study reported the effectiveness of treatment with Baerveldt GDD for aniridia, with a surgical success in 7 of 8 eyes over 11–39 months of follow up [21].

Two studies published so far have reported the results of AV implantation in aniridia-related glaucoma. Almousa and associates reported successful IOP control in seven of eight eyes over a mean follow up of 37.4 months [22]. In one eye, persistent vitreous hemorrhage and subsequent irreparable total retinal detachment occurred after the procedure. But, apart from this one, no other complication related to AV implantation, including tube exposure, were noted. In the second study, Demirok and associates implanted AV in six eyes, and the success rate was 66.6% at 12 months and 50.0% at the last follow up (range 12–36 months) [23]. In one patient, authors reported tube exposure at 1 month post operation and retinal detachment associated with vitreous hemorrhage. No other major complications were noted. In both studies presented above, there was no distinction between pediatric and adult patients.

The decrease in IOP and the number of antiglaucoma medications was significant at each follow-up time point in our study. The mean IOP at 36-month follow up was reduced by 40.2%. The surgical success rate was particularly high at 85.7%, which aligns with previously published results [22,23]. Furthermore, our study reported a low occurrence of major complications. We observed an IOP spike in two patients (28.6%) at one month postoperatively, which is common in GDD implantations. Nevertheless, at the following visit, IOP normalized. In all our patients, subconjunctival hemorrhage occurred both intraoperatively and postoperatively, which was related to the AV implantation procedure itself. We did not observe other major/minor intraoperative or postoperative complications, such as vitreoretinal hemorrhage, as reported in similar studies [22,23]. In our study group, none of the patients had tube exposure, which is one of the most threatening complications for the surgeon.

The current study has several limitations, including its retrospective, noncomparative design, the small number of cases, and the fact that it only involves adult patients. Nevertheless, it is the second largest clinical study and the most numerous adult study in the literature. Similar obstacles are common in aniridia studies due to the specificity of this condition.

Our results and the studies presented above reveal how challenging is to treat aniridic glaucoma. According to aniridia experts and a review of the literature, topical intraocular pressure lowering medications should be the first option in the treatment of aniridic glaucoma [24]. Prophylactic goniotomy could be considered when the rudimentary iris extends onto the trabecular meshwork and before glaucoma occurs. In cases of congenital or early-developing glaucoma, many clinicians recommend trabeculotomy. For more advanced stages of aniridic glaucoma, it appears that the GDD is the superior way to achieve that goal. Larger, randomized, and comparative studies are needed to determine the best surgical method for aniridia-related glaucoma.

5. Conclusions

The AV implantation procedure is relatively safe and well-tolerated for reducing IOP in adult aniridia patients with glaucoma in long-term follow up. These results should be validated through studies involving a larger patient cohort.

Author Contributions: Conceptualization, B.B. and D.T.; Methodology, B.B. and D.T.; Formal Analysis, D.T.; Investigation, B.B.; Resources, B.B.; Data Curation, B.B and D.T.; Writing—Original Draft Preparation, B.B.; Writing—Review & Editing, B.B., D.T., and E.W.; Visualization, B.B. and D.T..; Supervision, E.W.; Project Administration, B.B. and E.W. All authors have read and agreed to the published version of the manuscript.

Funding: This research received no external funding. The APC was funded by Medical University of Silesia in Katowice and University of Silesia in Katowice.

Institutional Review Board Statement: This study adhered to the principles outlined in the Declaration of Helsinki, and received approval from the Medical University of Silesia board (KNW/0022/KB1/131/16).

Informed Consent Statement: Informed consent was obtained from all subjects involved in the study.

Data Availability Statement: The datasets generated during and/or analyzed during the current study are available from the corresponding author on reasonable request.

Conflicts of Interest: The authors declare no conflict of interest.

Abbreviations

AV	Ahmed valve
IOP	Intraocular pressure
TSCPC	Diode laser transscleral cyclophotocoagulation
GDD	Glaucoma drainage device
IOP	Intraocular pressure
GAT	Goldmann applanation tonometer
SD	Standard Deviation

References

1. Gehring, W.J. The master control gene for morphogenesis and evolution of the eye. *Genes Cells* **1996**, *1*, 11–15. [CrossRef] [PubMed]
2. Lagali, N.; Wowra, B.; Fries, F.N.; Latta, L.; Moslemani, K.; Utheim, T.P.; Wylegala, E.; Seitz, B.; Käsmann-Kellner, B. PAX6 Mutational Status Determines Aniridia-Associated Keratopathy Phenotype. *Ophthalmology* **2020**, *127*, 273–275. [CrossRef]
3. Nelson, L.B.; Spaeth, G.L.; Nowinski, T.S.; Margo, C.E.; Jackson, L. Aniridia. A review. *Surv. Ophthalmol.* **1984**, *28*, 621–642. [CrossRef] [PubMed]
4. Gramer, E.; Reiter, C.; Gramer, G. Glaucoma and frequency of ocular and general diseases in 30 patients with Aniridia: A clinical study. *Eur. J. Ophthalmol.* **2011**, *22*, 104–110. [CrossRef] [PubMed]
5. Netland, P.A.; Scott, M.L.; Boyle, J.W.; Lauderdale, J.D. Ocular and systemic findings in a survey of aniridia subjects. *J. Am. Assoc. Pediatr. Ophthalmol. Strabismus* **2011**, *15*, 562–566. [CrossRef]
6. Tsai, J.H.; Derby, E.; Holland, E.J.; Khatana, A.K. Incidence and prevalence of glaucoma in severe ocular surface disease. *Cornea* **2006**, *25*, 530–532. [CrossRef]
7. Wiggins, R.E.; Tomey, K.F. The Results of Glaucoma Surgery in Aniridia. *Arch. Ophthalmol.* **1992**, *110*, 503–505. [CrossRef] [PubMed]
8. Chen, T.C.; Waltoii, D.S. Goniosurgery for prevention of aniridic glaucoma. *Arch. Ophthalmol.* **1999**, *117*, 1144–1148. [CrossRef]
9. Adachi, M.; Dickens, C.J.; Hetherington, J.; Hoskins, H.D.; Iwach, A.G.; Wong, P.C.; Nguyen, N.; Ma, A.S. Clinical experience of trabeculotomy for the surgical treatment of aniridic glaucoma. *Ophthalmology* **1997**, *104*, 2121–2125. [CrossRef]
10. Okada, K.; Mishima, H.K.; Masumoto, M.; Tsumamoto, Y.; Tsukamoto, H.; Takamatsu, M. Results of filtering surgery in young patients with aniridia. *Hiroshima J. Med. Sci.* **2000**, *49*, 135–138.
11. Durai, I.; Pallamparthy, S.; Puthuran, G.V.; Wijesinghe, H.K.; Uduman, M.S.; Krishnadas, S.R.; Robin, A.L.; Palmberg, P.; Gedde, S.J. Outcomes of Glaucoma Drainage Device Implantation and Trabeculectomy With Mitomycin C in Glaucoma Secondary to Aniridia. *Am. J. Ophthalmol.* **2021**, *227*, 173–181. [CrossRef] [PubMed]
12. Grant, W.M.; Walton, D.S. Progressive changes in the angle in congenital aniridia, with development of glaucoma. *Am. J. Ophthalmol.* **1974**, *78*, 842–847. [CrossRef] [PubMed]

13. Molteno, A.C.B.; Ancker, E.; Van Biljon, G. Surgical Technique for Advanced Juvenile Glaucoma. *Arch. Ophthalmol.* **1984**, *102*, 51–57. [CrossRef]
14. Kirwan, J.F.; Shah, P.; Khaw, P.T. Diode laser cyclophotocoagulation: Role in the management of refractory pediatric glaucomas. *Ophthalmology* **2002**, *109*, 316–323. [CrossRef]
15. Fieß, A.; Shah, P.; Sii, F.; Godfrey, F.; Abbott, J.; Bowman, R.; Bauer, J.; Dithmar, S.; Philippin, H. Trabeculectomy or Transscleral Cyclophotocoagulation as Initial Treatment of Secondary Childhood Glaucoma in Northern Tanzania. *J. Glaucoma* **2017**, *26*, 657–660. [CrossRef] [PubMed]
16. Wallace, D.K.; Plager, D.A.; Snyder, S.K.; Raiesdana, A.; Helveston, E.M.; Ellis, F.D. Surgical results of secondary glaucomas in childhood. *Ophthalmology* **1998**, *105*, 101–111. [CrossRef]
17. Shaarawy, T.M.; Sherwood, M.B.; Grehn, F. *Guidelines on Design and Reporting of Surgical Trials*; WGA Guidelines on Design and Reporting of Glaucoma Surgical Trials; World Glaucoma Association: Amsterdam, The Netherlands, 2009.
18. Wagle, N.S.; Freedman, S.F.; Buckley, E.G.; Davis, J.S.; Biglan, A.W. Long-term outcome of cyclocryotherapy for refractory pediatric glaucoma. *Ophthalmology* **1998**, *105*, 1921–1927. [CrossRef] [PubMed]
19. Walton, D.S. Aniridic glaucoma: The results of gonio-surgery to prevent and treat this problem. *Trans. Am. Ophthalmol. Soc.* **1986**, *84*, 59–70. [PubMed]
20. Billson, F.; Thomas, R.; Aylward, W. The use of two-stage molteno implants in developmental glaucoma. *J. Pediatr. Ophthalmol. Strabismus* **1989**, *26*, 3–8. [CrossRef]
21. Arroyave, C.P.; Scott, I.U.; Gedde, S.J.; Parrish, R.K.; Feuer, W.J. Use of glaucoma drainage devices in the management of glaucoma associated with aniridia. *Am. J. Ophthalmol.* **2003**, *135*, 155–159. [CrossRef]
22. Almousa, R.; Lake, D.B. Intraocular pressure control with Ahmed glaucoma drainage device in patients with cicatricial ocular surface disease-associated or aniridia-related glaucoma. *Int. Ophthalmol.* **2014**, *34*, 753–760. [CrossRef] [PubMed]
23. Demirok, G.S.; Ekşioğlu, Ü.; Yakın, M.; Kaderli, A.; Kaderli, S.T.; Örnek, F. Short- and long-term results of glaucoma valve implantation for aniridia-related glaucoma: A case series and literature review. *Turk. J. Ophthalmol.* **2019**, *49*, 183–187. [CrossRef] [PubMed]
24. Landsend, E.C.S.; Lagali, N.; Utheim, T.P. Congenital aniridia—A comprehensive review of clinical features and therapeutic approaches. *Surv. Ophthalmol.* **2021**, *66*, 1031–1050. [CrossRef] [PubMed]

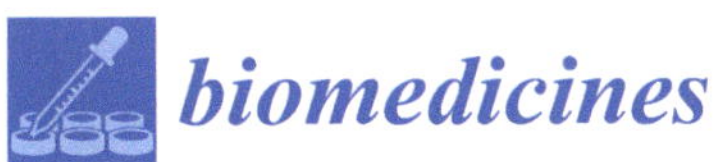

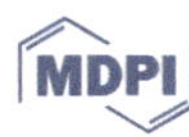

Article

The Preserflo MicroShunt Affects Microvascular Flow Density in Optical Coherence Tomography Angiography

Jens Julian Storp [1,*], Hannah Schatten [1,2], Friederike Elisabeth Vietmeier [1], Ralph-Laurent Merté [1], Larissa Lahme [1], Julian Alexander Zimmermann [1], Verena Anna Englmaier [1], Nicole Eter [1] and Viktoria Constanze Brücher [1]

1 Department of Ophthalmology, University of Muenster Medical Center, 48149 Muenster, Germany; friederikeelisabeth.vietmeier@ukmuenster.de (F.E.V.); ralph-laurent.merte@ukmuenster.de (R.-L.M.); larissa.lahme@ukmuenster.de (L.L.); julian.zimmermann@ukmuenster.de (J.A.Z.); verenaanna.englmaier@ukmuenster.de (V.A.E.); nicole.eter@ukmuenster.de (N.E.); viktoria.bruecher@ukmuenster.de (V.C.B.)

2 Augenklinik Roth am St. Josef-Hospital, 53225 Bonn, Germany

* Correspondence: jens.storp@ukmuenster.de; Tel.: +49-251-83-56001

Abstract: Intraocular pressure (IOP) lowering surgery has been shown to alter microvascular density in glaucoma patients. The aim of this study is to report changes in retinal flow density (FD) over the course of treatment with the Preserflo MicroShunt, using optical coherence tomography angiography (OCTA). 34 eyes from 34 patients who underwent Preserflo MicroShunt implantation were prospectively enrolled in this study. OCTA imaging was conducted at the superficial (SCP), deep (DCP) and radial peripapillary plexus (RPC) levels. The progression of FD and IOP was assessed at different time points from baseline to six months postoperatively for the entire patient population, as well as disease severity subgroups. The Preserflo MicroShunt achieved a significant reduction in IOP over the course of six months (median: 8 mmHg; $p < 0.01$). FD values of the SCP and DCP did not show significant fluctuations, even after adjusting for disease severity. FD of the RPC decreased significantly over the course of six months postoperatively from 42.31 at baseline to 39.59 at six months postoperatively ($p < 0.01$). The decrease in peripapillary FD was strongest in patients with advanced glaucoma (median: −3.58). These observations hint towards dysfunctional autoregulatory mechanisms in capillaries surrounding the optic nerve head in advanced glaucoma. In comparison, the microvascular structure of the macula appeared more resilient to changes in IOP.

Keywords: surgery; device; intraocular pressure; IOP; vessel density; MIGS; LIGS; glaucoma; severity

Citation: Storp, J.J.; Schatten, H.; Vietmeier, F.E.; Merté, R.-L.; Lahme, L.; Zimmermann, J.A.; Englmaier, V.A.; Eter, N.; Brücher, V.C. The Preserflo MicroShunt Affects Microvascular Flow Density in Optical Coherence Tomography Angiography. *Biomedicines* **2023**, *11*, 3254. https://doi.org/10.3390/biomedicines11123254

Academic Editor: Da-Wen Lu

Received: 1 November 2023
Revised: 28 November 2023
Accepted: 7 December 2023
Published: 8 December 2023

1. Introduction

Glaucoma is a global leading cause of blindness [1]. The "mechanical theory" of glaucoma progression regards intraocular pressure (IOP) as one of the main risk factors associated with the disease [2]. The majority of therapeutic interventions therefore target IOP reduction, which can be achieved by topical medication, non-penetrating procedures, or penetrating surgery. In the recent past, the need to reduce the postoperative care burden has given rise to new microinvasive approaches [3], which have been coined "MIGS" (microinvasive glaucoma surgery) or "LIGS" (less invasive glaucoma surgery). The Preserflo MicroShunt (Santen, Miami, FL, USA), an 8.5 mm long tubular structure with a 350 μm outer diameter and 70 μm lumen made from biocompatible (poly)styrene-block-isobutylene-block-styrene, represents a novel LIGS device and has been shown to effectively lower IOP in glaucoma patients [3–7].

The "mechanical theory", however, falls short in explaining the occurrence of normal-tension glaucoma and the fact that in some patients, simply lowering IOP does not halt the progression of the disease [1,8]. In response, the "vascular theory" of glaucoma development was proposed, according to which glaucoma is considered to result from inadequate blood supply to the eye. According to this theory, the development of glaucoma cannot be attributed solely to increased IOP but also to changes in systemic and microvascular perfusion [9,10].

Studies using optical coherence tomography angiography (OCTA), a new imaging technology that allows for the quantification of retinal microvasculature [11], have identified distinct changes in in glaucoma patients [12–18] and after IOP lowering surgery [19–24]. Bridging the gap between mechanical and vascular theories, these studies highlight the need for a comprehensive understanding of microvascular alterations attributed to less invasive glaucoma surgeries, particularly those involving devices like the Preserflo MicroShunt. Our study seeks to contribute to fill this gap in knowledge by quantifying longitudinal changes in retinal microvascular parameters associated with Preserflo MicroShunt implantation in glaucoma patients. Through this exploration, we aim to provide valuable insights into the microvascular dynamics influenced by this less invasive surgical approach, furthering our understanding of glaucoma management beyond the conventional mechanical paradigm.

This study aims to quantify longitudinal changes in retinal microvascular parameters associated with implantation of the Preserflo MicroShunt in glaucoma patients.

2. Materials and Methods

2.1. Design and Setting

All procedures were carried out in compliance with the 1964 Helsinki Declaration and its later amendments. This study was approved by the ethics committee of the Medical Association of Westfalen-Lippe and the University of Münster (No.: 2015-402-f-S). Data for this monocentric trial were collected from glaucoma patients visiting the Department of Ophthalmology at the University Hospital Münster, Germany, between August 2020 and November 2022. General patient information was retrieved from electronic patient files stored in the digital documentation system FIDUS (Arztservice Wente GmbH, Darmstadt, Germany).

2.2. Patient Examination

All patients older than 18 years of age, who were scheduled to receive Preserflo MicroShunt implantation due to glaucoma, were eligible for study inclusion. The following inclusion criteria were used: confirmed diagnosis of glaucoma, and the absence of any further retinal or neurological diseases. Individuals who had media opacities that precluded high-quality imaging, those with vitreoretinal or corneal disease, or who had undergone vitreoretinal or corneal surgery in the past were not allowed to participate in the study. Patients with previous glaucoma treatment, including surgery, were not excluded. If severe surgery-related complications that could distort retinal imaging, such as a central choroidal detachment or persistent hyphema, were present at the first follow-up, patients were excluded from the study.

In compliance with the guidelines of the World Glaucoma Association, all fellow eye surgeries were excluded from the database of this study [25].

All participants signed an informed consent form after having the study protocol thoroughly described to them, prior to enrolling. Patients were scheduled for re-visits at 1 month, 3 months, and 6 months after surgery. At baseline and each follow-up visit, all patients underwent a thorough ocular examination that included IOP assessment, refraction measures, slit lamp biomicroscopy, funduscopy, and OCTA imaging. At baseline, participants also received perimetric testing with the automated Humphrey visual field analyzer (HFA II, model 750, Carl Zeiss Meditec AG, Jena, Germany) with the standard program of the 30–2 Swedish interactive threshold algorithm (SITA fast). The occurrence of adverse events, as well as the frequency of postoperative 5-Fluorouracil (5-FU) injections were noted throughout the follow-up visits.

2.3. Surgical Procedure

To ensure that there is no conjunctival hyperemia on the day of surgery, patients at our clinic discontinue using all glaucoma eye drops four weeks before Preserflo implantation. Instead, they are given corticosteroid eye drops three days before surgery and oral azetacolamide for four weeks. They then receive intravenous acetazolamide and mannitol 2–3 h before surgery in an effort to reduce the pre- to postoperative pressure gradient. The subsequent surgery for implanting the Preserflo Microshunt has been thoroughly described elsewhere [5,26,27]. In brief, mitomycin-C (MMC) 0.2 mg/mL is given to the bare sclera for 3 min, by inserting sponges into the conjunctival flap after the conjunctiva and Tenon's capsule have been separated. A 2 mm deep scleral tunnel is formed using a 1 mm lance after rinsing with a balanced salt solution. A 25-gauge needle is then directed along this tract to enter the anterior chamber, producing a tunnel between the anterior chamber and the subconjunctival pocket located 3.5–4 mm from the limbus. The microshunt is retained inside the scleral pocket and introduced ab externo into the tunnel, with its tip reaching about 1–2 mm into the anterior chamber. Tenon's capsule and conjunctiva are sealed after the device's flow is verified by the appearance of drips at its outside end.

2.4. OCTA Imaging

OCTA technology has been thoroughly explained elsewhere [11]. In brief, OCTA devices apply a very high scanning rate to capture images of retinal vessels. In contrast to static tissue, blood movement in retinal vessels causes variations in signal amplitude between subsequent B-scans [11]. On the basis of these differences, the internal decorrelation algorithm generates en face views of the retinal microvasculature for different retinal layers and regions. In the present study, both the macula and the peripapillary sectors were measured. For OCTA imaging, the spectral-domain (SD) RTVue XR Avanti system (Angiovue/RTVue-XR Avanti, Optovue Inc., Fremont, CA, USA) was employed. Eyes were imaged without topical dilatation. The macula was angiographically imaged using 3 mm^2 scans, and papillary scans were performed using 4.5 mm^2 images. Imaging was conducted using the device's internal follow-up and tracking function to consistently map the same retinal region of each patient over the course of the study. The AngioVue algorithm automatically determined flow density (FD), which equals the ratio of bright pixels to the total number of pixels per scan, and is provided as a percentage value (%) for distinct retinal layers and sublocations.

OCTA imaging was conducted by an experienced examiner under identical circumstances for each patient and at the same site. Each papillary and macular slab underwent at least three consecutive images. The image with the greatest quality index (QI) among the three generated photos was chosen for study inclusion. If there were multiple photos with the same QI, one was randomly selected. Scans with artifacts or missing data were rejected. Images had to have a signal strength index (SSI) of 50.0 and a QI of 7. Manual sector segmentation was performed if necessary.

Each macular image contained FD data of the superficial (SCP) and deep macular plexus (DCP). In addition to these two, the FD values of the radial peripapilarry capillaries (RPCs) were extracted. Figure 1 depicts the OCT angiograms of the layers analyzed in the present study.

The FD values for the whole en face images of the macular and peripapillary plexus, as well as IOP development before and after Preserflo MicroShunt implantation, were analyzed longitudinally. Statistical analysis investigated fluctuations in FD and IOP over the course of the entire follow-up period, comparing baseline values to distinctive follow-up intervals: one month, three months, and six months after surgery. Further subgroup analyses investigated changes in FD and IOP in accordance with disease severity. The latter was determined through perimetric testing on the basis of the Hodapp–Parrish–Anderson classification [28]. Our rationale for investigating disparities based on disease severity stems from the well-established correlation between visual field loss and the severity of glaucoma. Despite the complexities associated with the non-linear nature of these changes, our primary objective is to address the inquiry into vascular alterations concerning glaucoma severity.

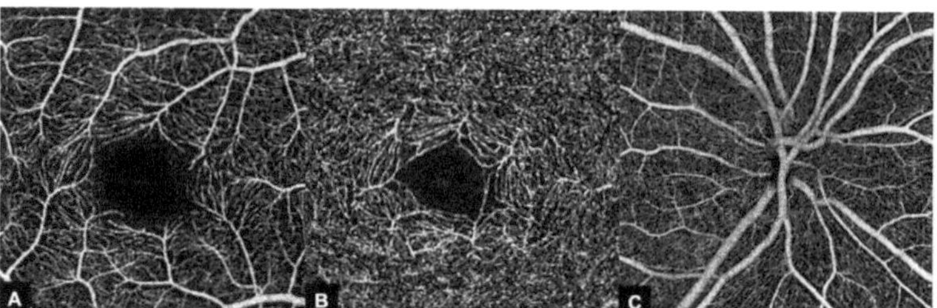

Figure 1. Representative en face angiograms of the regions analyzed using optical coherence tomography angiography (OCTA). (**A**): Superficial capillary plexus (SCP). (**B**): Deep capillary plexus (DCP). (**C**): (Peri)papillary capillary plexus with radial peripapillary capillaries (RPCs).

2.5. Statistical Analysis

Statistical analysis was carried out in IBM SPSS Statistics, version 28.0. The Shapiro–Wilk test was used to assess the distribution of the data. The data did not follow a normal distribution. Therefore, IOP and OCTA measures were evaluated using Wilcoxon signed-rank test. For the statistical calculations of IOP and OCTA metrics, only patients with complete datasets were included. Since the study was exploratory, no adjustment for multiple testing was applied. All analyses are exploratory and should be considered as such. All p-values less than 0.05 were regarded as statistically significant.

3. Results

34 eyes from 34 patients were included in this study. All patients were pseudophakic at time of study inclusion. Further patient characteristics are summarized in Table 1. The median follow-up time was 115 (interquartile range (IQR): 33–226) days.

Table 1. General patient characteristics.

Characteristics	Study Cohort
Eyes—*n*	34
Patients—*n*	34
Age (years)—median	67 (61–73)
Gender (M:F)—*n* (%)	17 (50%):17 (50%)
Study eye (R:L)—*n* (%)	16 (47%):18 (53%)
Disease severity groups—*n* (%)	
early	16 (47%)
moderate	3 (9%)
advanced	15 (44%)
Type of glaucoma—*n* (%)	
POAG	26 (76%)
PEX glaucoma	8 (24%)
Previous surgery—*n* (%)	
none	19 (56%)
total	15 (44%)
SLT	10 (29%)
SLT + MIGS	3 (9%)
TE	2 (6%)
Spherical equivalent	−1.63 (−2.38–0.38)
Visual acuity (LogMar)	0.2 (0.3–0)
Arterial hypertension—*n* (%)	12
treated—*n* (%)	10
Diabetes mellitus—*n* (%)	2
treated—*n* (%)	2

Data are presented as median (25–75% interquartile range), or as absolute and relative values. Abbreviations: *n* = number, % = percentage, M = male; F = female, R = right, L = left, POAG = primary open angle glaucoma, PEX = pseudoexfoliation, LogMar = logarithm of the minimum angle of resolution, SLT = selective laser trabeculoplasty, MIGS = microinvasive glaucoma surgery, TE = trabeculectomy.

3.1. IOP Development

The median IOP reduction for the entire study cohort over the follow-up period was 8 (IQR 3–12) mmHg ($p < 0.001$; Figure 2, Table 2). Based on disease severity, IOP reduction was greatest in patients with advanced glaucoma, followed by patients with moderate and early glaucoma (Table 2). Due to the small sample size, caution is advised when interpreting IOP development data for moderate glaucoma eyes.

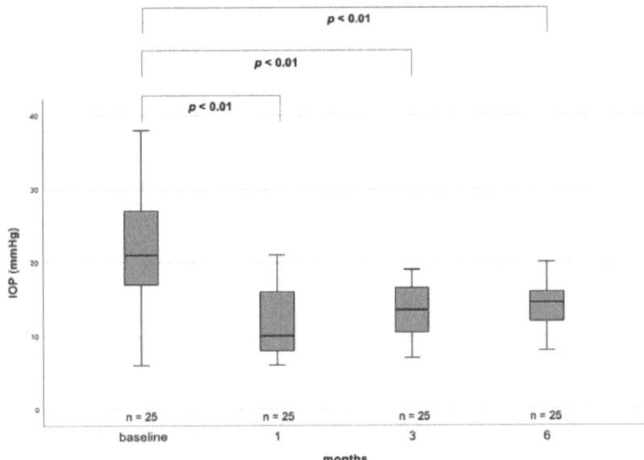

Figure 2. Boxplots showing IOP from baseline up to 6 months postoperatively for patients with complete datasets only. p-values for the difference between individual follow-up time points, as well as for the baseline-to-6-month comparison are presented and are derived from Wilcoxon signed-rank tests. p-values ≤ 0.05 are highlighted in bold. Note that distances between the time intervals are not to scale. IOP = intraocular pressure, mmHg = millimeters of mercury, n = number.

Table 2. IOP reduction at 6 months postoperatively in comparison to baseline for the entire patient population and by disease severity subgroups.

	IOP Baseline	**IOP 6 Months**	**IOP Reduction**
Total study population (mmHg)	$n = 34$ 22 (18–28)	$n = 25$ 15 (11–16)	$n = 25$ 8 (3–12)
Disease severity groups			
early (mmHg)	$n = 16$ 22 (18–25)	$n = 12$ 14 (9–16)	$n = 12$ 6 (3–7)
moderate (mmHg)	$n = 3$ 21 (19–25)	$n = 2$ 14 (13–15)	$n = 2$ 7 (6–7)
advanced (mmHg)	$n = 15$ 22 (18–27)	$n = 11$ 12 (9–15)	$n = 11$ 11 (6–14)

Data are presented as absolute numbers and median (25–75% IQR). Abbreviations: mmHg = millimeter mercury.

3.2. Postoperative Development

The median amount of supplemental medication dropped from 3 (IQR 3–4) at baseline to 1 (IQR 0–1) at follow-up ($p < 0.01$). 18 patients (53%) required supplemental medication after surgery and during the follow-up period. Of these, 11 patients (32%) administered carbonic anhydrase inhibitors, 6 (18%) took alpha agonists, and 1 (3%) continued therapy with carbonic anhydrase inhibitors and beta blockers.

Over the course of follow-up, 13 eyes (38%) were affected by hypotony (IOP $\leq$ 5 mmHg), with 6 eyes (18%) showing peripheral choroidal detachment. Central choroidal detachment was not observed in any patient. In all cases, hypotony resolved spontaneously, or with the support of topical steroid therapy during the first two weeks after surgery. 1 patient (3%) required revision surgery during the follow-up period to reposition the Preserflo Microshunt.

3.3. Injections of 5-FU

25 eyes (74%) received at least one subconjunctival injection of 5-FU during the follow-up period (range: 0–5; median: 2; interquartile range (IQR): 0–3).

3.4. Flow Density

FD of the SCP decreased from 32.54 (IQR 21.10–43.98) at baseline to 32.87 (IQR 24.42–41.32) at six months postoperatively; however, this change was not statistically significant ($p = 0.78$). Similarly, while FD at the three-month interval was significantly increased in the DCP compared to baseline, there was no significant change in DCP FD between baseline (44.82; IQR 36.72–52.92) and the six-month time point (46.82; IQR 40.89–52.75) ($p = 0.10$). On the contrary, FD of the RPC changed significantly over the course of follow-up from 42.31 (IQR 32.65–51.97) at baseline, to 37.29 (IQR 27.09–47.49) at the three-month interval ($p < 0.01$), to 39.59 (IQR 25.72–53.46) after six months postoperatively ($p < 0.01$) (Figure 3).

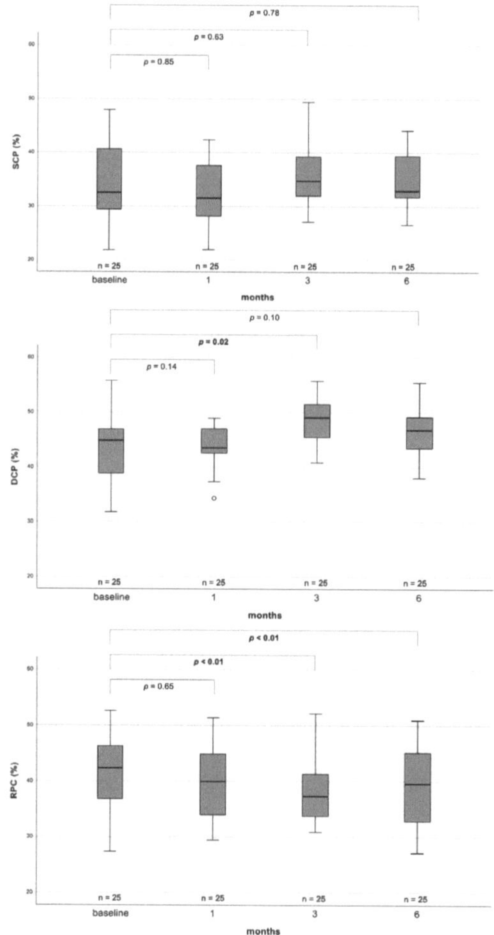

Figure 3. Boxplots depicting FD development from baseline up to 6 months postoperatively for patients with complete datasets only. p-values for the difference between baseline to individual follow-up time points are derived from Wilcoxon signed-rank tests. p-values ≤ 0.05 are highlighted in bold. Note that distances between the time intervals are not to scale. SCP = superficial capillary plexus, DCP = deep capillary plexus, RPC = radial peripapillary capillaries, n = number.

At the level of the SCP, the absence of substantial fluctuations in FD development remained, irrespective of disease severity. In the DCP of early glaucoma eyes, a significant increase in FD from baseline to month three with a subsequent reduction could be seen. The RPC showed a significant reduction of FD over the course of the entire follow-up period in eyes with advanced glaucoma, having a median FD of 37.73 (IQR 32.20–43.26) at baseline, which decreased to 34.15 (IQR 23.43–44.87) at six months postoperatively ($p < 0.01$). This was not seen in early disease eyes (baseline: 46.18; six months postoperatively: 45.34; $p = 0.18$) (Figure 4). Due to the small sample size, FD development for moderate glaucoma eyes is not displayed.

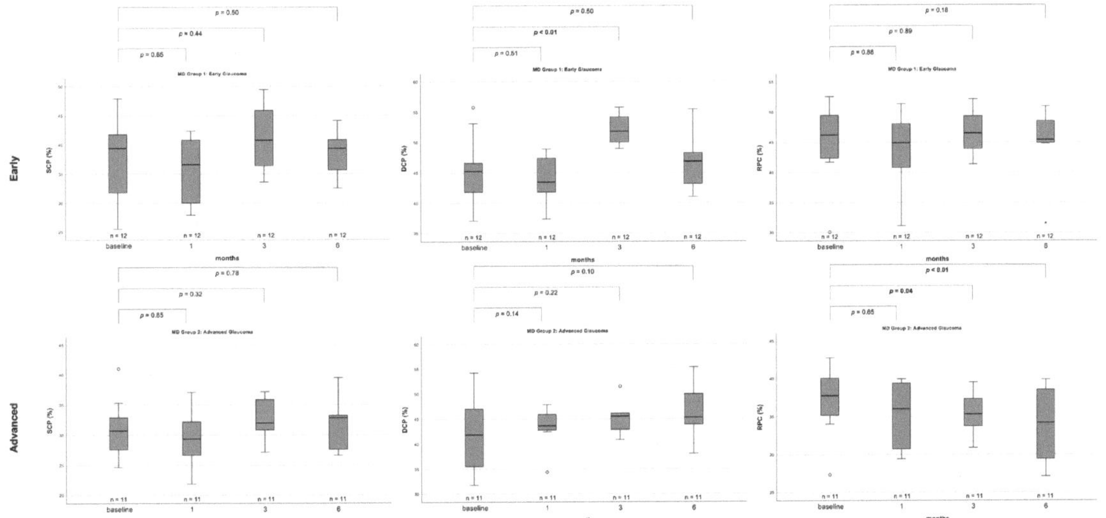

Figure 4. Boxplots depicting FD development from baseline up to 6 months postoperatively according to disease severity for patients with complete datasets only. Due to the small sample size, FD development for moderate glaucoma eyes is not displayed. p-values for the difference between baseline to individual follow-up time points are derived from Wilcoxon signed-rank tests. p-values ≤ 0.05 are highlighted in bold. Note that distances between the time intervals are not to scale. SCP = superficial capillary plexus, DCP = deep capillary plexus, RPC = radial peripapillary capillaries, n = number.

4. Discussion

The Preserflo MicroShunt has been shown to effectively lower IOP in glaucoma patients during long-term follow-up, irrespective of glaucoma subtype [5–7,29–32]. Recent studies have identified changes in retinal microvasculature related to IOP-lowering surgery in glaucoma patients [19–22,33]. This study represents the first trial to investigate changes in retinal FD in glaucoma patients related to treatment with the Preserflo MicroShunt.

In the present study, peripapillary FD in glaucoma eyes significantly decreased after the implantation of the Preserflo MicroShunt at the three- and six-month follow-up intervals. The reduction in FD was most apparent in eyes with advanced glaucomatous damage. FD of the macular layers, on the other hand, appeared less affected. Despite a temporary increase, FD of the DCP patients did not appear to be significantly altered at the latest follow-up in comparison to baseline, even when differentiating between disease severity groups. On the level of the SCP, no changes were detected throughout the follow-up period, even when differentiating between severity subgroups.

The exact relationship between IOP fluctuations and OCTA metrics has yet to be fully understood. The majority of studies in this field of research have investigated the effect of trabeculectomy on retinal vascular architecture [20,21,33]. The focus on this treatment can be attributed to the fact that trabeculectomy, being the gold standard for penetrating glaucoma surgery, is firstly, widely used in the treatment of glaucoma and secondly, expected to cause significant and lasting reductions in IOP, thus increasing the likelihood of detecting possible changes in retinal FD related to alterations in IOP. Recently, however, a few other works have investigated changes in retinal FD in less invasive glaucoma treatments [19,34]. The present study contributes to this area of expertise by providing the first data on the effect of the Preserflo MicroShunt, as one of the representatives of LIGS procedures.

The results from the current literature on microvascular changes after IOP-lowering interventions are as diverse as the treatment options for glaucoma. While some authors have attributed changes in FD to IOP fluctuations [34,35], others found no relation between IOP and changes in FD [16,36,37]. Some have described an increase in FD in certain retinal layers after IOP-lowering surgery [19–22,33], while others have contrarily described a decreasing effect or no effect at all [23,24,38,39]. The field of OCT angiographic research has, all in all, yielded non-unanimous results in clinical settings. It is, however, important to note that comparing trials investigating the effect of IOP reduction on FD is challenging, as different trials may apply different inclusion criteria, surgical techniques, and OCTA devices. Aside from clinical trials, an experimental approach by Patel et al. investigated the effect of big IOP changes on OCTA metrics. Patel et al. [40] evaluated the effect of IOP variations on retinal FD in six healthy Macaca mulatta (rhesus monkey) eyes. Every 10 min, they experimentally increased IOP by 10 mmHg, going up to a maximum of 60 mmHg before lowering it again. Each time they reached a 10 mmHg increment, OCTA imaging was conducted. Only when IOP reached 50 mmHg did the authors notice a statistically significant decline in FD, with a progressive restoration to baseline when IOP was once more lowered to 10 mmHg. This work strongly suggests a reciprocal relationship between IOP and retinal FD. At the same time, it implies that noticeable changes in FD only emerge at high IOP levels. This rationale explains the increase in FD after IOP-lowering interventions noticed by several authors [19,20,33,34], and it may also explain why others have not observed such trends. In these cases, the reduction in IOP may simply not have been big enough to cause significant changes in FD.

In the present study, retinal FD around the optic nerve head decreased significantly only in patients with advanced glaucoma. Eyes with early disease did not experience such changes. This observation could be related to differences in the amount of absolute IOP reduction in those subgroups. The IOP reduction over 6 months was smaller in early glaucoma eyes than in advanced glaucoma eyes, which could, in turn, translate into a lesser impact of IOP on FD in the early glaucoma subgroup. However, the findings by Patel et al. suggest that the differences in IOP reduction seen in this study between individual severity subgroups would most likely not be sufficient enough to cause a significant difference between these groups. On the other hand, they might lead to an increase in FD rather than a decrease. This suggests that the mere differences in IOP do not sufficiently explain the observations made in the present study. We believe that the changes observed can be better explained through the vascular autoregulatory mechanisms of the retina, which have been shown to dysfunction in glaucoma patients [41–43]. The findings of this trial fit with the current understanding of autoregulatory mechanisms in retinal perfusion, which sees a negative correlation between glaucoma severity and ocular blood flow [44]: eyes with early glaucomatous damage can still cope with moderate changes in IOP; however, advanced glaucomatous damage is associated with a reduced autoregulatory response to changes in IOP, which in this study, counterintuitively resulted in a reduction in FD around the optic disc. It can be postulated that we did not observe an increase in FD either because the deficient autoregulatory mechanisms in advanced glaucoma have led to a paradox reduction in FD in those eyes, or because autoregulatory mechanisms are delayed in advanced glaucoma, which would mean that a longer follow-up period could possibly reveal a postponed increase in FD.

While the question of the exact influence of glaucoma surgery on retinal microvasculature remains part of an ongoing discussion, the present study presents new data on the influence of a moderate IOP decrease on retinal FD. Belonging to LIGS, the reduction in IOP caused by the Preserflo MicroShunt is expected to be less than what would otherwise be anticipated from classical penetrating glaucoma surgery, such as trabeculectomy [3]. In this trial, the Preserflo MichroShunt achieved a median decrease in IOP of 8 (IQR 3–12) mmHg over a follow-up period of 6 months. This amount is comparable to previous studies [5–7]. The comparably short follow-up duration of only 6 months should, however, be taken into account when interpreting IOP development in the present analysis. Typically, IOP reduction is greatest directly after surgery, followed by a consecutive increase in IOP to a level that is lower than it used to be at baseline. This development was also seen in the analysis of the present study cohort and should be considered when comparing the results of this study to other IOP-lowering interventions.

The quantitative assessment of longitudinal changes in retinal microvascular parameters subsequent to Preserflo MicroShunt implantation yields valuable insights with potential implications for clinical practice. The identified microvascular alterations might function as potential biomarkers, providing critical information for predicting outcomes post-Preserflo implantation. Notably, the observed impact of surgery on the RPCs in patients with advanced glaucomatous damage suggests that preoperative analysis of this specific vascular layer could aid in decision-making, guiding the selection of appropriate candidates for Preserflo implantation. Considering instances in which the FD of the RPC is already low before surgery, caution against the risk of further reduction might be advised. In such cases, alternative IOP-modifying therapies could turn out to be more beneficial. Additionally, our findings contribute to a broader understanding of microvascular dynamics in less invasive glaucoma treatments, serving as a foundational basis for further research.

Limitations

This study has limitations, notably the lack of explicit assessment of ocular perfusion pressure and reliance on visual field grading for glaucoma severity. This hinders our ability to directly comment on autoregulatory mechanisms, introducing uncertainty in characterizing individual patients' vascular responses. In addition, although the design of this study minimizes the impact of differences in baseline characteristics between individuals on its outcomes by assessing intra-individual development of IOP and FD, possible confounding effects of baseline vessel diameter, as well as magnification errors, should be considered.

As recent studies have demonstrated, IOP is not expected to change significantly six months after Preserflo MicroShunt implantation [5–7,29]. Therefore, changes in retinal OCTA metrics related to sudden changes in IOP after the latest follow-up are not expected in this study population either. Yet, there have been reports describing late changes in retinal FD occurring beyond the follow-up duration of six months [22]. We therefore cannot fully rule out that further changes in retinal microvasculature in this study population might become visible in the future.

It is important to note that 53% of study participants required supplemental IOP-lowering medication after Preserflo surgery. These medications might have influenced FD values at the postoperative visits, as some studies demonstrated effects of antiglaucomatous medication on ocular blood flow [45–47].

In addition, this study only included patients with POAG and PEX glaucoma. Other glaucoma subtypes, such as normal-tension glaucoma, pigment dispersion glaucoma, or secondary glaucoma might yield different results, especially considering the fact that the exact mechanism between IOP fluctuations and FD alterations is not yet fully understood.

Further prospective studies with larger patient cohorts and longer follow-up periods investigating the effect of Preserflo MicroShunt implantation on retinal FD are needed to validate the results presented in this trial and elaborate on late effects of this treatment on OCTA metrics.

5. Conclusions

To summarize, while peripapillary FD in glaucoma eyes decreased significantly following Preserflo MicroShunt implantation, FD in the macular layers appeared to be less affected. While the FD of the RPCs for the entire population over six months saw a median reduction of −2.72, the decrease was greater in patients with advanced glaucoma (−3.58) than in patients with early glaucoma (−0.84). This observation might hint towards reduced autoregulatory responses in capillaries surrounding the optic nerve head in comparison to their macular counterparts—especially in eyes with an advanced disease state. It is still unclear whether these changes in FD ought to be considered a result of or a cause of glaucoma progression.

Author Contributions: Conceptualization, J.J.S., H.S., F.E.V., R.-L.M. and V.C.B.; data curation, J.J.S. and H.S.; formal analysis, J.J.S. and H.S.; investigation, J.J.S., H.S. and F.E.V.; methodology, J.J.S., H.S., F.E.V., R.-L.M., L.L. and V.C.B.; project administration, J.J.S. and V.C.B.; resources, N.E.; software, J.J.S., J.A.Z. and V.A.E.; supervision, R.-L.M. and V.C.B.; validation, J.J.S., J.A.Z. and V.A.E.; visualization, J.J.S.; writing—original draft, J.J.S.; writing—review and editing, J.J.S., H.S., F.E.V., L.L., J.A.Z., V.A.E., N.E. and V.C.B. All authors have read and agreed to the published version of the manuscript.

Funding: The authors acknowledge support from the Open Access Publication Fund of the University of Muenster.

Institutional Review Board Statement: The study was conducted in accordance with the Declaration of Helsinki and approved by the Ethics Committee of the University of Muenster, North Rhine Westphalia, Germany (No.: 2015-402-f-S).

Informed Consent Statement: Informed consent was obtained from all subjects involved in the study.

Data Availability Statement: Data are contained within the article.

Conflicts of Interest: The authors declare no conflict of interest.

References

1. Weinreb, R.N.; Aung, T.; Medeiros, F.A. The pathophysiology and treatment of glaucoma: A review. *JAMA* **2014**, *311*, 1901–1911. [CrossRef] [PubMed]
2. Fechtner, R.D.; Weinreb, R.N. Mechanisms of optic nerve damage in primary open angle glaucoma. *Surv. Ophthalmol.* **1994**, *39*, 23–42. [CrossRef] [PubMed]
3. Gambini, G.; Carlà, M.M.; Giannuzzi, F.; Caporossi, T.; De Vico, U.; Savastano, A.; Baldascino, A.; Rizzo, C.; Kilian, R.; Caporossi, A.; et al. PreserFlo® MicroShunt: An Overview of This Minimally Invasive Device for Open-Angle Glaucoma. *Vision* **2022**, *6*, 12. [CrossRef] [PubMed]
4. Green, W.; Lind, J.T.; Sheybani, A. Review of the Xen Gel Stent and InnFocus MicroShunt. *Curr. Opin. Ophthalmol.* **2018**, *29*, 162–170. [CrossRef] [PubMed]
5. Tanner, A.; Haddad, F.; Fajardo-Sanchez, J.; Nguyen, E.; Thong, K.X.; Ah-Moye, S.; Perl, N.; Abu-Bakra, M.; Kulkarni, A.; Trikha, S.; et al. One-year surgical outcomes of the PreserFlo MicroShunt in glaucoma: A multicentre analysis. *Br. J. Ophthalmol.* **2022**, *2021*, 320631. [CrossRef] [PubMed]
6. Durr, G.M.; Schlenker, M.B.; Samet, S.; Ahmed, I.I.K. One-year outcomes of stand-alone ab externo SIBS microshunt implantation in refractory glaucoma. *Br. J. Ophthalmol.* **2022**, *106*, 71–79. [CrossRef] [PubMed]
7. Storp, J.J.; Vietmeier, F.E.; Merté, R.-L.; Koch, R.; Zimmermann, J.A.; Eter, N.; Brücher, V.C. Long-Term Outcomes of the PRESERFLO MicroShunt Implant in a Heterogeneous Glaucoma Cohort. *J. Clin. Med.* **2023**, *12*, 4474. [CrossRef] [PubMed]
8. Flammer, J.; Mozaffarieh, M. What is the present pathogenetic concept of glaucomatous optic neuropathy? *Surv. Ophthalmol.* **2007**, *2*, 162–173. [CrossRef]
9. Flammer, J.; Orgül, S.; Costa, V.P.; Orzalesi, N.; Krieglstein, G.K.; Serra, L.M.; Renard, J.P.; Stefánsson, E. The impact of ocular blood flow in glaucoma. *Prog. Retin. Eye Res.* **2002**, *21*, 359–393. [CrossRef]
10. Flammer, J. The vascular concept of glaucoma. *Surv. Ophthalmol.* **1994**, *38*, 3–6. [CrossRef]
11. Spaide, R.F.; Fujimoto, J.G.; Waheed, N.K.; Sadda, S.R.; Staurenghi, G. Optical coherence tomography angiography. *Prog. Retin. Eye Res.* **2018**, *64*, 1–55. [CrossRef] [PubMed]
12. Alnawaiseh, M.; Lahme, L.; Müller, V.; Rosentreter, A.; Eter, N. Correlation of flow density, as measured using optical coherence tomography angiography, with structural and functional parameters in glaucoma patients. *Graefes Arch. Clin. Exp. Ophthalmol.* **2018**, *256*, 589–597. [CrossRef] [PubMed]
13. Rao, H.L.; Pradhan, Z.S.; Suh, M.H.; Moghimi, S.; Mansouri, K.; Weinreb, R.N. Optical Coherence Tomography Angiography in Glaucoma. *J. Glaucoma* **2020**, *29*, 312–321. [CrossRef] [PubMed]
14. WuDunn, D.; Takusagawa, H.L.; Sit, A.J.; Rosdahl, J.A.; Radhakrishnan, S.; Hoguet, A.; Han, Y.; Chen, T.C. OCT Angiography for the Diagnosis of Glaucoma: A Report by the American Academy of Ophthalmology. *Ophthalmology* **2021**, *128*, 1222–1235. [CrossRef] [PubMed]

15. Bojikian, K.D.; Chen, P.P.; Wen, J.C. Optical coherence tomography angiography in glaucoma. *Curr. Opin. Ophthalmol.* **2019**, *30*, 110–116. [CrossRef] [PubMed]
16. Müller, V.C.; Storp, J.J.; Kerschke, L.; Nelis, P.; Eter, N.; Alnawaiseh, M. Diurnal variations in flow density measured using optical coherence tomography angiography and the impact of heart rate, mean arterial pressure and intraocular pressure on flow density in primary open-angle glaucoma patients. *Acta Ophthalmol.* **2019**, *97*, 844–849. [CrossRef] [PubMed]
17. Zimmermann, J.A.; Storp, J.J.; Diener, R.; Danzer, M.F.; Esser, E.L.; Eter, N.; Brücher, V.C. Influence of Cilioretinal Arteries on Flow Density in Glaucoma Patients Measured Using Optical Coherence Tomography Angiography. *J. Clin. Med.* **2023**, *12*, 2458. [CrossRef]
18. Mannil, S.S.; Agarwal, A.; Conner, I.P.; Kumar, R.S. A comprehensive update on the use of optical coherence tomography angiography in glaucoma. *Int. Ophthalmol.* **2023**, *43*, 1785–1802. [CrossRef]
19. Alnawaiseh, M.; Müller, V.; Lahme, L.; Merté, R.-L.; Eter, N. Changes in Flow Density Measured Using Optical Coherence Tomography Angiography after iStent Insertion in Combination with Phacoemulsification in Patients with Open-Angle Glaucoma. *J. Ophthalmol.* **2018**, *2018*, 2890357. [CrossRef]
20. Miraftabi, A.; Jafari, S.; Nilforushan, N.; Abdolalizadeh, P.; Rakhshan, R. Effect of trabeculectomy on optic nerve head and macular vessel density: An optical coherence tomography angiography study. *Int. Ophthalmol.* **2021**, *41*, 2677–2688. [CrossRef]
21. Güngör, D.; Kayıkçıoğlu, Ö.R.; Altınışık, M.; Doğruya, S. Changes in optic nerve head and macula optical coherence tomography angiography parameters before and after trabeculectomy. *Jpn. J. Ophthalmol.* **2022**, *66*, 305–313. [CrossRef] [PubMed]
22. Ch'ng, T.W.; Gillmann, K.; Hoskens, K.; Rao, H.L.; Mermoud, A.; Mansouri, K. Effect of surgical intraocular pressure lowering on retinal structures—Nerve fibre layer, foveal avascular zone, peripapillary and macular vessel density: 1 year results. *Eye* **2020**, *34*, 562–571. [CrossRef] [PubMed]
23. Reitemeyer, E.; Pahlitzsch, M.; Cornelius, A.; Pilger, D.; Winterhalter, S.; Maier, A.B. Stabilization of macular, peripapillary and papillary vascular parameters after XEN and trabeculectomy visualized by the optical coherence tomography angiography. *Sci. Rep.* **2022**, *12*, 17251. [CrossRef] [PubMed]
24. Zéboulon, P.; Lévêque, P.M.; Brasnu, E.; Aragno, V.; Hamard, P.; Baudouin, C.; Labbé, A. Effect of Surgical Intraocular Pressure Lowering on Peripapillary and Macular Vessel Density in Glaucoma Patients: An Optical Coherence Tomography Angiography Study. *J. Glaucoma* **2017**, *26*, 466–472. [CrossRef] [PubMed]
25. Shaarawy, T.M.; Sherwood, M.B.; Grehn, F. *World Glaucoma Association Guidelines on Design & Reporting Glaucoma Trials*; Kugler Publications: Amsterdam, The Netherlands, 2009.
26. Schlenker, M.B.; Durr, G.M.; Michaelov, E.; Ahmed, I.I.K. Intermediate Outcomes of a Novel Standalone Ab Externo SIBS Microshunt with Mitomycin C. *Am. J. Ophthalmol.* **2020**, *215*, 141–153. [CrossRef] [PubMed]
27. Kerr, N.M.; Ahmed, I.I.K.; Pinchuk, L. Minimally Invasive Glaucoma Surgery. Springer: Singapore, 2021; PRESERFLO MicroShunt; pp. 91–103.
28. Hodapp, E.; Parrish, R.K.; Anderson, D.R. *Clinical Decisions in Glaucoma*; Mosby Incorporated: Maryland Heights, MO, USA, 1993.
29. Pillunat, K.R.; Herber, R.; Haase, M.A.; Jamke, M.; Jasper, C.S.; Pillunat, L.E. PRESERFLO™ MicroShunt versus trabeculectomy: First results on efficacy and safety. *Acta Ophthalmol.* **2022**, *100*, 779–790. [CrossRef] [PubMed]
30. Baker, N.D.; Barnebey, H.S.; Moster, M.R.; Stiles, M.C.; Vold, S.D.; Khatana, A.K.; Flowers, B.E.; Grover, D.S.; Strouthidis, N.G.; Panarelli, J.F.; et al. Ab-Externo MicroShunt versus Trabeculectomy in Primary Open-Angle Glaucoma: One-Year Results from a 2-Year Randomized, Multicenter Study. *Ophthalmology* **2021**, *128*, 1710–1721. [CrossRef]
31. Nobl, M.; Freissinger, S.; Kassumeh, S.; Priglinger, S.; Mackert, M.J. One-year outcomes of microshunt implantation in pseudoexfoliation glaucoma. *PLoS ONE* **2021**, *16*, 0256670. [CrossRef]
32. Batlle, J.F.; Corona, A.; Albuquerque, R. Long-term results of the PRESERFLO MicroShunt in patients with primary open-angle glaucoma from a single-center nonrandomized Study. *J. Glaucoma* **2021**, *30*, 281–286. [CrossRef]
33. Shin, J.W.; Sung, K.R.; Uhm, K.B.; Jo, J.; Moon, Y.; Song, M.K.; Song, J.Y. Peripapillary microvascular improvement and lamina cribrosa depth reduction after trabeculectomy in primary open-angle glaucoma. *Investig. Ophthalmol. Vis. Sci.* **2017**, *58*, 5993–5999. [CrossRef]
34. Holló, G. Influence of Large Intraocular Pressure Reduction on Peripapillary OCT Vessel Density in Ocular Hypertensive and Glaucoma Eyes. *J. Glaucoma* **2017**, *26*, 7–10. [CrossRef]
35. Wang, X.; Chen, J.; Kong, X.; Sun, X. Immediate Changes in Peripapillary Retinal Vasculature after Intraocular Pressure Elevation -an Optical Coherence Tomography Angiography Study. *Curr. Eye Res.* **2020**, *45*, 749–756. [CrossRef] [PubMed]
36. Zhang, Q.; Jonas, J.B.; Wang, Q.; Chan, S.Y.; Xu, L.; Wei, W.B.; Wang, Y.X. Optical coherence tomography angiography vessel density changes after acute intraocular pressure elevation. *Sci. Rep.* **2018**, *8*, 6024. [CrossRef]
37. Mansouri, K.; Rao, H.L.; Hoskens, K.; D'Alessandro, E.; Flores-Reyes, E.M.; Mermoud, A.; Weinreb, R.N. Diurnal variations of peripapillary and macular vessel density in glaucomatous eyes using optical coherence tomography angiography. *J. Glaucoma* **2018**, *27*, 336–341. [CrossRef] [PubMed]
38. Lommatzsch, C.; Rothaus, K.; Koch, J.M.; Heinz, C.; Grisanti, S. Retinal perfusion 6 months after trabeculectomy as measured by optical coherence tomography angiography. *Int. Ophthalmol.* **2019**, *39*, 2583–2594. [CrossRef] [PubMed]
39. Hong, J.W.; Sung, K.R.; Shin, J.W. Optical Coherence Tomography Angiography of the Retinal Circulation Following Trabeculectomy for Glaucoma. *J. Glaucoma* **2023**, *32*, 293–300. [CrossRef]

40. Patel, N.; McAllister, F.; Pardon, L.; Harwerth, R. The effects of graded intraocular pressure challenge on the optic nerve head. *Exp. Eye Res.* **2018**, *169*, 79–90. [CrossRef]
41. Luo, X.; Shen, Y.M.; Jiang, M.N.; Lou, X.F.; Shen, Y. Ocular Blood Flow Autoregulation Mechanisms and Methods. *J. Ophthalmol.* **2015**, *2015*, 864871. [CrossRef]
42. Pillunat, L.E.; Stodtmeister, R.; Wilmanns, I. Pressure compliance of the optic nerve head in low tension glaucoma. *Br. J. Ophthalmol.* **1987**, *71*, 181–187. [CrossRef]
43. Fuchsjäger-Mayrl, G.; Wally, B.; Georgopoulos, M.; Rainer, G.; Kircher, K.; Buehl, W.; Amoako-Mensah, T.; Eichler, H.G.; Vass, C.; Schmetterer, L. Ocular blood flow and systemic blood pressure in patients with primary open-angle glaucoma and ocular hypertension. *Investig. Ophthalmol. Vis. Sci.* **2004**, *45*, 834–839. [CrossRef]
44. Hwang, J.C.; Konduru, R.; Zhang, X.; Tan, O.; Francis, B.A.; Varma, R.; Sehi, M.; Greenfield, D.S.; Sadda, S.R.; Huang, D. Relationship among visual field, blood flow, and neural structure measurements in glaucoma. *Investig. Ophthalmol. Vis. Sci.* **2012**, *53*, 3020–3026. [CrossRef]
45. Feke, G.T.; Bex, P.J.; Taylor, C.P.; Rhee, D.J.; Turalba, A.V.; Chen, T.C.; Wand, M.; Pasquale, L.R. Effect of brimonidine on retinal vascular autoregulation and short-term visual function in normal tension glaucoma. *Am. J. Ophthalmol.* **2014**, *158*, 105–112. [CrossRef]
46. Tsuda, S.; Yokoyama, Y.; Chiba, N.; Aizawa, N.; Shiga, Y.; Yasuda, M.; Yokokura, S.; Otomo, T.; Fuse, N.; Nakazawa, T. Effect of topical tafluprost on optic nerve head blood flow in patients with myopic disc type. *J. Glaucoma* **2013**, *22*, 398–403. [CrossRef]
47. Siesky, B.; Harris, A.; Brizendine, E.; Marques, C.; Loh, J.; Mackey, J.; Overton, J.; Netland, P. Literature review and meta-analysis of topical carbonic anhydrase inhibitors and ocular blood flow. *Surv. Ophthalmol.* **2009**, *54*, 33–46. [CrossRef]

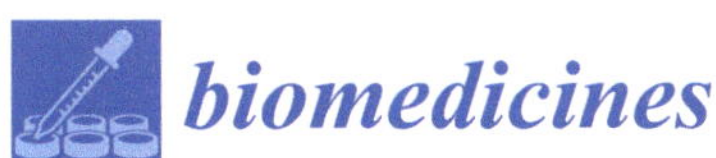

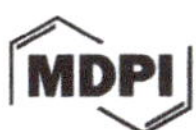

Article

Deep Learning Evaluation of Glaucoma Detection Using Fundus Photographs in Highly Myopic Populations

Yen-Ying Chiang [1], Ching-Long Chen [2] and Yi-Hao Chen [1,2,*]

[1] Graduate Institute of Life Sciences, National Defense Medical Center, Taipei 114, Taiwan; h200345@hotmail.com

[2] Department of Ophthalmology, Tri-Service General Hospital, National Defense Medical Center, Taipei 114, Taiwan; doc30881@mail.ndmctsgh.edu.tw

* Correspondence: doc30879@mail.ndmctsgh.edu.tw; Tel.: +886-2-87927163

Abstract: Objectives: This study aimed to use deep learning to identify glaucoma and normal eyes in groups with high myopia using fundus photographs. Methods: Patients who visited Tri-Services General Hospital from 1 November 2018 to 31 October 2022 were retrospectively reviewed. Patients with high myopia (spherical equivalent refraction of ≤ -6.0 D) were included in the current analysis. Meanwhile, patients with pathological myopia were excluded. The participants were then divided into the high myopia group and high myopia glaucoma group. We used two classification models with the convolutional block attention module (CBAM), an attention mechanism module that enhances the performance of convolutional neural networks (CNNs), to investigate glaucoma cases. The learning data of this experiment were evaluated through fivefold cross-validation. The images were categorized into training, validation, and test sets in a ratio of 6:2:2. Grad-CAM visual visualization improved the interpretability of the CNN results. The performance indicators for evaluating the model include the area under the receiver operating characteristic curve (AUC), sensitivity, and specificity. Results: A total of 3088 fundus photographs were used for the deep-learning model, including 1540 and 1548 fundus photographs for the high myopia glaucoma and high myopia groups, respectively. The average refractive power of the high myopia glaucoma group and the high myopia group were -8.83 ± 2.9 D and -8.73 ± 2.6 D, respectively ($p = 0.30$). Based on a fivefold cross-validation assessment, the ConvNeXt_Base+CBAM architecture had the best performance, with an AUC of 0.894, accuracy of 82.16%, sensitivity of 81.04%, specificity of 83.27%, and F1 score of 81.92%. Conclusions: Glaucoma in individuals with high myopia was identified from their fundus photographs.

Keywords: glaucoma; myopia; artificial intelligence; fundus photographs

Citation: Chiang, Y.-Y.; Chen, C.-L.; Chen, Y.-H. Deep Learning Evaluation of Glaucoma Detection Using Fundus Photographs in Highly Myopic Populations. *Biomedicines* **2024**, *12*, 1394. https://doi.org/10.3390/biomedicines12071394

Academic Editor: Masaru Takeuchi

Received: 28 April 2024
Revised: 14 June 2024
Accepted: 19 June 2024
Published: 23 June 2024

Correction Statement: This article has been republished with a minor change. The change does not affect the scientific content of the article and further details are available within the backmatter of the website version of this article.

1. Introduction

In recent years, the prevalence of myopia has increased rapidly particularly in East and Southeast Asian countries, such as Singapore, China, Taiwan, Hong Kong, Japan, and South Korea [1]. Based on surveys, since 2015 [2], approximately 1.406 billion people (22.9% of the total population) globally can develop myopia. Further, approximately 163 million people (2.7% of the total population) have high myopia (spherical equivalent refraction [SER] of <-5.0 D). According to the development trend of high myopia, considering environmental and lifestyle changes, the incidence of high myopia worldwide can reach approximately 10% by 2050. Thus, it is a public health issue that cannot be ignored. Glaucoma is a progressive optic neuropathy [3]. Injured optic nerve causing visual field loss is commonly irreversible [4,5]. Globally, >76 million people are diagnosed with glaucoma, which reduces the quality of life, impairs vision, and has an increasing incidence [6,7]. The severity of visual field defects will further increase with age [8,9]. Patients with glaucoma require long-term treatment and examination to avoid continued degradation and loss of visual field. Myopia is an important risk factor for glaucoma. The risk of developing glaucoma increases alongside myopia severity [10,11]. A meta-analysis study by Ahnul Ha et al. included seven studies reporting risk estimates for high myopia and revealed that the pooled odds ratio for developing glaucoma was 4.142 (95% confidence interval [CI]: 2.567–6.685) [12]. As the population of individuals with high myopia increases, it is extremely important to accurately diagnose glaucoma. However, clinicians often encounter challenges when diagnosing patients with glaucoma who present with high myopia. This is caused by the structure and function similarities between glaucoma and myopia [13].

Axial elongation because of high myopia changes the retinal structure and function, including morphology similar to that seen in patients with glaucoma, such as disc size, shape, neuroretinal rim shape, and pallor [14,15]. As high myopia worsens, the axial length of the eye elongates, and the optic disc stretches horizontally into an oval shape on fundus photography. Further, the condition may cause sagittal rotation of the optic disc, which is referred to as "tilted disc". The normal optic disc shape and glaucoma are vertically elliptical. The cup-to-disc ratio in nonglaucoma high myopia is approximately 1.5 times higher than that without myopia [16]. However, previous research has shown that the optic disc size is not an important risk factor for the development of glaucoma [17]. In myopia, the height between the neuroretinal edge and the base of the optic cup is reduced by flattening the optic cup. Simultaneously, the Bruch's membrane opening expands, and the retinal edge becomes thinner. The neuroretinal edge loss in glaucoma progresses as inferotemporal, supratemporal, infranasal, and supranasal as the disease progresses [18–20]. High myopic glaucoma is more difficult to diagnose because of the abnormal shape of the optic retinal edge, which no longer conforms to the inferior–superior–nasal–temporal rule [21,22]. High myopia and glaucoma cause thinning of the retinal nerve fiber layer. High myopia is mainly caused by the excessive elongation of the eyeball, and RNFL thinning is mainly observed in the superior and inferior temporal regions. Meanwhile, glaucoma is attributed to optic nerve damage caused by increased intraocular pressure. Further, the thickness of the RNFL and ganglion cell complex decreases significantly over time [23,24]. According to the progression of visual field defects in myopia and glaucoma, non-myopic glaucoma usually manifests as Bjerrum area defects and nasal steps in the early stage. Further, central visual field defects develop over time. In the early stage of myopic glaucoma, central or paracentral darkening is more common [25]. High myopia can be interpreted as false-positive glaucoma when diagnosing glaucoma [26,27]. Fundus photography, optical coherence tomography (OCT) is usually required to compare the results of long-term tracking changes with those of visual field examination. Therefore, diagnosing glaucoma in highly myopic eyes is difficult.

In recent years, artificial intelligence has made significant progress in the field of medical imaging. In particular, the application of convolutional neural networks (CNNs) is extremely suitable for processing spatial patterns and performing tasks, such as image classification and object detection, thereby promoting the development of deep-learning technology for image classification and pattern recognition [28]. Deep-learning algorithms require a large amount of data for training, which is particularly challenging when clinical data are limited. At this point, transfer learning can often leverage models pretrained on the dataset, thereby reducing training time and improving performance [29]. Several ophthalmologic diseases, such as diabetic retinopathy [30], glaucoma [31,32], macular degeneration [33], and myopia [34], have been evaluated via artificial intelligence medical imaging. The artificial intelligence-assisted diagnosis of glaucoma mainly involves analyzing OCT, visual field test results, and fundus photography. Fundus photography has significant advantages in related applications as they are accessible, have a high quality, and are cost-effective [35].

In the study by Li et al. [36], ophthalmologists classified 48,116 fundus photographs. Glaucoma was defined as a vertical cup-to-disc ratio of $\geq$0.7. In the Inception-v3 architecture, the AUC was 0.986, the accuracy was 92.9%, the sensitivity was 95.6%, and the specificity was 92.0%. In the study by Kim et al. [37], 747 myopic healthy eyes and 1860 myopic glaucoma eyes were included, using macular vertical OCT to evaluate the glaucoma diagnostic ability of patients with high myopia. In the EfficientNet architecture, the external test dataset showed an AUC of 0.984 using macular vertical OCT scans and an AUC of 0.983 using individual data combinations. Asaoka et al. analyzed the visual field of the first diagnosis of evident glaucoma and the visual field of healthy people. Deep learning can be used to predict the development trend of glaucoma and achieve good outcomes (AUC: 92.6%) [38]. Regarding fundus photography medical imaging detection of glaucoma, previous studies focused more on the cutting of the optic disc and the structure of the optic nerve head, although they all have excellent performance [38–42]. However, fundus photos with a viewing angle of 45° are not always used, and other signs in the eye map may be ignored.

Previous deep-learning studies have used non-highly myopic or OCT parameters for deep learning, or overly focused on the optic nerve head structure. Moreover, currently, no study has utilized fundus photos for evaluating high myopia glaucoma. Herein, several novel issues were explored. First, this is the study to specifically use fundus photographs for detecting glaucoma in patients with high myopia. Second, we develop a deep-learning framework incorporating convolutional block attention modules (CBAMs) to enhance the performance of CNN glaucoma detection. Finally, the use of Grad-CAM visualization improves the interpretability of CNN results and helps comprehend how the model makes predictions. The use of fundus photographs can prevent issues related to the inability to convert data between different machines such as OCT. The fundus photographs are also available easily and are time-saving [39,40]. This study aimed to use deep learning to detect glaucoma on the fundus photographs of individuals with high myopia. We believe that this method can assist ophthalmologists in achieving an accurate diagnosis or other professionals, such as optometrists, family physicians, and non-ophthalmologists, in making early referrals.

2. Materials and Methods

2.1. Ethics, Consent, and Permissions

This study obtained ethical approval from the research ethics committee of the Tri-Service General Hospital (TSGHIRB No. C202305105) and adhered to the principles of the Declaration of Helsinki.

2.2. Datasets Collection

We retrospectively reviewed patients who visited Tri-Services General Hospital from 1 November 2018 to 31 October 2022. Initially, there were 35,327 patients with 126,955 fundus photographs. All patients underwent visual acuity assessment, refractive error, and slit-lamp biomicroscopy. All patients with high myopia underwent non-mydriatic fundus photography (AFC-330; Nideck Co. Ltd., Gamagori, Aichi, Japan), whereas all patients with glaucoma underwent central 24-2 threshold testing using a standard Humphrey Field Analyzer (Carl Zeiss Meditec, Dublin, CA, USA) and optical coherence tomography (RTVue-100; Optovue Inc., Fremont, CA, USA). OCT was used to measure optic disc cupping, circumpapillary retinal nerve fiber layer thickness, and macular layer thickness. All clinical records were deidentified and anonymized before analysis in this study.

The inclusion criteria for people with high myopia were (1) age of >20 years at baseline examination and (2) SER of ≤ -6.0 D [41]. SER is a measure of the refractive error of the eye and is calculated using the following formula: spherical power + 0.5 * (cylindrical power). This study excludes patients with pathological myopia, those who have undergone cataract surgery, refractive surgery, diabetes, and macular degeneration, any other ocular or systemic disease affecting the retinal nerve fiber layer, and other diseases impacting the visual field (e.g., neuroophthalmic disease, uveitis, retinal, or choroidal disease, trauma), as well as those with severe media opacity that interferes with fundus photography or OCT image acquisition. High myopia includes axial myopia and refractive myopia, and the axial length of the eye is not used as a single inclusion criterion.

Patients with glaucoma were selected after excluding those who did not meet the criteria. All patients with glaucoma were diagnosed after long-term follow-up by professional ophthalmologists. The inclusion criteria for patients with glaucoma were as follows: first, changes that indicate glaucomatous optic nerve or nerve fiber layer defects, such as increased narrowing of the neuroretinal rim (change in a sector of the neuroretinal rim from narrow to complete loss or from a homogeneous neuroretinal rim to a narrow sector) and a significant expansion of a retinal nerve fiber layer defect on OCT. Second, automated visual field testing showed glaucomatous visual field progression defined using the Anderson–Patella criteria, i.e., the Glaucoma Hemifield Test (GHT) result was outside normal limits. There was a cluster of three or more non-edge points in the typical location of the glaucoma, all of which were depressed on the pattern deviation plot at a p value of <5%, with at least one of these points depressed at a p value of <1%. In addition, the corrected pattern standard deviation was abnormal at a p value of <5%. All patients with glaucoma are receiving antiglaucoma treatment, such as the following eye drops: beta blockers, alpha-2 adrenergic agonists, prostaglandin analogs, and carbonic anhydrase inhibitors. Finally, they were categorized into high myopia and high myopia with glaucoma groups. Different image categories are described in the Supplementary Material. Figure 1 shows the Flowchart of patient inclusion and exclusion.

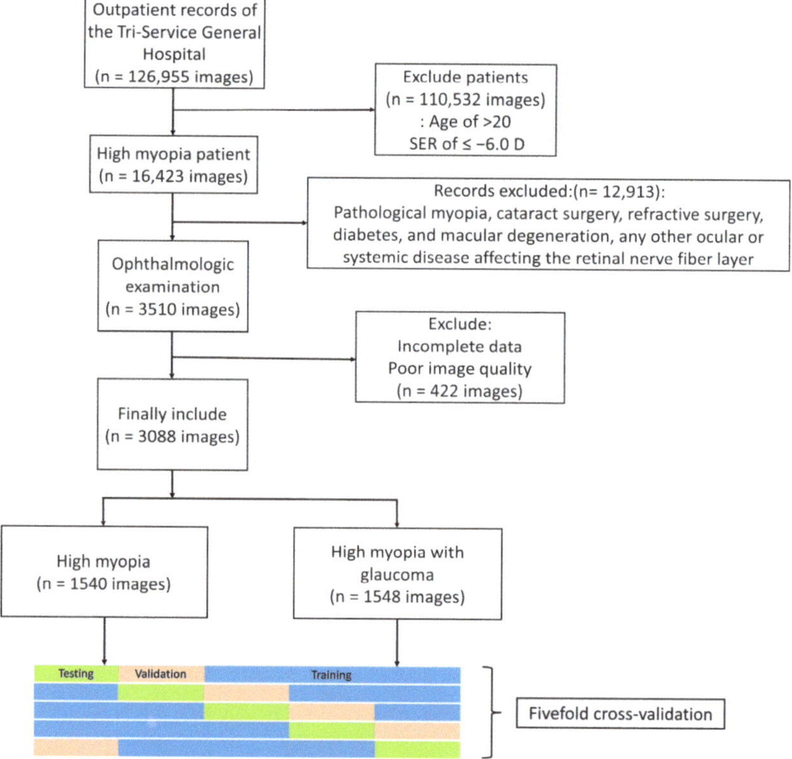

Figure 1. Flowchart of patient inclusion and exclusion.

2.3. Model Building

A CNN retrieves image features for classification tasks through its deep structure, which greatly improves the accuracy and efficiency of disease diagnosis in medical image classification [42]. Our study used two CNN architecture models: EfficientNet_V2-S [43], which was proposed by Tan and Le in 2021, and ConvNeXt_Base [44], which was introduced by Liu et al. in 2022. Additionally, we used transfer learning. Previous literature has revealed that pretrained parameters improve classification capabilities more quickly. The weights are derived from pretraining on the ImageNet visual recognition challenge dataset [45]. The last layer of the model (the fully connected layer) is replaced, and the output is ultimately classified into two categories. The training setup for all model architectures features a batch size of 8 across 30 epochs. Initially, the learning rate starts from 0.01 and decays by 0.3 times every 6 epochs. This configuration used the Cross-Entropy Loss function and the AdamW [46] optimizer with a learning rate of 10^{-5} and weight decay of 10^{-5}. Additionally, it includes a StepLR scheduler with a step size of 10 and incorporates a dropout rate of 0.2.

The CBAM (Figure 2) is used in the model to improve the performance of the CNN to improve the accuracy of target detection and object classification. The attention mechanism module [47] CBAM sequentially applies channel and spatial attention mechanisms to progressively refine the attention distribution of feature maps.

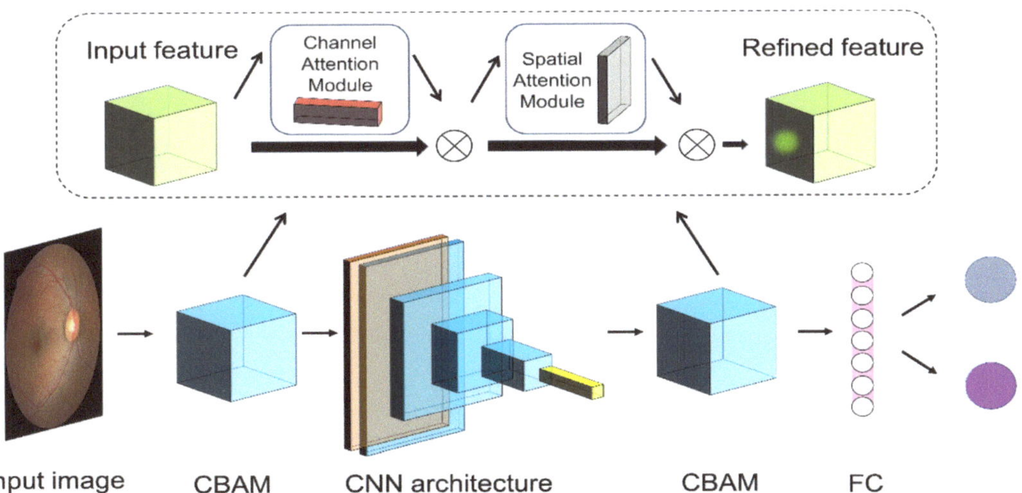

Figure 2. Convolutional neural network (CNN) and the convolutional block attention module (CBAM) attention mechanism. The image is input after preprocessing. Different CNN architectures were replaced.

The channel attention mechanism assigns a weight to each channel, emphasizing important channels and suppressing less important ones. This is expressed as follows:

$$M_c(F) = \sigma(MLP(AvgPool\ (F)) + MLP(MaxPool(F)) \quad (1)$$

F denotes the input feature map. $AvgPool$ and $MaxPool$ indicate the average and max pooling operations across the channel dimension, which capture the channels' global statistical information. MLP stands for multilayer perceptron. The symbol σ signifies the sigmoid activation function, which produces the channel attention weights M_c.

The spatial attention mechanism emphasizes important spatial regions within the feature maps. This is expressed as follows:

$$M_s(F) = \sigma\left(f^{7\times7}\ ([AvgPool(F);\ MaxPool(F)])\right) \quad (2)$$

F indicates the input feature map. First, the feature map independently undergoes average and max pooling across each channel, followed by stacking the two pooling results along the channel dimension. $f^{7\times7}$ represents a convolution operation with a 7×7 kernel, capturing contextual information in the spatial domain. Finally, the sigmoid function σ generates the spatial attention weights M_S.

2.4. Image Preprocessing

We evaluated the learning data for this experiment through fivefold cross-validation. The dataset is randomly divided into five equal subset sizes in the fivefold cross-validation, and the images are categorized into training, validation, and test sets in a ratio of 6:2:2 (Figure 3). Fundus photographs of each patient are not repeated. Each image will appear in only one of the subsets and will not be repeated. In particular, it only exists in the training set, but not in the validation or test sets. The image was resized to $3 \times 224 \times 224$ and augmented with data, including horizontal flipping and random rotation within 20°. The execution system uses an Intel Core i7-11370H 3.3 GHz (TSMC, Hisnchu, Taiwan) processor with 40 GB memory and an NVIDIA GeForce RTX-3070 with 8 GB DDR6 (Asus, Taipei, Taiwan) distinct graphics card. The implementation of the deep neural network is based on the PyTorch platform version 2.1.0+cu121.

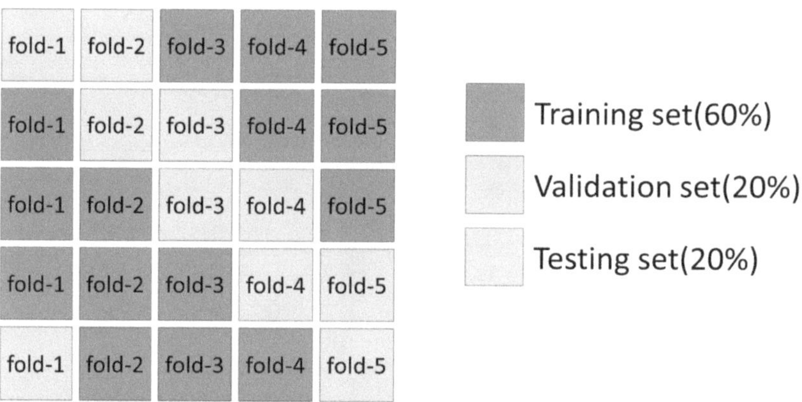

Figure 3. Fivefold cross-validation.

2.5. Visualization of the Imaging Features

Heatmap visualization using Grad-CAM [48] improves the comprehensibility of CNN outcomes. Every image produces heat maps that highlight the areas of focus for the deep-learning model. This method involves calculating the derivative of the CNN architecture's final convolutional layer output relative to each pixel of the input image. Pixels in the image with a higher influence appear nearer to the red spectrum on the heatmap, whereas those with a lesser influence are aligned closer to the blue spectrum.

2.6. Statistical Methods

Statistical Package for the Social Sciences version 22.0 (Chicago, IL, USA) was used for statistical analyses. Demographic comparisons between patients with high myopia group and those with high myopia glaucoma group were performed using independent t-tests or chi-square tests. p values of 0.05 were considered statistically significant. The metrics used to assess the model's efficacy encompass the area under the curve (AUC) of the receiver operating characteristic (ROC), accuracy, sensitivity, specificity, and F1 score. The ROC curve depicts the balance between sensitivity and the complement of the false positive rate (1—specificity). The AUC under the ROC curve was computed. An AUC value of 1.0 signifies flawless differentiation, whereas a value of 0.5 indicates discrimination equivalent to random chance. Accuracy is a metric that measures the proportion of correctly predicted instances among the total instances in a classification model. The F1 score is a metric that combines precision and sensitivity to evaluate the performance of a classification model, with values ranging from 0 to 1, where a higher score indicates a better model performance. The results of the fivefold cross-validation are averaged to assess generalizability.

3. Results

This study initially included 35,327 patients with 126,955 fundus photographs and 16,423 images with high myopia. After excluding patients who did not meet the conditions (n = 12,913) and those with poor image quality (n = 422), 1637 met the criteria. In total, there were 3088 fundus images, including those of 796 patients in the high myopia glaucoma group, with 1540 fundus images. Women accounted for 48.77% and 59.04% in the high myopia glaucoma and high myopia groups, respectively, in terms of gender ($p < 0.001$). The average age was 47.6 ± 12.0 and 46.4 ± 14.2 (p = 0.01). The average diopter was −8.83 ± 2.9 D and −8.73 ± 2.6 D (p = 0.30) (Table 1). The OCT parameters of the high myopia glaucoma group were as follows: average RNFL, 78.17 ± 15.2 μm; rim area, 0.9 ± 1.4 mm^2; disc area, 2.20 ± 2.9 mm^2; cup volume, 0.38 ± 0.38 mm^3; and average C/D area ratio, 0.71 ± 3.2. The VF parameters of the high myopia glaucoma group were as follows: average MD, −6.15 ± 7.5 dB and average VFI, 84.88% ± 22.6% (Table 1). Table 2 shows the number of images in the training, validation, and test sets in the fivefold cross-validation.

Table 1. Baseline demographics and clinical characteristics.

Variables	HM Glaucoma	HM	p Value
Patient	796	841	-
Eye (n)	1540	1548	-
Age (year)	47.6 ± 12.0	46.4 ± 14.2	**0.01**
Female (%)	48.77	59.04	**<0.001**
SE (diopter)	−8.83 ± 2.9	−8.73 ± 2.6	0.30
OCT parameters			
Average RNFL (um)	78.17 ± 15.2	-	-
Rim area (mm^2)	0.9 ± 1.4	-	-
Disc area (mm^2)	2.20 ± 2.9	-	-
Cup volume (mm^3)	0.38 ± 0.38	-	-
Average C/D area ratio	0.71 ± 3.2	-	-
VF parameters			
Average MD (dB)	−6.15 ± 7.5	-	-
Average VFI (%)	84.88 ± 22.6	-	-

RNFL: retinal nerve fiber layer; VF: visual field; VFI: visual field index; C/D: cup/disc. All data are presented as mean ± standard deviation, unless otherwise stated. Statistically significant values are denoted in bold.

Table 2. Fivefold cross-validation data distribution.

	Train		Validation		Test	
	HMG	HM	HMG	HM	HMG	HM
Fold-1	924	930	308	309	308	309
Fold-2	924	930	308	309	308	309
Fold-3	924	930	308	309	308	309
Fold-4	924	927	308	312	308	309
Fold-5	924	927	308	309	308	312

HMG: high myopia glaucoma; HM: high myopia.

Table 3 presents the classification performance of the various learning networks. The two different model architectures, EfficientNet_V2-S and ConvNeXt_Base, demonstrated AUCs of 0.86 and 0.870, accuracy of 79.34% and 78.85%, sensitivities of 79.22% and 74.67%, and specificities of 79.46% and 83.01%, F1 score of 79.27% and 77.89%, respectively. The results of using CBAM in the model architecture (EfficientNet_V2-S+CBAM and ConvNeXt_Base+CBAM) indicated AUCs of 0.885 and 0.894, accuracy of 81.38% and 82.16%, sensitivities of 76.56% and 81.04%, and specificities of 86.18% and 83.27%, F1 score of 80.40% and 81.92%, respectively. The results after using CBAM in the model architecture and adding patient characteristics (EfficientNet_V2-S+CBAM+Meta and ConvNeXt_Base+CBAM+Meta) showed AUCs of 0.879 and 0.893, accuracy of 80.38% and 81.77%, sensitivities of 77.62% and 77.60%, and specificities of 84.11% and 85.95%, F1 score of 79.57% and 80.93%, respectively. Figure 4 illustrates the ROC curves and AUC values of various learning networks.

Table 3. Classification performance of convolutional neural networks.

Model	AUC	Accuracy	Sensitivity	Specificity	F1 Score
EfficientNet_V2-S	0.861	79.34%	79.22%	79.46%	79.27%
ConvNeXt_Base	0.870	78.85%	74.67%	83.01%	77.89%
EfficientNet_V2-S+CBAM	0.885	81.38%	76.56%	86.18%	80.40%
ConvNeXt_Base+CBAM	0.894	82.16%	81.04%	83.27%	81.92%
EfficientNet_V2-S+CBAM+Meta	0.879	80.38%	76.62%	84.11%	79.57%
ConvNeXt_Base+CBAM+Meta	0.893	81.77%	77.60%	85.92%	80.93%

Meta, gender, age, and diopter.

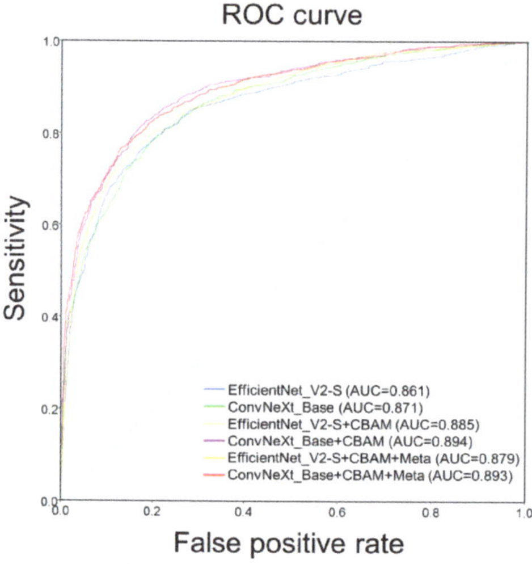

Figure 4. Operating characteristic curve of each classifier under different CNN architectures.

Figure 5 shows the confusion matrix of each classifier under different CNN architectures. The confusion matrices of EfficientNet_V2-S and ConvNeXt_Base were as follows: TP = 1220, 1150 images; FN = 320, 390 images; FP = 318, 263 images; and TN = 1230, 1285 images, respectively. The confusion matrices of EfficientNet_V2-S+CBAM and ConvNeXt_Base+CBAM were as follows: TP = 1179, 1248 images; FN = 361, 292 images; FP = 214, 259 images; and TN = 1334, 1289 images, respectively. The coefficient matrices of EfficientNet_V2-S+CBAM+Meta and ConvNeXt_Base+CBAM+Meta were as follows: TP = 1180, 1195 images; FN = 360, 345 images; FP = 246, 218 images; and TN = 1302, 1330 images, respectively. Figure 6 shows the visual image heat map under the ConvNeXt_Base+CBAM architecture. The upper row (a, b) shows high myopia and the lower row (c, d) exhibits high myopia glaucoma.

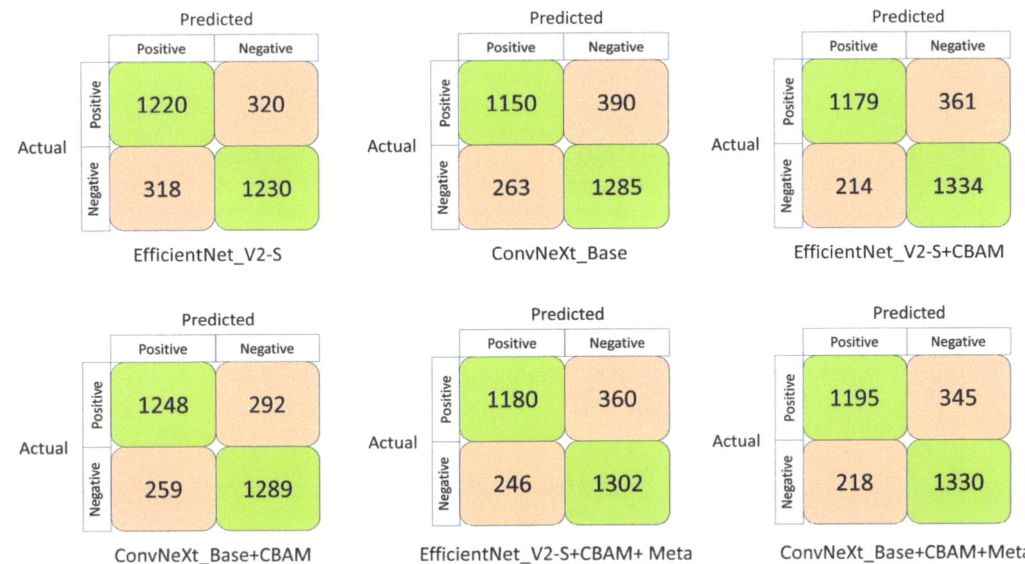

Figure 5. Confusion matrix of each classifier under different CNN architectures.

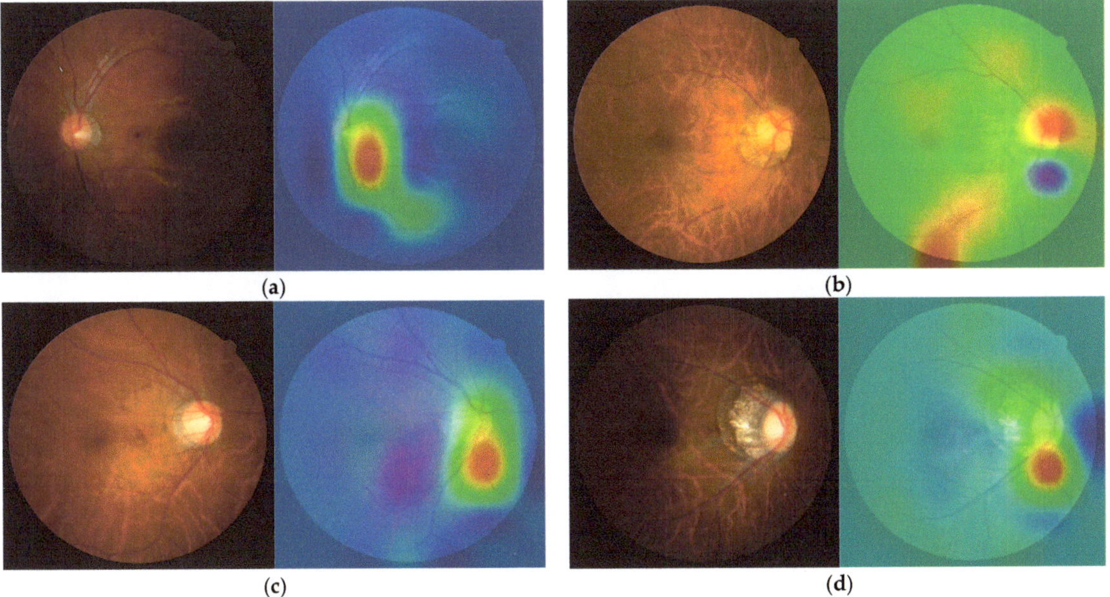

Figure 6. (**a**–**d**) Visual image heat maps. (**a**) Highly myopic left eye: diopter = −8.00 D, average RNFL = 105 µm, average C/D area ratio = 0.34, average MD = 0.78 dB, and normal GHT. (**b**) Highly myopic right eye: diopter = −8.50 D, average RNFL = 101 µm, average C/D area ratio = 0.41, average MD = 1.32 dB, and normal GHT. (**c**) High myopic glaucoma in the right eye: diopter = −10.25 D, average RNFL = 81 µm, average C/D area ratio = 0.56, average MD = −2.50 dB, and GHT outside the normal limits. (**d**) High myopic glaucoma in the right eye: diopter = −7.00 D, average RNFL = 76 µm, average C/D area ratio = 0.36, average MD = −2.21 dB, and GHT outside normal limits.

4. Discussion

This study investigates glaucoma through fundus photographs of highly myopic individuals and reveals good results in CNN deep learning. Glaucoma is the second leading cause of blindness globally after cataracts [49,50]. Screening for glaucoma is essential. OCT and visual field examination require ample time; thus, our study uses deep learning to provide a simple way to screen for glaucoma. This study indicates two differences. First, the use of fivefold cross-validation does not only use the model performance validation for a single test set, so the generalization ability and reliability of the model can be effectively improved during the training process. Second, we placed the CBAM behind the image input layer and in front of the fully connected layer, two positions used to enhance features. EfficientNet_V2-S and ConvNeXt_Base use ImageNet pretrained weights, with AUCs of 0.861 and 0.870, respectively. Table 3 shows that ConvNeXt_Base demonstrated a better performance. The use of CBAM demonstrated the AUC values of 0.885 and 0.894 in the EfficientNet_V2-S+CBAM and ConvNeXt_Base+CBAM models, respectively, indicating that CBAM improves model accuracy and exhibits good performance, which is consistent with previous research results [47]. EfficientNet_V2-S+CBAM+Meta and ConvNeXt_Base+CBAM+Meta added with more patient characteristics, including gender, age, and diopter, demonstrated AUC values of 0.879 and 0.893, respectively. Surprisingly, model performance decreased after adding patient characteristics. A significant difference in the male-to-female ratio was found between the high myopia group and the high myopia glaucoma group ($p < 0.001$), but the model performance did not improve after adding gender characteristics, and it did not affect the model performance in this study.

Although the incidence of high myopia is low, deep learning requires a large amount of data to improve performance of the model. Hence, pretraining was used, and it was combined with CBAM. Based on previous research [51–54], we utilized CNN models with different architectures, such as EfficientNet_V2-S, ConvNeXt_Base, ResNet50, and ViT_B_16. The model with a higher accuracy in ImageNet Top-1 image classification was used as a basis for the initial training. Finally, EfficientNet_V2-S and ConvNeXt_Base, which have a better performance, were selected as the final model architecture. Among the models, ConvNeXt_Base+CBAM had the highest sensitivity. Thus, it can be useful in providing assistance to professional ophthalmologists to obtain an accurate diagnosis. However, ConvNeXt_Base+CBAM and EfficientNet_V2-S+CBAM differ, EfficientNet_V2-S+CBAM has the best sensitivity and can assist other professionals, such as optometrists, family physicians, and non-ophthalmologists in screening patients who may have high myopia glaucoma.

Li et al. [36] and Cho et al. [55] included a C/D ratio of >0.7 to evaluate glaucoma and normal eyes. The AUCs of large-scale data sets were 0.986 and 0.975, both of which had a good performance. Previous studies have shown that a C/D ratio of >0.7 is characteristic of glaucoma [56], which may be one of the reasons why the model can improve glaucoma diagnosis. Among the inclusion conditions of this study, patients with high myopia and glaucoma were not restricted to a C/D ratio of >0.7. The C/D ratio of patients with high myopia is larger than that of people with normal eyes [14]; therefore, this is not specifically included in the condition. Shibata et al. [54] included only 55 patients with high myopia in a deep learning study. The images of high myopia with glaucoma can be diverse, and our research data can be more reliable when the number of images increases. Islam et al. [57] used four different deep-learning algorithms to diagnose glaucoma from cropped eye cup and fundus photographs. Among them, EfficientNet_b3 had the best test results, with an AUC score of 0.9512. In addition, satisfactory results were achieved using the U-net model for blood vessel segmentation on the full-eye color base map. However, although the cropped eye cup image can increase the training speed, it will sacrifice the possible sign impact of the images around the fundus. Therefore, the use of the whole fundus in our study can include more imaging parameters. Due to the black box effect in deep learning, we cannot fully understand the internal mechanism of the model. However, the accuracy of image diagnosis can be improved using the Grad-CAM technology. Further, an improved image quality can help improve diagnostic accuracy. In addition, we tried to verify the results of the ConvNeXt_Base+CBAM training model with the external data REFUGE test set. [58] The result had an AUC of 0.921, showing a certain degree of accuracy. We have demonstrated the use of deep learning to detect high myopic glaucoma, but there is still room for improvement. Kim et al. [37] used OCT data and combined demographic and ophthalmic characteristics, such as age, sex, axial length, and MD, to detect high myopic glaucoma. Therefore, a large amount of data resources and good results, with an AUC of 0.995, can be achieved. However, due to high equipment requirements, it is not easy to quickly screen and widely promote this method in clinical practice.

The study performed a Grad-CAM visual analysis of fundus photographs. The red areas in Figure 6a,c represent the pixels that contribute the most to the diagnostic results. Most pixels are located in the cup/disc area and neuroretinal rim and a few are located in the center of the macula, blood vessels, and other locations. This is consistent with the findings of ophthalmologists check when diagnosing glaucoma. In particular, the thermal imaging in parts of Figure 6a,b also focuses on the RNFL area. Additionally, it focuses on the highly myopic checkerboard-shaped fundus in Figure 6b,d.

In particular, this study excluded patients with pathological myopia, as there is a close relation between pathological myopia and glaucoma. Pathological myopia is defined as the presence of a myopic macula that is equal to or worse than diffuse chorioretinal atrophy. For local lesions [59], fundus features may be challenging to assess because the optic disc is severely tilted, deformed, and the optic nerve become thin. These features are similar to the pathological features of glaucoma, thereby making diagnosis more difficult. Future studies should consider including this patient population to completely evaluate the efficacy of deep-learning techniques in glaucoma diagnosis.

To the best of our knowledge, this is the first deep learning study to detect high myopic glaucoma from a large number of fundus photographs. Diagnosing glaucoma in ophthalmology requires multiple reference data and structural changes (intraocular pressure, OCT data, visual field data, fundus photographs, etc.), and diagnosis is only made after long-term observation. According to the myopia rate prediction report for 2050 [2], the incidence rate of high myopia among older adults will increase annually, and more people will develop age-related glaucoma. Consequently, glaucoma in highly myopic eyes will be challenging to diagnose and, currently, is a major public health issue. Our research used deep-learning methods and the fundus photography technology to address this difficulty. AI-assisted diagnosis can be applied in the field of ophthalmology in the future. For example, it can help non-ophthalmologists, such as optometrists and family physicians, make referrals or directly assist ophthalmologists in making accurate and rapid diagnoses. Overall, our study provides a feasible option for deep learning of fundus photographs to differentiate high myopia from glaucoma.

This study has some limitations. First, this study only included one ethnic group of Asians, and thus results should be interpreted with caution when applied to other ethnic groups. Second, we have not classified the degree of glaucoma. Different degrees of glaucoma are structurally different. Third, our data included no externally verified fundus photographs data; therefore, we cannot infer other image types, which reduce the generalization ability of the model. Fourth, there are insufficient OCT and visual field parameters in the high myopia group based on a medical record review. Although we have been extremely cautious in screening, these cases may still be misclassified. It is possible to increase sensitivity; however, glaucoma specialists should examine more eyes. Finally, patients with pathological myopia were excluded from the study. Hence, more clinicians will find it challenging to distinguish pathological myopia from glaucoma. Therefore, future studies should focus on this direction.

5. Conclusions

Glaucoma in individuals with high myopia was identified from their fundus photographs.

Supplementary Materials: The following supporting information can be downloaded at: https://www.mdpi.com/article/10.3390/biomedicines12071394/s1, Figure (a),(b): High Myopia; Figure (c),(d): Glaucoma.

Author Contributions: Conceptualization, Y.-Y.C. and Y.-H.C.; methodology, Y.-Y.C., C.-L.C. and Y.-H.C.; software, Y.-Y.C.; formal analysis, C.-L.C.; writing—original draft preparation, Y.-Y.C.; writing—review and editing, Y.-H.C.; visualization, Y.-Y.C.; supervision, C.-L.C. and Y.-H.C.; Writing—review and editing Y.-Y.C., C.-L.C. and Y.-H.C. All authors have read and agreed to the published version of the manuscript.

Funding: This study was supported by Tri-Service General Hospital, Taipei, Taiwan, Grant Numbers: TSGH-E-113269.

Institutional Review Board Statement: The study was conducted in accordance with the Declaration of Helsinki, and approved by the research ethics committee of the Tri-Service General Hospital (TSGHIRB No. C202305105) and date of approval 9 September 2023.

Informed Consent Statement: Patient consent was waived due to the retrospective nature of the study and the de-identification of personal identifiers.

Data Availability Statement: The present data belong to and are stored at the Tri-Service General Hospital and cannot be shared without permission.

Conflicts of Interest: The authors declare no conflicts of interest.

References

1. George, A.S.; George, A.H.; Shahul, A. The Myopia Epidemic: A Growing Public Health Crisis Impacting Children Worldwide. *Partn. Univers. Int. Res. J.* **2023**, *2*, 120–138.
2. Holden, B.A.; Fricke, T.R.; Wilson, D.A.; Jong, M.; Naidoo, K.S.; Sankaridurg, P.; Wong, T.Y.; Naduvilath, T.J.; Resnikoff, S. Global Prevalence of Myopia and High Myopia and Temporal Trends from 2000 through 2050. *Ophthalmology* **2016**, *123*, 1036–1042. [CrossRef] [PubMed]
3. Spaeth, G.L. European Glaucoma Society Terminology and Guidelines for Glaucoma. *Br. J. Ophthalmol.* **2021**, *105* (Suppl. S1), 1–169. [CrossRef]
4. Flammer, J.; Mozaffarieh, M. What Is the Present Pathogenetic Concept of Glaucomatous Optic Neuropathy? *Surv. Ophthalmol.* **2007**, *52*, S162–S173. [CrossRef] [PubMed]
5. Schacknow, P.N.; Samples, J.R. *The Glaucoma Book: A Practical, Evidence-Based Approach to Patient Care*; Springer Science & Business Media: New York, NY, USA, 2010.
6. Tham, Y.-C.; Li, X.; Wong, T.Y.; Quigley, H.A.; Aung, T.; Cheng, C.-Y. Global Prevalence of Glaucoma and Projections of Glaucoma Burden through 2040: A Systematic Review and Meta-Analysis. *Ophthalmology* **2014**, *121*, 2081–2090. [CrossRef] [PubMed]
7. Quigley, H.A.; Broman, A.T. The number of people with glaucoma worldwide in 2010 and 2020. *Br. J. Ophthalmol.* **2006**, *90*, 262–267. [CrossRef] [PubMed]
8. Guedes, G.; Tsai, J.C.; Loewen, N.A. Glaucoma and aging. *Curr. Aging Sci.* **2011**, *4*, 110–117. [CrossRef] [PubMed]
9. Choi, E.Y.; Wong, R.C.S.; Thein, T.; Pasquale, L.R.; Shen, L.Q.; Wang, M.; Li, D.; Jin, Q.; Wang, H.; Baniasadi, N.; et al. The Effect of Ametropia on Glaucomatous Visual Field Loss. *J. Clin. Med.* **2021**, *10*, 2796. [CrossRef] [PubMed]
10. Marcus, M.W.; de Vries, M.M.; Montolio, F.G.J.; Jansonius, N.M. Myopia as a Risk Factor for Open-Angle Glaucoma: A Systematic Review and Meta-Analysis. *Ophthalmology* **2011**, *118*, 1989–1994.e2. [CrossRef] [PubMed]
11. Haarman, A.E.G.; Enthoven, C.A.; Tideman, J.W.L.; Tedja, M.S.; Verhoeven, V.J.M.; Klaver, C.C.W. The Complications of Myopia: A Review and Meta-Analysis. *Investig. Ophthalmol. Vis. Sci.* **2020**, *61*, 49. [CrossRef]
12. Ha, A.; Kim, C.Y.; Shim, S.R.; Chang, I.B.; Kim, Y.K. Degree of myopia and glaucoma risk: A dose-response meta-analysis. *Am. J. Ophthalmol.* **2022**, *236*, 107–119. [CrossRef] [PubMed]
13. Tan, N.Y.Q.; Sng, C.C.A.; Jonas, J.B.; Wong, T.Y.; Jansonius, N.M.; Ang, M. Glaucoma in myopia: Diagnostic dilemmas. *Br. J. Ophthalmol.* **2019**, *103*, 1347–1355. [CrossRef] [PubMed]
14. Lan, Y.W.; Chang, S.Y.; Sun, F.J.; Hsieh, J.W. Different Disc Characteristics Associated With High Myopia and the Location of Glaucomatous Damage in Primary Open-Angle Glaucoma and Normal-Tension Glaucoma. *J. Glaucoma* **2019**, *28*, 519–528. [CrossRef] [PubMed]
15. Lu, Y.; Ji, Z.; Jia, J.; Shi, R.; Liu, Y.; Shu, Q.; Lu, F.; Ge, T.; He, Y. Progress in clinical characteristics of high myopia with primary open-angle glaucoma. *Biotechnol. Genet. Eng. Rev.* **2023**, 1–20. [CrossRef] [PubMed]
16. Dichtl, A.; Jonas, J.B.; Naumann, G.O. Histomorphometry of the optic disc in highly myopic eyes with absolute secondary angle closure glaucoma. *Br. J. Ophthalmol.* **1998**, *82*, 286–289. [CrossRef] [PubMed]
17. Hoffmann, E.M.; Zangwill, L.M.; Crowston, J.G.; Weinreb, R.N. Optic disk size and glaucoma. *Surv. Ophthalmol.* **2007**, *52*, 32–49. [CrossRef] [PubMed]

18. Quigley, H.A.; Addicks, E.M.; Green, W.R.; Maumenee, A. Optic nerve damage in human glaucoma: II. The site of injury and susceptibility to damage. *Arch. Ophthalmol.* **1981**, *99*, 635–649. [CrossRef] [PubMed]
19. Tuulonen, A.; Airaksinen, P.J. Initial glaucomatous optic disk and retinal nerve fiber layer abnormalities and their progression. *Am. J. Ophthalmol.* **1991**, *111*, 485–490. [CrossRef] [PubMed]
20. Jonas, J.B.; Fernández, M.C.; Stürmer, J. Pattern of glaucomatous neuroretinal rim loss. *Ophthalmology* **1993**, *100*, 63–68. [CrossRef] [PubMed]
21. Jonas, J.B.; Wang, Y.X.; Dong, L.; Panda-Jonas, S. High Myopia and Glaucoma-Like Optic Neuropathy. *Asia Pac. J. Ophthalmol.* **2020**, *9*, 234–238. [CrossRef] [PubMed]
22. Qiu, K.; Wang, G.; Lu, X.; Zhang, R.; Sun, L.; Zhang, M. Application of the ISNT rules on retinal nerve fibre layer thickness and neuroretinal rim area in healthy myopic eyes. *Acta Ophthalmol.* **2018**, *96*, 161–167. [CrossRef] [PubMed]
23. Zhang, Y.; Wen, W.; Sun, X. Comparison of Several Parameters in Two Optical Coherence Tomography Systems for Detecting Glaucomatous Defects in High Myopia. *Investig. Ophthalmol. Vis. Sci.* **2016**, *57*, 4910–4915. [CrossRef] [PubMed]
24. Hung, K.C.; Wu, P.C.; Poon, Y.C.; Chang, H.W.; Lai, I.C.; Tsai, J.C.; Lin, P.W.; Teng, M.C. Macular Diagnostic Ability in OCT for Assessing Glaucoma in High Myopia. *Optom. Vis. Sci.* **2016**, *93*, 126–135. [CrossRef] [PubMed]
25. Kimura, Y.; Hangai, M.; Morooka, S.; Takayama, K.; Nakano, N.; Nukada, M.; Ikeda, H.O.; Akagi, T.; Yoshimura, N. Retinal nerve fiber layer defects in highly myopic eyes with early glaucoma. *Investig. Ophthalmol. Vis. Sci.* **2012**, *53*, 6472–6478. [CrossRef] [PubMed]
26. Lin, P.W.; Chang, H.W.; Poon, Y.C. Retinal Thickness Asymmetry in Highly Myopic Eyes with Early Stage of Normal-Tension Glaucoma. *J. Ophthalmol.* **2021**, *2021*, 6660631. [CrossRef] [PubMed]
27. Vinod, K.; Salim, S. Addressing Glaucoma in Myopic Eyes: Diagnostic and Surgical Challenges. *Bioengineering* **2023**, *10*, 1260. [CrossRef] [PubMed]
28. Li, Z.; Liu, F.; Yang, W.; Peng, S.; Zhou, J. A survey of convolutional neural networks: Analysis, applications, and prospects. *IEEE Trans. Neural Netw. Learn. Syst.* **2021**, *33*, 6999–7019. [CrossRef] [PubMed]
29. Weiss, K.; Khoshgoftaar, T.M.; Wang, D. A survey of transfer learning. *J. Big Data* **2016**, *3*, 1–40. [CrossRef]
30. Alyoubi, W.L.; Shalash, W.M.; Abulkhair, M.F. Diabetic retinopathy detection through deep learning techniques: A review. *Inform. Med. Unlocked* **2020**, *20*, 100377. [CrossRef]
31. Abbas, Q. Glaucoma-deep: Detection of glaucoma eye disease on retinal fundus images using deep learning. *Int. J. Adv. Comput. Sci. Appl.* **2017**, *8*, 41–45. [CrossRef]
32. Nunez, R.; Harris, A.; Ibrahim, O.; Keller, J.; Wikle, C.K.; Robinson, E.; Zukerman, R.; Siesky, B.; Verticchio, A.; Rowe, L.; et al. Artificial Intelligence to Aid Glaucoma Diagnosis and Monitoring: State of the Art and New Directions. *Photonics* **2022**, *9*, 810. [CrossRef] [PubMed]
33. Peng, Y.; Dharssi, S.; Chen, Q.; Keenan, T.D.; Agrón, E.; Wong, W.T.; Chew, E.Y.; Lu, Z. DeepSeeNet: A deep learning model for automated classification of patient-based age-related macular degeneration severity from color fundus photographs. *Ophthalmology* **2019**, *126*, 565–575. [CrossRef] [PubMed]
34. Du, R.; Xie, S.; Fang, Y.; Igarashi-Yokoi, T.; Moriyama, M.; Ogata, S.; Tsunoda, T.; Kamatani, T.; Yamamoto, S.; Cheng, C.-Y. Deep learning approach for automated detection of myopic maculopathy and pathologic myopia in fundus images. *Ophthalmol. Retin.* **2021**, *5*, 1235–1244. [CrossRef] [PubMed]
35. Bragança, C.P.; Torres, J.M.; Macedo, L.O.; Soares, C.P.d.A. Advancements in Glaucoma Diagnosis: The Role of AI in Medical Imaging. *Diagnostics* **2024**, *14*, 530. [CrossRef] [PubMed]
36. Li, Z.; He, Y.; Keel, S.; Meng, W.; Chang, R.T.; He, M. Efficacy of a Deep Learning System for Detecting Glaucomatous Optic Neuropathy Based on Color Fundus Photographs. *Ophthalmology* **2018**, *125*, 1199–1206. [CrossRef] [PubMed]
37. Kim, J.-A.; Yoon, H.; Lee, D.; Kim, M.; Choi, J.; Lee, E.J.; Kim, T.-W. Development of a deep learning system to detect glaucoma using macular vertical optical coherence tomography scans of myopic eyes. *Sci. Rep.* **2023**, *13*, 8040. [CrossRef] [PubMed]
38. Asaoka, R.; Murata, H.; Iwase, A.; Araie, M. Detecting Preperimetric Glaucoma with Standard Automated Perimetry Using a Deep Learning Classifier. *Ophthalmology* **2016**, *123*, 1974–1980. [CrossRef] [PubMed]
39. Thakur, S.; Dinh, L.L.; Lavanya, R.; Quek, T.C.; Liu, Y.; Cheng, C.-Y. Use of artificial intelligence in forecasting glaucoma progression. *Taiwan J. Ophthalmol.* **2023**, *13*, 168–183. [PubMed]
40. Anton, A.; Nolivos, K.; Pazos, M.; Fatti, G.; Ayala, M.E.; Martínez-Prats, E.; Peral, O.; Poposki, V.; Tsiroukis, E.; Morilla-Grasa, A.; et al. Diagnostic Accuracy and Detection Rate of Glaucoma Screening with Optic Disk Photos, Optical Coherence Tomography Images, and Telemedicine. *J. Clin. Med.* **2022**, *11*, 216. [CrossRef] [PubMed]
41. Flitcroft, D.I.; He, M.; Jonas, J.B.; Jong, M.; Naidoo, K.; Ohno-Matsui, K.; Rahi, J.; Resnikoff, S.; Vitale, S.; Yannuzzi, L. IMI–Defining and classifying myopia: A proposed set of standards for clinical and epidemiologic studies. *Investig. Ophthalmol. Vis. Sci.* **2019**, *60*, M20–M30. [CrossRef] [PubMed]
42. Abdulnabi, A.H.; Wang, G.; Lu, J.; Jia, K. Multi-task CNN model for attribute prediction. *IEEE Trans. Multimed.* **2015**, *17*, 1949–1959. [CrossRef]
43. Wang, W.; Jiang, X.; Yuan, H.; Chen, J.; Wang, X.; Huang, Z. Research on Algorithm for Authenticating the Authenticity of Calligraphy Works Based on Improved EfficientNet Network. *Appl. Sci.* **2023**, *14*, 295. [CrossRef]
44. Liu, Z.; Mao, H.; Wu, C.-Y.; Feichtenhofer, C.; Darrell, T.; Xie, S. A convnet for the 2020s. In Proceedings of the IEEE/CVF Conference on Computer Vision and Pattern Recognition, New Orleans, LA, USA, 18–24 June 2022; pp. 11976–11986.

45. Deng, J.; Dong, W.; Socher, R.; Li, L.-J.; Li, K.; Fei-Fei, L. Imagenet: A large-scale hierarchical image database. In Proceedings of the 2009 IEEE Conference on Computer Vision and Pattern Recognition, Miami, FL, USA, 20–25 June 2009; pp. 248–255.
46. Loshchilov, I.; Hutter, F. Decoupled Weight Decay Regularization. *arXiv* **2019**, arXiv:1711.05101.
47. Woo, S.; Park, J.; Lee, J.-Y.; Kweon, I.S. Cbam: Convolutional block attention module. In Proceedings of the European Conference on Computer Vision (ECCV), Munich, Germany, 8–14 September 2018; pp. 3–19.
48. Selvaraju, R.R.; Cogswell, M.; Das, A.; Vedantam, R.; Parikh, D.; Batra, D. Grad-cam: Visual explanations from deep networks via gradient-based localization. In Proceedings of the IEEE International Conference on Computer Vision, Venice, Italy, 22–29 October 2017; pp. 618–626.
49. Zhang, N.; Wang, J.; Li, Y.; Jiang, B. Prevalence of primary open angle glaucoma in the last 20 years: A meta-analysis and systematic review. *Sci. Rep.* **2021**, *11*, 13762. [CrossRef] [PubMed]
50. Blindness, G.B.D.; Vision Impairment, C.; Vision Loss Expert Group of the Global Burden of Disease, S. Causes of blindness and vision impairment in 2020 and trends over 30 years, and prevalence of avoidable blindness in relation to VISION 2020: The Right to Sight: An analysis for the Global Burden of Disease Study. *Lancet Glob. Health* **2021**, *9*, e144–e160. [CrossRef]
51. Alghamdi, M.; Abdel-Mottaleb, M. A comparative study of deep learning models for diagnosing glaucoma from fundus images. *IEEE Access* **2021**, *9*, 23894–23906. [CrossRef]
52. Chen, D.; Ran, E.A.; Tan, T.F.; Ramachandran, R.; Li, F.; Cheung, C.; Yousefi, S.; Tham, C.C.Y.; Ting, D.S.W.; Zhang, X.; et al. Applications of Artificial Intelligence and Deep Learning in Glaucoma. *Asia-Pac. J. Ophthalmol.* **2023**, *12*, 80–93. [CrossRef] [PubMed]
53. Zedan, M.J.M.; Zulkifley, M.A.; Ibrahim, A.A.; Moubark, A.M.; Kamari, N.A.M.; Abdani, S.R. Automated Glaucoma Screening and Diagnosis Based on Retinal Fundus Images Using Deep Learning Approaches: A Comprehensive Review. *Diagnostics* **2023**, *13*, 2180. [CrossRef] [PubMed]
54. Shibata, N.; Tanito, M.; Mitsuhashi, K.; Fujino, Y.; Matsuura, M.; Murata, H.; Asaoka, R. Development of a deep residual learning algorithm to screen for glaucoma from fundus photography. *Sci. Rep.* **2018**, *8*, 14665. [CrossRef] [PubMed]
55. Cho, H.; Hwang, Y.H.; Chung, J.K.; Lee, K.B.; Park, J.S.; Kim, H.-G.; Jeong, J.H. Deep Learning Ensemble Method for Classifying Glaucoma Stages Using Fundus Photographs and Convolutional Neural Networks. *Curr. Eye Res.* **2021**, *46*, 1516–1524. [CrossRef] [PubMed]
56. Ng, M.; Sample, P.A.; Pascual, J.P.; Zangwill, L.M.; Girkin, C.A.; Liebmann, J.M.; Weinreb, R.N.; Racette, L. Comparison of visual field severity classification systems for glaucoma. *J. Glaucoma* **2012**, *21*, 551. [CrossRef] [PubMed]
57. Islam, M.T.; Mashfu, S.T.; Faisal, A.; Siam, S.C.; Naheen, I.T.; Khan, R. Deep learning-based glaucoma detection with cropped optic cup and disc and blood vessel segmentation. *IEEE Access* **2021**, *10*, 2828–2841. [CrossRef]
58. Orlando, J.I.; Fu, H.; Barbosa Breda, J.; van Keer, K.; Bathula, D.R.; Diaz-Pinto, A.; Fang, R.; Heng, P.-A.; Kim, J.; Lee, J.; et al. REFUGE Challenge: A unified framework for evaluating automated methods for glaucoma assessment from fundus photographs. *Med. Image Anal.* **2020**, *59*, 101570. [CrossRef] [PubMed]
59. Ohno-Matsui, K. Pathologic Myopia. *Asia-Pac. J. Ophthalmol.* **2016**, *5*, 415–423. [CrossRef] [PubMed]

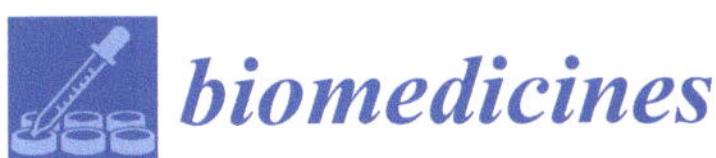

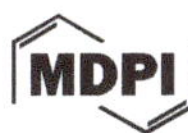

Article

Diagnosis of Glaucoma Based on Few-Shot Learning with Wide-Field Optical Coherence Tomography Angiography

Kyoung Ok Yang [1,†], Jung Min Lee [2,†], Younji Shin [3], In Young Yoon [3], Jun Won Choi [3,4,*] and Won June Lee [2,5,*]

1 Department of Artificial Intelligence, Hanyang University, Seoul 04763, Republic of Korea; koyang@spa.hanyang.ac.kr
2 Department of Ophthalmology, Hanyang University Seoul Hospital, Seoul 04763, Republic of Korea; jjungmin250@gmail.com
3 Department of Electrical Engineering, Hanyang University, Seoul 04763, Republic of Korea; yjshin@spa.hanyang.ac.kr (Y.S.); inyoungyoon@spa.hanyang.ac.kr (I.Y.Y.)
4 Department of Electrical and Computer Engineering, College of Liberal Studies, Seoul National University, Seoul 08826, Republic of Korea
5 Department of Ophthalmology, Hanyang University College of Medicine, Seoul 04763, Republic of Korea
* Correspondence: junwchoi@snu.ac.kr (J.W.C.); wonjunelee@hanyang.ac.kr (W.J.L.); Tel.: +82-2-880-8487 (J.W.C.); +82-2-2290-8570 (W.J.L.)
† These authors contributed equally to this work.

Abstract: This study evaluated the utility of incorporating deep learning into the relatively novel imaging technique of wide-field optical coherence tomography angiography (WF-OCTA) for glaucoma diagnosis. To overcome the challenge of limited data associated with this emerging imaging, the application of few-shot learning (FSL) was explored, and the advantages observed during its implementation were examined. A total of 195 eyes, comprising 82 normal controls and 113 patients with glaucoma, were examined in this study. The system was trained using FSL instead of traditional supervised learning. Model training can be presented in two distinct ways. Glaucoma feature detection was performed using ResNet18 as a feature extractor. To implement FSL, the ProtoNet algorithm was utilized to perform task-independent classification. Using this trained model, the performance of WF-OCTA through the FSL technique was evaluated. We trained the WF-OCTA validation method with 10 normal and 10 glaucoma images and subsequently examined the glaucoma detection effectiveness. FSL using the WF-OCTA image achieved an area under the receiver operating characteristic curve (AUC) of 0.93 (95% confidence interval (CI): 0.912–0.954) and an accuracy of 81%. In contrast, supervised learning using WF-OCTA images produced worse results than FSL, with an AUC of 0.80 (95% CI: 0.778–0.823) and an accuracy of 50% (p-values < 0.05). Furthermore, the FSL method using WF-OCTA images demonstrated improvement over the conventional OCT parameter-based results (all p-values < 0.05). This study demonstrated the effectiveness of applying deep learning to WF-OCTA for glaucoma diagnosis, highlighting the potential of WF-OCTA images in glaucoma diagnostics. Additionally, it showed that FSL could overcome the limitations associated with a small dataset and is expected to be applicable in various clinical settings.

Keywords: deep learning; image processing; glaucoma; diagnostic ability; few-shot learning

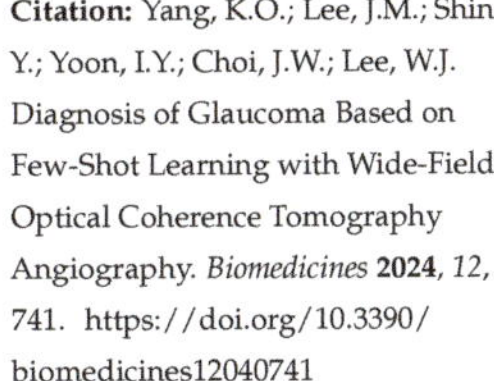

Citation: Yang, K.O.; Lee, J.M.; Shin, Y.; Yoon, I.Y.; Choi, J.W.; Lee, W.J. Diagnosis of Glaucoma Based on Few-Shot Learning with Wide-Field Optical Coherence Tomography Angiography. *Biomedicines* **2024**, *12*, 741. https://doi.org/10.3390/biomedicines12040741

Academic Editor: Da-Wen Lu

Received: 22 February 2024
Revised: 15 March 2024
Accepted: 16 March 2024
Published: 27 March 2024

1. Introduction

Glaucoma refers to a disease that involves specific morphologic changes in the optic nerve resulting in functional changes in the visual field due to loss of the retinal nerve fiber layer (RNFL) [1,2]. Disc photography, optical coherence tomography (OCT) [3–9], and OCT angiography (OCTA) are among the various imaging devices used for diagnosing glaucoma. The diagnostic data are presented as images or numerical values, depending on the instrument used. Among these techniques, OCTA is a non-invasive imaging method that assesses the vasculature of the retina and optic nerve without the need for dye injection [10,11]. Changes in vessel density in OCTA align with functional and structural alterations detected through visual field exams and OCT scans, providing good consistency and effectively distinguishing between the glaucomatous and the normal eyes.

Wide-field OCTA (WF-OCTA), which overcomes the limited field of view in traditional OCTA, is emerging as one of the new diagnostic imaging approaches for retinal disease and glaucoma [12–16]. WF-OCTA's scanning capabilities have been improved with technical advancements, such as swept-source OCT (SS-OCT), now allowing the examination of large areas of the posterior pole, encompassing both the optic nerve head and macula. Notably, when examining pathologic eyes with structural distortion of the optic disc, such as high myopia or retinal diseases, including epiretinal membrane and peripapillary retinoschisis, errors may occur in measuring conventional RNFL thickness maps. Additionally, WF-OCTA displays broader angiographic data in comparison to conventional imaging. This could potentially enhance the accuracy of glaucoma diagnosis, especially when other pathological alterations in the eyes complicate the process.

This study evaluates the accuracy of a deep-learning (DL) algorithm using WF-OCTA for identifying glaucoma. DL image classification is being assessed as a pre-diagnostic tool before human diagnosis. Sufficient data are crucial for effectively training DL networks for image classification in medical imaging diagnosis. Insufficient data can result in issues like overfitting and underfitting. Collecting sufficient medical data for training is a challenge due to limited data availability and privacy concerns. Furthermore, the clinical stage of WF-OCTA—the technology utilized in this study—creates difficulties in obtaining adequate data.

In recent years, few-shot learning (FSL) has emerged as a promising approach in DL, particularly in scenarios where limited annotated data are available. Unlike traditional supervised learning methods, which rely on large, labeled datasets for training, FSL enables models to generalize to new tasks with only a small amount of annotated data, mimicking human learning processes with limited examples [17]. The relationship between dataset size and accuracy in machine learning, including FSL, is complex. While larger datasets typically offer more diverse examples for model training, several factors impact this relationship. High-quality, well-annotated data are crucial for training accurate models, and task complexity and model architecture also influence performance [18]. Imbalanced data distributions and the use of regularization techniques further shape the interplay between dataset size and accuracy [19]. In the context of FSL, dataset size plays a crucial role in model performance. Although FSL techniques can handle limited data scenarios, increasing the dataset size can significantly enhance performance, especially if the additional data includes rare cases or provides greater diversity [20]. It is essential to understand these dynamics to optimize model performance and effectively utilize available data resources.

In such situations, implementing the FSL [21–23] approach may be a way to overcome this challenge. FSL methodology permits machine learning from a small number of samples, usually less than 10. Therefore, this study assessed the diagnostic potential of WF-OCTA for detecting glaucoma using an FSL approach to overcome data scarcity.

2. Materials and Methods

This study's protocol was approved by the Institutional Review Board (IRB) of Hanyang University Hospital, Seoul, Republic of Korea (IRB number: HYUH 2021-07-036). This study was designed in accordance with the tenets of the Declaration of Helsinki for biomedical research. The need for participant consent for retrospective data assessment was waived by the ethics committee.

2.1. Study Design and Participants

In this retrospective, comparative study, a total of 195 eyes were examined at Hanyang University Seoul Hospital Glaucoma Clinic between December 2021 and December 2022. Of these, 82 eyes were affected with glaucoma, and 113 controls were without glaucoma.

All participants underwent WF-OCTA imaging with the same SS-OCT device (Topcon, DRI OCT Triton), and the glaucoma was diagnosed by a glaucoma specialist. Diagnosis of glaucoma and selection of the control group were performed similarly to that in previous studies (Supplementary Materials) [24,25]. To eliminate ambiguity, this study excluded patients with high myopia (sph < −6.0D), retinal diseases, and glaucoma suspect states without definite visual field impairment or RNFL defects.

2.2. WF-OCTA

The wide-field 12 × 12 mm OCTA scan generates an en-face image of retinal vessels through various segmented layers. The SS-WF-OCTA scans volumes centered on the retina within a 12 × 12 mm field of view at a scan rate of 100,000 A-scans per second, offering a lateral resolution of 20 um. The device's built-in software corrects actual refraction to prevent refractometric degradation. The report of the WF-OCTA scan for the 12 × 12 area overlaps with the RNFL or ganglion cell–inner plexiform layer (GCIPL)/ganglion cell complex (GCC) thickness map on the WF-OCTA image.

Figure 1 displays (A) the OCT RNFL thickness map used in pre-training and the three types of WF-OCTA images in the FSL, (B) a combination of WF-OCTA and RNFL thickness map (Combi 1), (C) a combination of WF-OCTA and GCC thickness map (Combi 2), and (D) WF-OCTA itself (black and white). Apart from the WF-OCTA, this work evaluated the vessel density using optic disc OCTA (4.5 × 4.5 mm). The vessel density of the superficial capillary plexus (SCP) was assessed in four groups, superior, nasal, inferior, and temporal, to determine whether the vessel density had decreased.

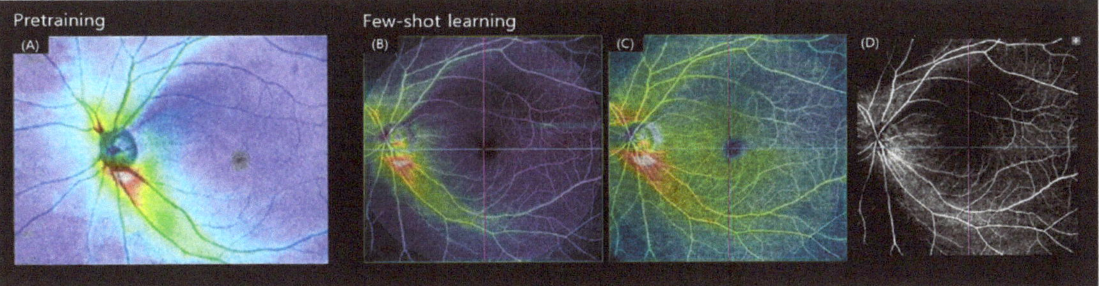

Figure 1. Dataset examples for pre-training and FSL: (**A**) SS-OCT RNFL thickness map (12 × 9 mm) used in pretraining, (**B**) WF-OCTA-RNFL Combi, (**C**) WF-OCTA-GCC Combi, and (**D**) WF-OCTA used for FSL.

2.3. DL Techniques: Image Classification on Medical Diagnosis

Medical image classification is pivotal in clinical treatment and early diagnosis. However, traditional methods have demonstrated limited performance and often require significant time and effort to identify and select features for classification. DL methods have surpassed the performance of some existing models and streamlined the design process through a data-driven approach. In particular, the supervised learning (SL) method using DL networks has achieved great success in various image classification tasks [26–28]. As the parameters of DL networks for image classification tend to be large, a large amount of training data is required to train networks. However, when it comes to medical image classification, the preparation of extensive training datasets demands costly and time-consuming manual annotations by medical professionals. Moreover, the distribution of medical data can be significantly imbalanced. Acquiring a vast amount of normal data might be easy; however, obtaining negative samples is challenging due to the rarity of certain disease cases. To address this issue, a training approach capable of accurately diagnosing diseases with a very limited amount of data was required. FSL aims to make predictions in situations where only a few examples are available for each class [29]. This study presents an effective glaucoma detection method leveraging the FSL method.

Data used in FSL can be broadly classified into three categories: training set, support set, and query set [30] (Figure 2). Additionally, the 'class' used in FSL refers to the group of objects that the model is trying to learn and distinguish from other classes. FSL initially learns how to distinguish between classes through the training set with a large amount of data. Then, through the support set, FSL learns from only a small amount of data for each class that is not present in the training set. When a query sample is input, the system compares which class of the support set is most similar to the answer.

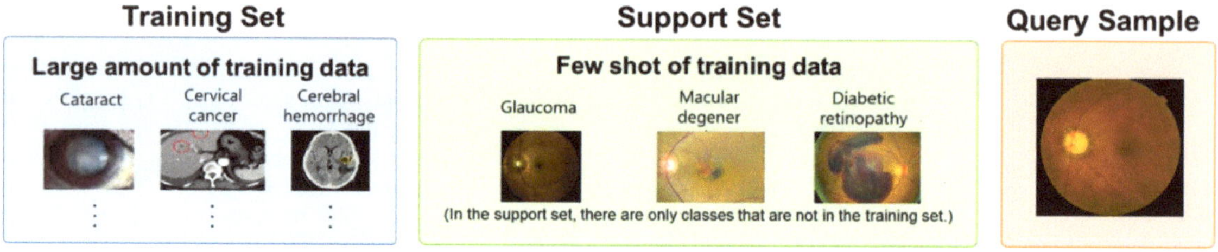

Figure 2. Categorization of datasets in FSL. The training set is used to train a deep-learning network to extract task-specific features from images. The support set is a small set of data points (e.g., 1, 2, 5, 10, etc.) used for training an FSL model for a new task. The query sample is data to evaluate the effectiveness of a network trained on a limited dataset.

ProtoNet [31] is an FSL method that uses a prototype that represents each class or concept as a central reference point in the feature space. During training, the model learns to create a prototype from a few labeled examples, using DL networks such as convolutional neural networks to extract meaningful features from the input data. The prototype is computed as the average feature vector of the supporting examples belonging to each class, and during the inference step, the model compares the query example to the prototype and assigns it to the class with the closest prototype. ProtoNet utilizes a metric learning objective function, enabling effective learning with limited data. This capability allows the model to differentiate between various classes and apply to new instances.

2.4. DL Techniques: Proposed Method

This study proposes a ProtoNet-based network for predicting WF-OCTA through DL. The ProtoNet-based network comprises a feature-extracting backbone network and a true/false classifying clustering module. The backbone network varies based on the size and type of data in both networks. Moreover, ResNet18 was deployed as our backbone network [27].

ResNet18 is trained on a very large dataset, such as ImageNet [32] (1.2 million images stored in 1000 categories), using a pre-trained model [33]. We can utilize the pre-trained model as an initialization or a fixed feature extractor and employ the transfer learning method [34]. Transfer learning is a DL method in which a model trained for one task is repurposed for a related second task. We utilized the weight of the backbone network by applying this fine-tuning of the transfer learning method with SS-OCT images [24,25] using ResNet18 pre-trained with ImageNet (Figure S1). For pre-training, the SS-OCT RNFL thickness map (12 × 9 mm) of glaucoma and normal groups was used (Figure 1). The data from the patient group in our existing study (*Journal of Glaucoma*) was used [25], and a total of 417 eyes with glaucoma and 258 normal eyes were included.

From this point forward, this discussion focuses on the process of acquiring knowledge about ProtoNet's clustering module through training and testing. To train the clustering module, Mini-ImageNet [35], a modified version of ImageNet for FSL, was utilized. Training with WF-OCTA introduces a potential risk of overfitting, as the model may become too specialized in WF-OCTA data. As each patient demonstrates different glaucoma symptoms in the data, overfitting the training data increases the risk of incorrect predictions for new patients. To mitigate this, we trained ProtoNet on Mini-ImageNet to establish a general understanding of the difference between similarity and dissimilarity.

Finally, the network's performance on WF-OCTA data was evaluated in the test or inference phase. We trained the neural network on WF-OCTA data from 10 patients with glaucoma and 10 normal individuals, forming a support set. Few-shot training, in this case, refers to the adaptation of a pre-existing network to a new task with minimal input, specifically for glaucoma. Subsequently, we supplemented the set with 100 unseen data points, referred to as the query set, and evaluated whether each data point represented glaucoma or not. The schematic diagram is presented in Figure 3.

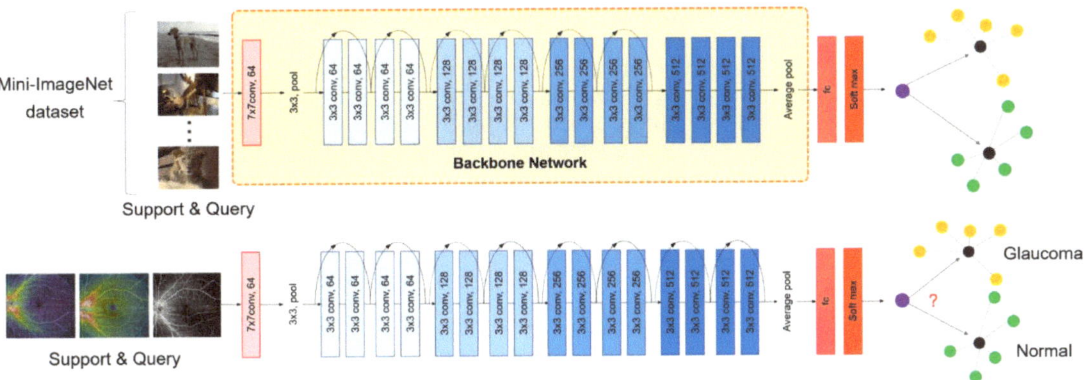

Figure 3. Implementation of FSL for WF-OCTA integration. This study employed FSL to integrate WF-OCTA into an AI algorithm. ResNet18 served as the backbone network, trained on ophthalmic images to capture relevant features. The ProtoNet algorithm facilitated feature clustering and classification. Training utilized the Mini-ImageNet benchmark dataset. The WF-OCTA data were split into support and query sets for validation.

2.5. Statistical Analysis

This study compared the diagnostic performance between FSL conducted with pre-training on different images and Mini-ImageNet and conventional SL using a limited number of WF-OCTA images. Furthermore, this study extended the comparison to evaluate the diagnostic capabilities of numerical values (parameters) commonly used in traditional OCT and OCTA.

To assess the diagnostic capability for detecting the presence or absence of glaucoma, we computed the area under the receiver operating characteristic curve (AUC) and accuracy. Additionally, AUC with a 95% confidence interval (95% CI) was employed while varying the cutoff value for the probability of glaucoma. The method described by DeLong et al. [36] was utilized to compare AUC values among different parameters. Accuracy served as a metric for the precision in classifying the stages of glaucoma. The proportion of correctly classified data from the entire dataset used for testing was also estimated. p-values < 0.05 were considered statistically significant. Values are presented as mean $\pm$ standard deviation. Statistical tests were conducted using SPSS version 24 (IBM Inc., Armonk, NY, USA), MedCalc Version 19.1.3 (MedCalc Software, Ostend, Belgium), and the PyTorch Version 1.12.0 in Python (Facebook AI Research Lab, Menlo Park, CA, USA) [37].

3. Results

Demographics and ocular characteristics of the support set and query set are summarized in Table S1. The median age was 58.4 $\pm$ 15.8. No statistically significant differences were observed in spherical equivalent, axial length, and intraocular pressure, regardless of the presence of glaucoma. Both glaucoma and control groups were evenly composed with similar numerical values of other ocular characteristics such as MD (dB), VFI (%), RNFL, GCIPL, and GCC thickness (μm).

In the experiment, 20 WF-OCTA images, consisting of 10 glaucoma and 10 normal datasets, were examined. Additionally, 100 WF-OCTA images of 50 glaucoma and 50 normal datasets were classified in FSL experiments with 1, 2, 5, and 10 shots by default. Shot refers to the number of data points used to adapt training to a new task. For example, if it is one shot, it means that the model only looks at one glaucoma data and one normal data and fits 100 data. Table S2 demonstrates the WF-OCTA image accuracy value and the AUC. The results clearly display that as the number of shots increases, so does the accuracy. The comparison was based on 10 shots.

We were interested in the feasibility of using SL to predict WF-OCTA even with a limited amount of data. To investigate this point, we conducted a performance verification and comparison between the existing SL method using ResNet18 and the proposed method with the WF-OCTA data. For SL, we trained with a total of 20 WF-OCTA data and tested with 100 WF-OCTA data. Therefore, Figure 4 and Table 1 demonstrate that SL does not learn with an accuracy of 50%. Additionally, the accuracy and the AUC value are high for FSL, and the *p*-value is set at 0.05 for all results, which is significant.

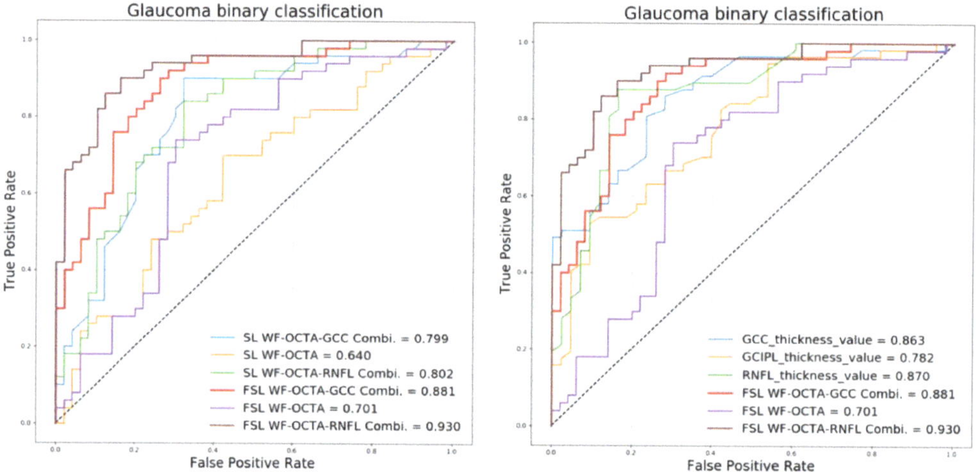

Figure 4. Receiver operating curves for glaucoma diagnostic methods. Left is FSL vs. SL with WF-OCTA images. FSL shows a higher AUC. The right is a classification of glaucoma vs. normal cases. FSL WF-OCTA RNFL Combi and FSL WF-OCTA GCC Combi achieve the highest AUC (0.930 and 0.881). These outperform conventional thickness values (RNFL, GCC, and GCIPL thickness AUC: 0.870, 0.863, and 0.782).

Table 1. Comparison of accuracy and area under the receiver operating characteristic curve between few-shot learning and supervised learning.

WF-OCTA	FSL			SL			FSL vs. SL: *p*-Value		
	RNFL Combi	**GCC Combi**	**Alone**	**RNFL Combi**	**GCC Combi**	**Alone**	**RNFL Combi**	**GCC Combi**	**Alone**
Accuracy (%)	81	80	68	50	50	50	<0.05	<0.05	<0.05
AUC	0.930	0.881	0.701	0.802	0.799	0.640	<0.05	<0.05	<0.05

FSL = few-shot learning; SL = supervised learning; WF-OCTA = wide-field optical coherence tomography angiography; AUC = area under the receiver operating characteristic curve; RNFL = retinal nerve fiber layer; GCC = ganglion cell complex.

This study also compared our method with existing methods based on peripapillary RNFL, macular GCIPL, and macular GCC thickness values, which are widely used in the glaucoma field.

As displayed in Table 2, the AUC values demonstrate that the performance of WF-OCTA Combis adopting FSL is significantly higher than those of thickness values, and the respective *p*-values are significant at 0.05 or less.

Table 2. Comparison of accuracy and area under the receiver operating characteristic curve between few-shot learning and conventional thickness value (*p*-values are expressed in the table below).

		FSL			Thickness Value		
		WF OCTA_ RNFL Combi	**WF OCTA_ GCC Combi**	**WF-OCTA**	**RNFL**	**GCC**	**GCIPL**
	AUC	**0.930**	**0.881**	**0.701**	**0.870**	**0.863**	**0.782**
FSL	WF OCTA_RNFL Combi	NA	<0.05	<0.05	<0.05	<0.05	<0.05
	WF OCTA_GCC Combi	<0.05	NA	<0.05	<0.05	<0.05	<0.05
	WF-OCTA	<0.05	<0.05	NA	<0.05	<0.05	<0.05
Thickness Value	RNFL	<0.05	<0.05	<0.05	NA	0.83	0.49
	GCC	<0.05	<0.05	<0.05	0.83	NA	0.37
	GCIPL	<0.05	<0.05	<0.05	0.49	0.37	NA

FSL = few-shot learning; AUC = area under the receiver operating characteristic curve; WF-OCTA = wide-field optical coherence tomography angiography; RNFL = retinal nerve fiber layer; GCC = ganglion cell complex; GCIPL = ganglion cell–inner plexiform layer.

4. Discussion

In this study, the effectiveness of WF-OCTA as an image diagnostic modality for glaucoma diagnosis is investigated using DL algorithms, and an FSL method is also introduced to overcome the difficulties of data collection for WF-OCTA. Although many previous studies have applied artificial intelligence (AI) to images such as OCT and SS-OCT to diagnose glaucoma, no studies have been conducted on WF-OCTA images. Therefore, the application of DL to WF-OCTA images is the first of its kind.

In the field of ophthalmology, various attempts have been made to use small-shot learning as an automatic diagnostic evaluation method for images. Quellec et al. applied FSL to the detection of rare conditions such as papilledema or anterior ischemic optic neuropathy from the OPHDIAT diabetic retinopathy screening program [38]. Kim et al. introduced a novel approach for the development of an effective computational model for early diagnosis of glaucoma, relying solely on a single type of image (high-resolution fundus images) using FSL, employing a matching network older than ProtoNet [39]. Han et al. used FSL for ophthalmic disease screening, focusing primarily on enhancing data by fusion or aggregation of various data types rather than relying on a small amount of data [40].

First of all, comparing FSL and SL, the diagnostic power of FSL demonstrated better performance. The reason SL does not perform is because of an error called underfitting that occurs due to the small amount of image data (like WF-OCTA). This means that to examine the effectiveness of using AI in this situation, FSL, rather than the existing methodology SL, must be used as another methodology that can improve performance. This does not serve as a comparison to establish the superiority of SL over FSL; instead, it underscores the importance of FSL as a fitting methodology in specific circumstances. FSL was utilized to construct models by incorporating various data sources, including open benchmark data, to verify its effectiveness for WF-OCTA data.

This study conducted experiments on the FSL method utilizing an algorithm called ProtoNet, which transforms data into prototypes and clusters them, making them suitable for displaying particularity distributions. To adjust the ProtoNet for the FSL algorithm for this study, we identified two stages. The first step involves extracting features, which capture critical image elements to be evaluated, followed by classification, which determines whether results are positive or negative. The feature extractor was trained using RNFL and the transfer learning method [41], which utilized an existing ophthalmic medical image. This resulted in an effective feature extractor for ophthalmic medical images. To reduce potential task dependence, the model was trained on ImageNet during the classification process. Additionally, the use of distinct datasets for training both sections of the network aimed to maximize its benefits.

The FSL method employed in this study has the potential to significantly impact real-world medical applications. We think this is the result of improving FSL's capabilities through the aforementioned efforts. FSL can be useful in cases where there are not enough images available for training due to the rarity of the disease or the release of new image types in the future. As new images will continue to be introduced with the development of technology, incorporating FSL will help research and evaluate the diagnostic power at the time of introduction of such images.

This study also compared the FSL of WF-OCTA with existing methods based on peripapillary RNFL, macular GCIPL, and macular GCC thickness values, which are widely used parameters in glaucoma. Application of WF-OCTA data to FSL, especially in WF-OCTA Combi data, demonstrated that this method surpasses conventional numeric parameter-based diagnosis. Nevertheless, WF-OCTA (not combi, alone, grayscale) exhibits decreased performance compared to the other two images. The reason for this discrepancy lies in the fact that the RNFL image used for feature training is in RGB format, while the other two images are in RGB format, and WF-OCTA is a grayscale image, thus degrading the feature extraction performance due to different channels. To enhance the efficiency of WF-OCTA (grayscale), acquire enough grayscale glaucoma images to train the feature extractor or use additional shots to increase the accuracy of the network. We expect that increasing the number of attempts beyond 10 may potentially enhance the algorithm's performance in future research.

WF-OCTA offers several distinct advantages in detecting RNFL defects for glaucoma diagnosis [42]. First, WF-OCTA visualizes a wider area (12 $\times$ 12 mm) compared to the existing OCT RNFL thickness map (12 $\times$ 9 mm). This may also be useful in assessing peripheral regions and detecting abnormalities that can be missed in conventional imaging. Second, visualization of blood flow dynamics improves the accuracy of glaucoma diagnosis in cases with other ocular pathologies where the existing thickness map is compromised by retinal diseases such as ERM or peripapillary retinoschisis. Particularly in cases of high myopia, where RNFL defects may not be clearly observed in the red-free fundus photo, WF-OCTA can be helpful [15,43]. By providing angiographic information across a broader field than conventional imaging, WF-OCTA has the potential to enhance glaucoma diagnosis.

However, the current active clinical utilization of WF-OCTA can be limited due to some disadvantages. WF-OCTA takes a long time to acquire, requires cooperation, and can make imaging difficult for older patients, especially those with tremors. Moreover, deviation maps cannot be created, and the current embedded software only offers a combination map with RNLF, GCC, and GCIPL thickness maps since the normative database of OCTA values has not been established yet. These may make the active clinical utilization of WF-OCTA challenging.

Nevertheless, when diagnosing glaucoma becomes challenging due to other pathological changes in the eye, such as high myopia or retinal diseases, WF-OCTA can serve as a valuable adjunctive imaging technique. This study's findings demonstrate that WF-OCTA could offer a valuable alternative to the current RNFL method for diagnosing glaucoma, especially in patients with co-existing ocular conditions. Therefore, we believe that it can be readily applied in clinical settings, particularly in cooperative patients who can endure relatively long examination times. With the assistance of FSL, the accuracy of WF-OCTA for glaucoma diagnosis could further improve, leading to significant advancements in the diagnosis and treatment of glaucoma. Moreover, FSL could be clinically applicable not only in glaucoma management but also in relatively less prevalent conditions like inherited retinal diseases or neuro-ophthalmic diseases.

This study has certain limitations. First, the advantages of FSL could have been demonstrated more accurately if we had used a wide fundus photo or OCT RNFL thickness map instead of WF-OCTA. However, this study tried to demonstrate the advantages of both FSL (new DL algorithm) and WF-OCTA (newly introduced imaging method). Second, 100 OCT RNFL thickness map images were used for feature extraction, which is still too small for pre-training. Third, it would have been more intriguing if we could compare the accuracy between diagnosis by the physician and the FSL. Fourth, OCT RNFL thickness maps were used for the training set, which are very similar to the images used in the support set (WF-OCTA). Our future studies plan to address the accuracy when using images with lower similarity as the training set.

5. Conclusions

This study demonstrated the effectiveness of applying DL to WF-OCTA for glaucoma diagnosis, highlighting the potential of WF-OCTA images in glaucoma diagnostics. Additionally, the application of FSL was shown to overcome the limitation of small dataset size. Utilizing FSL with imaging techniques characterized by limited data can be effective, and its applicability in various clinical settings is anticipated.

Supplementary Materials: The following supporting information can be downloaded at https://www.mdpi.com/article/10.3390/biomedicines12040741/s1. Supplementary Material: Diagnosis of glaucoma and selection of control group. Figure S1: Training ResNet18 weight by using SS-OCT data to train ResNet18. Table S1: Demographic and clinical characteristics of eyes and patients in the training vs. test samples. It is written that there are 95 sheets in the training overall, but in the actual experiment, 20 sheets are randomly selected and used. Table S2: Comparison of shot, accuracy, and area under the receiver operating characteristic curve results as a function of number of shots.

Author Contributions: Conceptualization, J.W.C. and W.J.L.; methodology, W.J.L.; software, J.W.C.; validation, Y.S., K.O.Y., J.M.L. and I.Y.Y.; formal analysis, Y.S., K.O.Y. and W.J.L.; investigation, Y.S., K.O.Y. and W.J.L.; resources, W.J.L.; data curation, Y.S., K.O.Y. and W.J.L.; writing—original draft preparation, Y.S., K.O.Y. and J.M.L.; writing—review and editing, W.J.L.; visualization, Y.S., K.O.Y. and J.M.L.; supervision, J.W.C. and W.J.L.; project administration, W.J.L.; funding acquisition, W.J.L. All authors have read and agreed to the published version of the manuscript.

Funding: This research was supported by the Bio and Medical Technology Development Program of the National Research Foundation (NRF), funded by the Korean Government (MSIT) (No. NRF-2022R1A2C1092176).

Institutional Review Board Statement: This study was conducted in accordance with the Declaration of Helsinki and approved by the Institutional Review Board of Hanyang University Hospital (IRB number: HYUH 2021-07-036, date of approval: 2021.07.27).

Informed Consent Statement: Informed consent was obtained from all subjects involved in this study.

Data Availability Statement: Data are available upon reasonable request.

Conflicts of Interest: The authors declare no conflicts of interest.

References

1. Weinreb, R.N.; Aung, T.; Medeiros, F.A. The pathophysiology and treatment of glaucoma: A review. *JAMA* **2014**, *311*, 1901–1911. [CrossRef] [PubMed]
2. Kwon, Y.H.; Fingert, J.H.; Kuehn, M.H.; Alward, W.L. Primary open-angle glaucoma. *N. Engl. J. Med.* **2009**, *360*, 1113–1124. [CrossRef] [PubMed]
3. Bussel, I.I.; Wollstein, G.; Schuman, J.S. OCT for glaucoma diagnosis, screening and detection of glaucoma progression. *Br. J. Ophthalmol.* **2014**, *98* (Suppl. S2), ii15–ii19. [CrossRef] [PubMed]
4. Grewal, D.S.; Tanna, A.P. Diagnosis of glaucoma and detection of glaucoma progression using spectral domain optical coherence tomography. *Curr. Opin. Ophthalmol.* **2013**, *24*, 150–161. [CrossRef]

5. Vessani, R.M.; Moritz, R.; Batis, L.; Zagui, R.B.; Bernardoni, S.; Susanna, R. Comparison of quantitative imaging devices and subjective optic nerve head assessment by general ophthalmologists to differentiate normal from glaucomatous eyes. *J. Glaucoma* **2009**, *18*, 253–261. [CrossRef]
6. Sung, K.R.; Kim, J.S.; Wollstein, G.; Folio, L.; Kook, M.S.; Schuman, J.S. Imaging of the retinal nerve fibre layer with spectral domain optical coherence tomography for glaucoma diagnosis. *Br. J. Ophthalmol.* **2011**, *95*, 909–914. [CrossRef]
7. Mwanza, J.-C.; Warren, J.L.; Budenz, D.L. Combining spectral domain optical coherence tomography structural parameters for the diagnosis of glaucoma with early visual field loss. *Investig. Ophthalmol. Vis. Sci.* **2013**, *54*, 8393–8400. [CrossRef]
8. Lisboa, R.; Mansouri, K.; Zangwill, L.M.; Weinreb, R.N.; Medeiros, F.A. Likelihood ratios for glaucoma diagnosis using spectral-domain optical coherence tomography. *Am. J. Ophthalmol.* **2013**, *156*, 918–926.e2. [CrossRef]
9. Greaney, M.J.; Hoffman, D.C.; Garway-Heath, D.F.; Nakla, M.; Coleman, A.L.; Caprioli, J. Comparison of optic nerve imaging methods to distinguish normal eyes from those with glaucoma. *Investig. Ophthalmol. Vis. Sci.* **2002**, *43*, 140–145.
10. Rao, H.L.; Pradhan, Z.S.; Suh, M.H.; Moghimi, S.; Mansouri, K.; Weinreb, R.N. Optical Coherence Tomography Angiography in Glaucoma. *J. Glaucoma* **2020**, *29*, 312–321. [CrossRef] [PubMed]
11. Werner, A.C.; Shen, L.Q. A Review of OCT Angiography in Glaucoma. *Semin. Ophthalmol.* **2019**, *34*, 279–286. [CrossRef] [PubMed]
12. Grewal, D.S.; Agarwal, M.; Munk, M.R. Wide Field Optical Coherence Tomography and Optical Coherence Tomography Angiography in Uveitis. *Ocul. Immunol. Inflamm.* **2022**, *32*, 105–115. [CrossRef] [PubMed]
13. Hamada, M.; Hirai, K.; Wakabayashi, T.; Ishida, Y.; Fukushima, M.; Kamei, M.; Tsuboi, K. Real-world utility of wide-field OCT angiography to detect retinal neovascularization in eyes with proliferative diabetic retinopathy. *Ophthalmol. Retina*, 2023; *in press*. [CrossRef]
14. Hirano, T.; Hoshiyama, K.; Takahashi, Y.; Murata, T. Wide-field swept-source OCT angiography (23 × 20 mm) for detecting retinal neovascularization in eyes with proliferative diabetic retinopathy. *Graefes Arch. Clin. Exp. Ophthalmol.* **2023**, *261*, 339–344. [CrossRef] [PubMed]
15. Kim, Y.J.; Na, K.I.; Lim, H.W.; Seong, M.; Lee, W.J. Combined wide-field optical coherence tomography angiography density map for high myopic glaucoma detection. *Sci. Rep.* **2021**, *11*, 22034. [CrossRef] [PubMed]
16. Munsell, M.K.; Garg, I.; Duich, M.; Zeng, R.; Baldwin, G.; Wescott, H.E.; Koch, T.; Wang, K.L.; Patel, N.A.; Miller, J.B. A normative database of wide-field swept-source optical coherence tomography angiography quantitative metrics in a large cohort of healthy adults. *Graefes Arch. Clin. Exp. Ophthalmol.* **2023**, *261*, 1835–1859. [CrossRef] [PubMed]
17. Lake, B.M.; Salakhutdinov, R.; Tenenbaum, J.B. Human-level concept learning through probabilistic program induction. *Science* **2015**, *350*, 1332–1338. [CrossRef] [PubMed]
18. Bishop, C.M.; Nasrabadi, N.M. *Pattern Recognition and Machine Learning*; Springer: New York, NY, USA, 2006; Volume 4, p. 738.
19. He, H.; Garcia, E.A. Learning from imbalanced data. *IEEE Trans. Knowl. Data Eng.* **2009**, *21*, 1263–1284.
20. Chen, W.Y.; Liu, Y.C.; Kira, Z.; Wang YC, F.; Huang, J.B. A closer look at few-shot classification. *arXiv* **2019**, arXiv:1904.04232.
21. Miller, E.G.; Matsakis, N.E.; Viola, P.A. Learning from one example through shared densities on transforms. In Proceedings of the IEEE Conference on Computer Vision and Pattern Recognition, CVPR 2000 (Cat. No. PR00662), Hilton Head, SC, USA, 13–15 June 2000; pp. 464–471.
22. Lake, B.; Salakhutdinov, R.; Gross, J.; Tenenbaum, J. One shot learning of simple visual concepts. In Proceedings of the Annual Meeting of the Cognitive Science Society, Boston, MA, USA, 20–23 July 2011.
23. Koch, G.; Zemel, R.; Salakhutdinov, R. *Siamese Neural Networks for One-Shot Image Recognition*; ICML Deep Learning Workshop: Lille, France, 2015.
24. Shin, Y.; Cho, H.; Shin, Y.U.; Seong, M.; Choi, J.W.; Lee, W.J. Comparison between deep-learning-based ultra-wide-field fundus imaging and true-colour confocal scanning for diagnosing glaucoma. *J. Clin. Med.* **2022**, *11*, 3168. [CrossRef]
25. Shin, Y.; Cho, H.; Jeong, H.C.; Seong, M.; Choi, J.W.; Lee, W.J. Deep Learning-based Diagnosis of Glaucoma Using Wide-field Optical Coherence Tomography Images. *J. Glaucoma* **2021**, *30*, 803–812. [CrossRef]
26. Szegedy, C.; Liu, W.; Jia, Y.; Sermanet, P.; Reed, S.; Anguelov, D.; Erhan, D.; Vanhoucke, V.; Rabinovich, A. Going deeper with convolutions. In Proceedings of the IEEE Conference on Computer Vision and Pattern Recognition, Boston, MA, USA, 7–12 June 2015; pp. 1–9.
27. He, K.; Zhang, X.; Ren, S.; Sun, J. Deep residual learning for image recognition. In Proceedings of the IEEE Conference on Computer Vision and Pattern Recognition, Las Vegas, NV, USA, 26 June–July 1 2016; pp. 770–778.
28. Xie, S.; Girshick, R.; Dollár, P.; Tu, Z.; He, K. Aggregated residual transformations for deep neural networks. In Proceedings of the IEEE Conference on Computer Vision and Pattern Recognition, Honolulu, HI, USA, 21–26 July 2017; pp. 1492–1500.
29. Wang, Y.; Yao, Q.; Kwok, J.T.; Ni, L.M. Generalizing from a few examples: A survey on few-shot learning. *ACM Comput. Surv.* **2020**, *53*, 1–34. [CrossRef]
30. Song, Y.; Wang, T.; Cai, P.; Mondal, S.K.; Sahoo, J.P. A comprehensive survey of few-shot learning: Evolution, applications, challenges, and opportunities. *ACM Comput. Surv.* **2023**, *55*, 1–40. [CrossRef]
31. Snell, J.; Swersky, K.; Zemel, R. Prototypical networks for few-shot learning. *Adv. Neural Inf. Process. Syst.* **2017**, *30*.
32. Deng, J.; Dong, W.; Socher, R.; Li, L.-J.; Li, K.; Fei-Fei, L. Imagenet: A large-scale hierarchical image database. In Proceedings of the 2009 IEEE Conference on Computer Vision and Pattern Recognition, Miami, FL, USA, 20–25 June 2009; pp. 248–255.
33. Han, X.; Zhang, Z.; Ding, N.; Gu, Y.; Liu, X.; Huo, Y.; Qiu, J.; Yao, Y.; Zhang, A.; Zhang, L.; et al. Pre-trained models: Past, present and future. *AI Open* **2021**, *2*, 225–250. [CrossRef]

34. Pan, S.J.; Yang, Q. A survey on transfer learning. *IEEE Trans. Knowl. Data Eng.* **2009**, *22*, 1345–1359. [CrossRef]
35. Vinyals, O.; Blundell, C.; Lillicrap, T.; Wierstra, D. Matching networks for one shot learning. *Adv. Neural Inf. Process. Syst.* **2016**, *29*.
36. DeLong, E.R.; DeLong, D.M.; Clarke-Pearson, D.L. Comparing the areas under two or more correlated receiver operating characteristic curves: A nonparametric approach. *Biometrics* **1988**, *44*, 837–845. [CrossRef]
37. Paszke, A.; Gross, S.; Chintala, S.; Chanan, G.; Yang, E.; DeVito, Z.; Lin, Z.; Desmaison, A.; Antiga, L.; Lerer, A. Automatic Differentiation in Pytorch. 2017. Available online: https://openreview.net/pdf/25b8eee6c373d48b84e5e9c6e10e7cbbbce4ac73.pdf?ref=blog.premai.io (accessed on 29 October 2017).
38. Quellec, G.; Lamard, M.; Conze, P.-H.; Massin, P.; Cochener, B. Automatic detection of rare pathologies in fundus photographs using few-shot learning. *Med. Image Anal.* **2020**, *61*, 101660. [CrossRef]
39. Kim, M.; Zuallaert, J.; De Neve, W. Few-shot learning using a small-sized dataset of high- resolution FUNDUS images for glaucoma diagnosis. In Proceedings of the 2nd International Workshop on Multimedia for Personal Health and Health Care, Mountain View, CA, USA, 23 October 2017; pp. 89–92.
40. Han, Z.K.; Xing, H.; Yang, B.; Hong, C.Y. A few-shot learning-based eye diseases screening method. *Eur. Rev. Med. Pharmacol. Sci.* **2022**, *26*, 8660–8674. [CrossRef]
41. Zhuang, F.; Qi, Z.; Duan, K.; Xi, D.; Zhu, Y.; Zhu, H.; Xiong, H.; He, Q. A comprehensive survey on transfer learning. *Proc. IEEE* **2020**, *109*, 43–76. [CrossRef]
42. Hong, R.K.; Kim, J.H.; Toh, G.; Na, K.I.; Seong, M.; Lee, W.J. Diagnostic performance of wide-field optical coherence tomography angiography for high myopic glaucoma. *Sci. Rep.* **2024**, *14*, 367. [CrossRef]
43. Kim, H.; Park, H.M.; Jeong, H.C.; Moon, S.Y.; Cho, H.; Lim, H.W.; Seong, M.; Park, J.; Lee, W.J. Wide-field optical coherence tomography deviation map for early glaucoma detection. *Br. J. Ophthalmol.* **2023**, *107*, 49–55. [CrossRef]

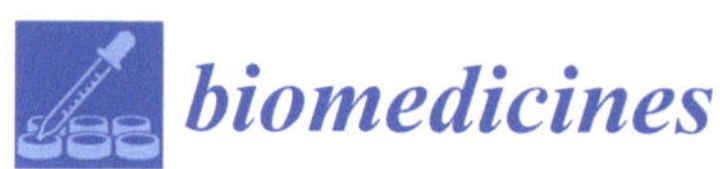

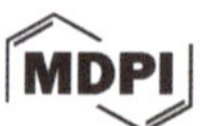

Article

Adding Genetics to the Risk Factors Model Improved Accuracy for Detecting Visual Field Progression in Newly Diagnosed Exfoliation Glaucoma Patients

Marcelo Ayala [1,2,3]

[1] Department of Clinical Neuroscience, Institute of Neuroscience and Physiology, Sahlgrenska Academy, University of Gothenburg, 40530 Gothenburg, Sweden; marcelo.ayala@vgregion.se
[2] Eye Department, Region Västra Götaland, Skaraborg Hospital/Skövde, 54142 Skövde, Sweden
[3] Department of Clinical Neuroscience, Karolinska Institute, 17165 Stockholm, Sweden

Abstract: Background: This study aims to determine whether including genetics as a risk factor for progression will improve the accuracy of the models used in newly diagnosed exfoliation glaucoma patients. Methods: This was a prospective cohort study. This study included only patients who were newly diagnosed with exfoliation glaucoma and received treatment upon inclusion. Blood samples were taken from all patients at inclusion to test for the single nucleotide polymorphisms (SNPs) *LOXL-1* rs2165241 and rs1048661. Results: This study found that the frequency of SNPs, as well as intraocular pressure (IOP), mean deviation (MD), and visual field index (VFI) values at diagnosis, were significant predictors of visual field deterioration ($p \leq 0.001$). This study showed that interaction terms, including SNPs, were highly significant ($p \leq 0.001$). Furthermore, logistic regression analysis also showed highly significant results for interaction terms when SNPs were included ($p \leq 0.001$). Finally, the area under the curve (AUC) analysis showed an increased value of around 10–20% when SNPs were included. Conclusions: Adding genetic factors to the well-known clinical risk factors can increase the accuracy of models for predicting visual field deterioration in exfoliation glaucoma patients. However, further studies are needed to investigate the role of other genes in this process.

Keywords: genetics; exfoliation glaucoma; visual fields; cohort studies; intraocular pressure; models

Citation: Ayala, M. Adding Genetics to the Risk Factors Model Improved Accuracy for Detecting Visual Field Progression in Newly Diagnosed Exfoliation Glaucoma Patients. *Biomedicines* **2024**, *12*, 1225. https://doi.org/10.3390/biomedicines12061225

Academic Editor: Da-Wen Lu

Received: 25 April 2024
Revised: 16 May 2024
Accepted: 24 May 2024
Published: 31 May 2024

1. Introduction

Glaucoma is a set of eye disorders that gradually damage the optic nerve and often cause permanent loss of the visual field. The condition usually results from high intraocular pressure (IOP) but can also occur with normal or low IOP. Glaucoma affects millions of people globally and is a major cause of blindness, which poses a significant public health challenge [1]. There are several types of glaucoma, with primary open-angle glaucoma being the most common worldwide. However, in Scandinavia, exfoliation glaucoma is the most widespread type [2]. Exfoliation glaucoma (EXFG) is a specific form of glaucoma that is characterized by the presence of exfoliation material in the anterior chamber of the eye. This material is often described as flaky, white deposits accumulating on different eye structures. This accumulation leads to increased IOP and damage to the optic nerve [3,4].

Exfoliation glaucoma is associated with the shedding of abnormal extracellular material in the eye's anterior segment. Although the exact cause of exfoliation glaucoma is not fully understood, genetic factors have been demonstrated to contribute to its development. The Lysyl Oxidase Like 1 (*LOXL-1*) gene is the most studied gene related to EXFG [5]. The *LOXL-1* gene encodes for the lysozyme oxidase enzyme, involved in elastin biogenesis and collagen cross-linking [6]. In a previous article, the authors demonstrated the association between three single nucleotides (SNPs) and the presence of exfoliation glaucoma in a Swedish population [7]. Furthermore, two SNPs (rs2165241 and rs1048661) have been linked to an increased risk of visual field deterioration [8].

Several factors can contribute to the development of glaucoma. While some risk factors are beyond an individual's control, it is essential to be aware of them to diagnose the condition early and manage it effectively. These risk factors include age, family history, ethnicity, increased IOP, and exfoliation [9–11]. However, simply having one or more of these risk factors does not necessarily mean that an individual will develop glaucoma. Conversely, some people may develop the condition despite having no apparent risk factors. As a result, individuals with one or more risk factors must undergo regular eye examinations to detect and manage glaucoma early. With early intervention, it may be possible to slow down or even prevent further vision loss associated with this condition.

This study aimed to evaluate the potential impact of incorporating genetics as a risk factor in the models utilized for newly diagnosed exfoliation glaucoma patients. This study is expected to produce valuable insights into the potential benefits of incorporating genetic factors into the exfoliation glaucoma diagnostic framework.

2. Materials and Methods

This study observed patients diagnosed with EXFG and was conducted as a non-randomized prospective cohort study. Patients who visited the Ophthalmology Department at Skaraborg Hospital, Skövde, Sweden, between 1 January 2012 and 31 December 2017 were included in this study. This study followed the Strengthening the Reporting of Observational studies in Epidemiology (STROBE) guidelines for reporting observational studies [12] (Supplementary Table S1). Before enrolling in this study, all participants were provided with both written and oral information. This study was approved by the Regional Ethical Committee at the University of Gothenburg (DN:119-12) and followed the principles of the Helsinki Declaration.

This study's methodology was previously published and involved patients who were recently diagnosed with exfoliation glaucoma (EXFG) [13,14]. To summarize, all patients underwent an ophthalmological exam conducted by the same ophthalmologist (MA). At the time of diagnosis (inclusion), various variables were measured, including age, sex, IOP (using a Goldmann applanation tonometer), central corneal thickness (CCT), visual acuity (determined with the Snellen chart), gonioscopy, cup-to-disc ratio (C/D-ratio) of the optic nerve, and visual field using the Humphrey Field Analyzer (Carl-Zeiss, Straße 22, 73447 Oberkochen, Germany) using the 24-2 strategy of the Swedish Interactive Threshold Algorithm (SITA fast). Additionally, all patients completed a questionnaire about their medical history, which included diabetes, hypertension, smoking, medication intake, and family history of glaucoma.

As part of this study, all patients were given eye drops to decrease their IOP and maintain it at $\leq$20 mmHg. The patient's visual acuity, IOP, medication count (i.e., eye drops), and visual field were evaluated at every appointment (every six months). The patients were closely monitored in accordance with the Swedish Guidelines for Glaucoma Care [15]. In cases where the desired IOP level could not be attained, the number of medications was incremented and/or selective laser trabeculoplasty (SLT) was performed.

2.1. Endpoints

This study's primary objective was to ascertain the progression of the visual field employing highly reliable visual fields. The reliable visual fields were defined as those that displayed $\leq$15% false positives and fewer than 20% fixation losses. To ensure accuracy, only visual fields with an MD (mean deviation) between 0 and −16 dB were included. Including visual fields with significant damage can lead to "ceiling effects" and may not represent actual damage [16].

This study measured visual field progression using three parameters: mean deviation (MD), visual field index (VFI), and the guided progression analysis (GPA). MD estimates the overall level of visual field sensitivity in decibels (dB), with normal visual fields around 0 dB and significantly damaged visual fields around −20 dB. The VFI, on the other hand, is based on MD values but is more specific in detecting glaucoma damage. It emphasizes central parts of the visual field and is less affected by cataract development. The VFI calculates visual fields in percentages, with a normal visual field showing 100%.

The Guided Progression Analysis (GPA) system classifies the visual field progression as absent, possible, or likely. This study combined the possible and likely categories to form a single outcome of progression versus no progression. This simplified the outcome variable into a dichotomy of visual field progression.

2.2. Genetic Analysis

Each patient underwent venipuncture to extract blood samples as part of the inclusion process. Standard procedures were then followed to extract DNA from the samples. Subsequently, LGC Genomics (Hoddesdon, Herts, UK) utilized the KASPar PCR SNP genotyping system to genotype two specific SNPs (rs2165241 and rs1048661) in the *LOXL1* gene. The genotyping process yielded a success rate of over 95% for all SNPs and demonstrated adherence to the Hardy–Weinberg equilibrium. The genetic variants identified in the patients were analyzed using an additive genetic model, which was determined to be the most appropriate model for this study [7]. In this model, the non-risk homozygous genotype was assigned a value of 0, the heterozygous genotype was assigned a value of 1, and the high-risk homozygous genotype was assigned a value of 2.

2.3. Statistics

This study's statistical analyses were performed using IBM's SPSS software (29.0.1.1) (Armonk, NY 10504, USA). Initially, a single linear regression analysis was conducted on all predictor variables, and only statistically significant predictors ($p \leq 0.05$) were selected for further analysis. The Kolmogorov–Smirnov test was used to assess the normality of these predictors, and Pearson's coefficients were used to study correlations between them.

All significant predictors from the initial regression were utilized in the next step, where three strategies were applied with the same predictors. The first method involved a linear regression analysis to test the continuous outcome variables MD and VFI. The regression analysis also calculated the R^2 value and "B-coefficient". The model was adjusted for covariates. General Linear Models in SPSS were used to calculate interaction terms.

The second method was a logistic regression analysis for the binary outcome variable GPA, which also provided the R^2 and the "Exp B coefficient". Another accuracy value was shown by the regression analysis, namely the prediction accuracy (PA) from the "classification table". All regression models and R^2 values were adjusted for covariates.

The third method was a receiver operator curve with the area under the curve (AUC). The AUC was calculated based on the results from the logistic regression analysis. A predictive curve for interactions between predictors was calculated based on probability calculations from the logistic regression analysis.

Lastly, a power analysis for MD values based on linear regression was conducted. It revealed that a sample size of at least 81 experimental subjects was necessary to detect a 10% difference in MD over three years with a power of 0.80 and a significance level of 0.05.

3. Results

In this study, a total of 96 patients were included. Regrettably, 16 patients had to be excluded from this study as they did not meet the inclusion criteria. The reasons for exclusion varied, ranging from having undergone glaucoma surgery to poor adherence to check-up visits and low-quality visual fields. These exclusions were necessary to ensure this study's accuracy and reliability, as factors such as glaucoma surgery could have influenced this study's outcome. At the same time, poor adherence to check-up visits and low-quality visual fields could have affected the reliability of the results.

The cohort's general characteristics were previously published [13,14]. To summarize, the patients included in this study were approximately 70 years old, with an almost equal distribution of male and female participants. Their visual acuity upon inclusion averaged 0.8 (Snellen units), and their mean IOP was relatively high at 32.52 mmHg. Out of the

96 patients, 66 had EXFG in one eye only, while 30 had it in both eyes. By the six-month check-up, the IOP values had decreased to 21.19 mmHg, and at the last IOP control three years later, the IOP was at 17.94 mmHg.

Upon inclusion, a significant correlation was found between IOP and MD values, as indicated by the Pearson's coefficient ($p = 0.001$, r = 0.51). Similar results were observed for the correlation between IOP and VFI values at inclusion (Pearson's coefficient: $p = 0.001$, r = 0.55). The correlation between MD and VFI values at inclusion was high (Pearson's coefficient; *p*-, r = 0.92). Moreover, Pearson's test was used to examine the correlation between two SNPs, *LOXL1*_rs2165241 and *LOXL1*_rs1048661, which revealed a significant correlation between the two SNPs (*p*-, r = 0.66).

We conducted an analysis of all variables using univariate linear regression for the endpoints, MD and VFI, at the end of this study. Our results revealed that several variables exhibited significant results, including SNPs, IOP, MD, and VFI at diagnosis, the number of medications, and SLT treatment during the three-year follow-up. Additionally, predictors IOP, MD, and VFI at diagnosis were normally distributed according to the Kolmogorov–Smirnov test (with *p*-values of 0.10, 0.17, and 0.25, respectively). To further validate our findings, we retested the predictors in a multivariate analysis with MD and VFI at the end of this study as endpoints. Even in the multivariate analysis, the predictors (SNPs, IOP, MD, and VFI at diagnosis) remained significant predictors for visual field deterioration. However, we observed that the interaction terms of IOP*MD at diagnosis and IOP*VFI at diagnosis were not significant. Conversely, the interaction terms, including IOP, MD, and VFI at diagnosis and the SNPs, were all highly significant. For additional information, please refer to Table 1.

Table 1. Multivariate analysis using the MD, VFI, and IOP values at diagnosis and the SNPs (*LOXL1*_rs2165241 and *LOXL1*_rs1048661) as predictors and MD and VFI at three years' follow-up as outcomes.

Outcomes \ Predictors	MD			VFI		
	B Coeff. [95% CI]	$R^{2\,(1)}$	*p*	B Coeff. [95% CI]	$R^{2\,(1)}$	*p*
IOP at diagnosis [1]	−0.49 [−0.67, −0.31]	0.34	2×10^{-3} *	−1.19 [−1.74, −0.64]	0.37	4×10^{-4} *
MD at diagnosis [1]	1.08 [0.98–1.19]	0.55	3×10^{-3} *	N.A.	N.A.	N.A.
VFI at diagnosis [1]	N.A.	N.A.	N.A.	1.09 [1.01–1.17]	0.58	2×10^{-4} *
LOXL1_rs2165241 [1]	0.78 [0.01–1.55]	0.41	0.01 *	1.04 [0.44–1.64]	0.43	6×10^{-4} *
LOXL1_rs1048661 [1]	1.05 [0.25–1.85]	0.42	8×10^{-3} *	1.13 [0.52–1.75]	0.44	2×10^{-4} *
IOP * MD at diagnosis [2]	N.A.	N.A.	0.89	N.A.	N.A.	N.A.
IOP * VFI at diagnosis [2]	N.A.	N.A.	N.A.	N.A.	N.A.	0.55
LOXL1_rs2165241 * IOP at diagnosis [2]	0.26 [0.12–0.34]	0.78	3×10^{-6} *	0.12 [0.08–0.14]	0.82	4×10^{-7} *
LOXL1_rs1048661 * IOP at diagnosis [2]	0.31 [0.25–0.36]	0.79	2×10^{-7} *	0.22 [0.12–0.28]	0.83	5×10^{-8} *
LOXL1_rs2165241 * MD at diagnosis [2]	0.82 [0.75–0.89]	0.85	6×10^{-5} *	N.A.	N.A.	N.A.
LOXL1_rs1048661 * MD at diagnosis [2]	0.94 [0.88–0.99]	0.86	4×10^{-6} *	N.A.	N.A.	N.A.
LOXL1_rs2165241 * VFI at diagnosis [2]	N.A.	N.A.	N.A.	1.06 [0.99–1.13]	0.88	3×10^{-8} *
LOXL1_rs1048661 * VFI at diagnosis [2]	N.A.	N.A.	N.A.	1.08 [1.01–1.15]	0.89	4×10^{-9} *

MD: Mean deviation. VFI: Visual field index. IOP: Intraocular pressure. SLT: Selective laser trabeculoplasty. [1] Adjusted for SLT treatment and the number of medications. [2] Interaction terms were calculated using the General Linear Models strategy in SPSS. Also adjusted for SLT treatment and the number of medications. The (1) are the adjusted values so it's the same than 1. The * are the significants values.

A logistic regression analysis was performed to investigate the relationship between GPA results during the three-year follow-up period and various variables, including

IOP, MD, and VFI at diagnosis, as well as the two specific SNPs (*LOXL1*_rs2165241 and *LOXL1*_rs1048661). The results indicated that all these factors remained significant predictors of GPA outcomes. Interestingly, the two SNPs exhibited different levels of accuracy, with *LOXL1*_rs2165241 showing better performance than *LOXL1*_rs1048661 (R^2 values of 0.43 and 0.19, respectively) and higher prediction accuracy (PA values of 76% and 65%, respectively).

Although the interaction terms of IOP*MD at diagnosis were nearly significant (p = 0.04), the interaction term of IOP*VFI at diagnosis was not significant (p = 0.24), likely due to the presence of collinearity between predictors. Nevertheless, all interaction terms, including those related to the SNPs, showed high levels of significance and improved accuracy. Please see Table 2 for further details and information.

Table 2. Logistic regression analysis using the MD, VFI, and IOP values at diagnosis and the SNPs (*LOXL1*_rs2165241 and *LOXL1*_rs1048661) as predictors and GPA at three years' follow-up as the outcome.

Predictors / Outcomes	GPA			
	Exp(B) Coeff. [95% CI]	**$R^{2\,(2)}$**	**PA (%)**	***p***
IOP at diagnosis [1]	1.10 [1.09–1.12]	0.09	62	0.01 *
MD at diagnosis [1]	0.77 [0.67–0.9]	0.24	71	5×10^{-4} *
VFI at diagnosis [1]	0.93 [0.89–0.98]	0.25	70	3×10^{-3} *
***LOXL1*_ rs2165241** [1]	6.2 [3.06–12.56]	0.43	76	4×10^{-7} *
***LOXL1*_ rs1048661** [1]	2.6 [1.54–4.57]	0.19	65	3×10^{-4} *
IOP * MD at diagnosis [1]	0.99 [0.98–1]	0.32	72	0.04 *
IOP * VFI at diagnosis [1]	N.A.	N.A.	N.A.	0.24
***LOXL1*_ rs2165241 * IOP at diagnosis** [1]	1.05 [1.03–1.08]	0.45	77	3×10^{-8} *
***LOXL1*_ rs1048661 * IOP at diagnosis** [1]	1.03 [1.01–1.05]	0.24	65	5×10^{-5} *
***LOXL1*_ rs2165241 * MD at diagnosis** [1]	0.69 [0.59–0.81]	0.54	80	7×10^{-6} *
***LOXL1*_ rs1048661 * MD at diagnosis** [1]	0.82 [0.74–0.9]	0.36	74	1×10^{-4} *
***LOXL1*_ rs2165241 * VFI at diagnosis** [1]	1.02 [1.01–1.03]	0.34	78	5×10^{-6} *
***LOXL1*_ rs1048661 * VFI at diagnosis** [1]	1.01 [1–1.02]	0.26	72	4×10^{-3} *

GPA: Guided glaucoma progression. PA: Prediction accuracy (classification table). MD: Mean deviation. VFI: Visual field index. IOP: Intraocular pressure. SLT: Selective laser trabeculoplasty. [1] Adjusted for SLT treatment and the number of medications. [(2)] Adjusted R^2: Nagelkerke R square. The * are the significants values.

During the analysis, we used the area under curve (AUC) to evaluate the performance of our predictors. All the AUCs showed significant results. At the time of diagnosis, the predictors IOP, MD, and VFI had AUC values of 0.70, 0.80, and 0.79, respectively, indicating a good predictive performance. The AUC values increased by around 10–15% when genetics were included. For more information, please refer to Table 3.

Table 3. Summary of the results obtained from the analysis of the area under the curve (AUC).

	AUC [95% CI]	p	Sensitivity	Specificity
IOP at diagnosis	0.70 [0.59–0.82]	3×10^{-4}	0.70	0.67
***LOXL1*_ rs2165241**	0.80 [0.72–0.90]	1.6×10^{-8}	0.92	0.58
IOP at diagnosis * *LOXL1*_rs2165241	0.85 [0.77–0.92]	2.3×10^{-12}	0.80	0.73
***LOXL1*_ rs1048661**	0.71 [0.60–0.81]	1.8×10^{-4}	0.78	0.55
IOP at diagnosis * *LOXL1*_rs1048661	0.77 [0.67–0.86]	4×10^{-8}	0.75	0.71
MD at diagnosis	0.8 [0.7–0.89]	1.5×10^{-8}	0.78	0.76
MD at diagnosis * *LOXL1*_rs2165241	0.90 [0.84–0.96]	2.2×10^{-14}	0.82	0.64
MD at diagnosis * *LOXL1*_rs1048661	0.82 [0.73–0.90]	5.4×10^{-13}	0.78	0.76
VFI at diagnosis	0.79 [0.69–0.88]	8.5×10^{-9}	0.75	0.70
VFI at diagnosis * *LOXL1*_rs2165241	0.91 [0.85–0.97]	3.2×10^{-15}	0.82	0.65
VFI at diagnosis * *LOXL1*_rs1048661	0.81 [0.70–0.88]	3.7×10^{-10}	0.78	0.64

Table 3. *Cont.*

IOP: Intraocular pressure. MD: Mean deviation. VFI: Visual field index.

The evaluation of AUCs showed significant outcomes for all predictors, with the predictive curve (interaction term) surpassing each individual predictor. We utilized IBM's SPSS software (29.0.1.1) (Armonk, NY 10504, USA) to plot the data on a graph, generating Figures 1–6 that depict these curves.

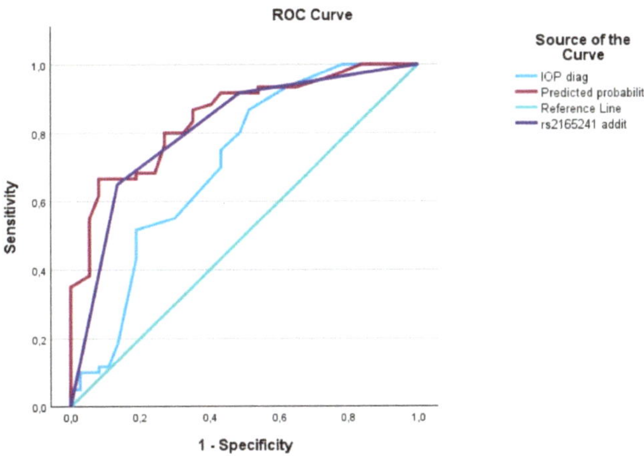

Figure 1. The AUC analysis of IOP at diagnosis and *LOXL1*_rs2165241. The IOP at diagnosis (---) was 0.70 [0.59–0.82], the *LOXL1*_rs2165241 (---) was 0.80 [0.72–0.90], and the interaction between IOP at diagnosis and *LOXL1*_rs2165241 (predicted curve) (---) was 0.85 [0.77–0.92].

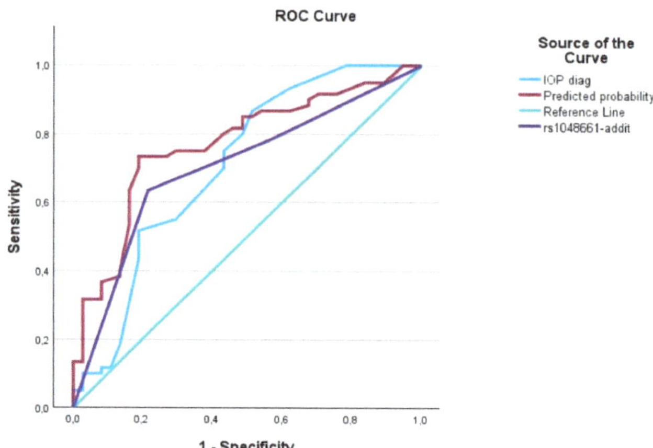

Figure 2. The AUC analysis of IOP at diagnosis and *LOXL1*_rs1048661. The IOP at diagnosis (---) was 0.70 [0.59–0.82], the *LOXL1*_rs1048661 (---) was 0.71 [0.60–0.81], and the interaction between IOP at diagnosis and *LOXL1*_rs1046661 (predicted curve) (---) was 0.77 [0.67–0.86].

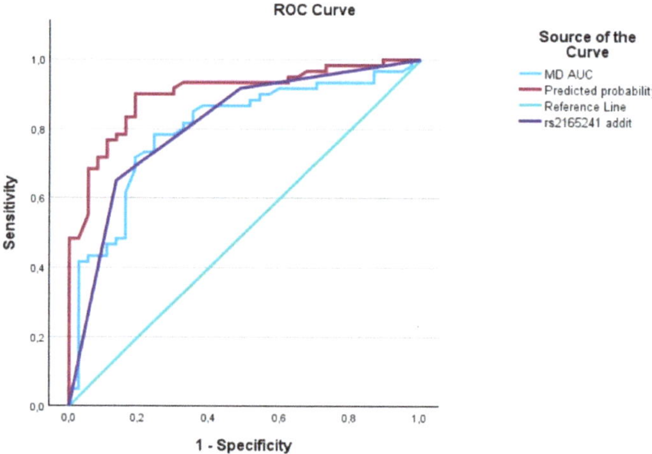

Figure 3. The AUC analysis of MD at diagnosis and *LOXL1*_rs2165241. The MD at diagnosis (---) was 0.8 [0.7–0.89], the *LOXL1*_rs2165241 (---) was 0.80 [0.72–0.90], and the interaction between IOP at diagnosis and *LOXL1*_rs2165241 (predicted curve) (---) was 0.90 [0.84–0.96].

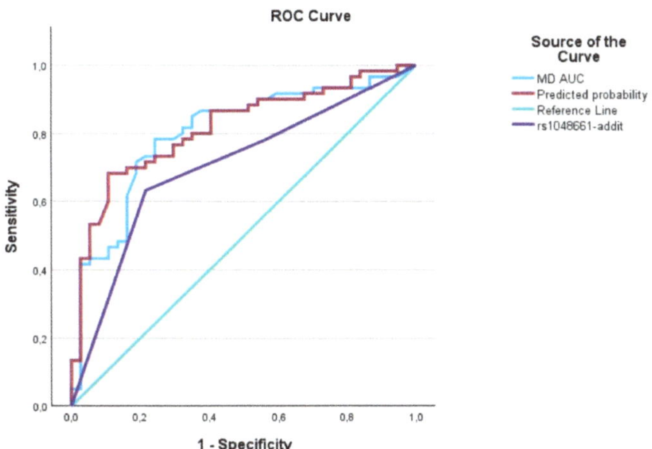

Figure 4. The AUC analysis of MD at diagnosis and *LOXL1*_rs1048661. The MD at diagnosis (---) was 0.8 [0.7–0.89], the *LOXL1*_rs1048661 (---) was 0.71 [0.60–0.81], and the interaction between MD at diagnosis and *LOXL1*_rs1046661 (predicted curve) (---) was 0.82 [0.73–0.90].

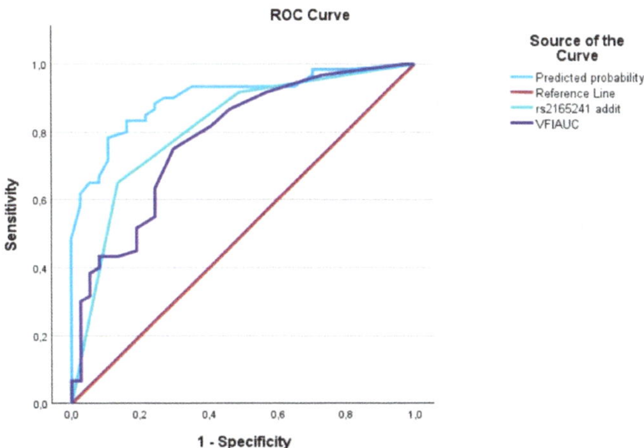

Figure 5. The AUC analysis of VFI at diagnosis and *LOXL1*_rs216524. The VFI at diagnosis (---) was 0.79 [0.69–0.88], the *LOXL1*_rs2165241 (---) was 0.80 [0.72–0.90], and the interaction between VFI at diagnosis and *LOXL1*_rs2165241 (predicted curve) (---) was 0.91 [0.85–0.97].

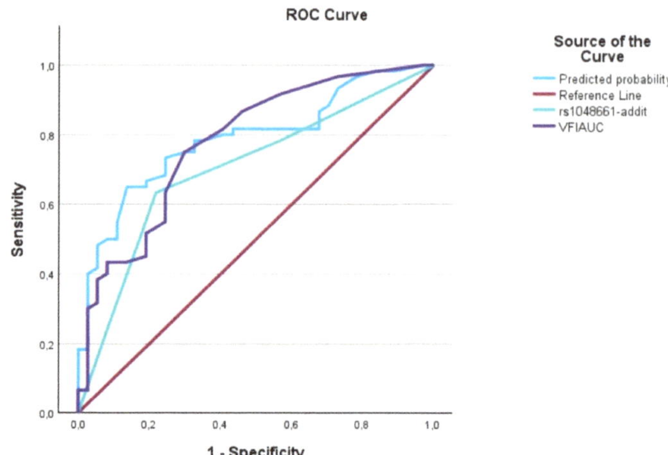

Figure 6. The AUC analysis of VFI at diagnosis and *LOXL1*_rs1048661. The VFI at diagnosis (---) was 0.79 [0.69–0.88], the *LOXL1*_rs1048661 (---) was 0.71 [0.60–0.81], and the interaction between VFI at diagnosis and *LOXL1*_rs2165241 (predicted curve) (---) was 0.81 [0.70–0.88].

4. Discussion

In this study, we evaluated visual field deterioration in patients with newly diagnosed exfoliation glaucoma using three different strategies: MD, VFI, and GPA. The models showed increased accuracy when genetics were included as a risk factor. This finding was consistent across all three strategies and was observed in both linear and logistic regression models. Additionally, the AUC analysis confirmed these results.

This study found that clinical predictors such as IOP/MD and VFI at diagnosis were highly associated with glaucoma progression. This association was present in both linear and logistic regression analyses. However, when interaction terms were built using IOP and MD or VFI at diagnosis as predictors, the association was not significant. In the case of linear regression, the *p*-values were 0.89 and 0.55. In the case of logistic regression, a slight significance was found when MD was included in the interaction term ($p = 0.04$), but this was not observed when VFI was included ($p = 0.24$). These non-significant results may be due to collinearity between the predictors. The Pearson's coefficient confirmed this, showing a significant correlation between IOP and MD ($p = 0.001$, $r = 0.51$). Similar results were observed for the correlation between IOP and VFI values at the time of inclusion (Pearson's coefficient: $p = 0.001$, $r = 0.55$). In summary, this study suggested that patients diagnosed with high IOP tended to have more advanced visual field damage than those with low IOP.

When evaluating the accuracy of linear regression models, it is essential to consider the R^2 value. This value measures the percentage of variance in the effect variable that can be explained by the predictor variable. A higher R^2 value indicates a better fit. However, there is no defined cut-off value, so it is crucial to interpret R^2 values clinically. In our study, we calculated adjusted R^2 values due to multiple predictor variables in the multivariate linear regression. The IOP at diagnosis resulted in R^2 values of around 0.34–0.37, while MD and VFI were around 0.55–0.58. The SNPs showed R^2 values of 0.41–0.44. However, when we combined clinical predictors with SNPs in interaction terms, we saw an increase in the adjusted R^2 values to 0.78–0.89, almost doubling the model accuracy. We also saw an increase in the R^2 values for logistic regression analysis when combining SNPs with clinical predictors.

According to the logistic regression analysis, including SNPs increased predictive accuracy (PA). *LOXL1*_rs2165241, combined with MD/VFI at diagnosis, showed the highest PA values of 80% and 78%. On the other hand, when the other SNP (*LOXL1*_rs1048661) was included, PA values of 74% and 72% were obtained. PA values increased around 5–10% when the SNPs were added to the model. The AUC analysis also indicated a good prediction accuracy for all the predictors. The combination terms of MD/VFI * *LOXL1*_rs2165241 showed the highest AUC values (around 0.90), demonstrating an excellent prediction capacity. However, when *LOXL1*_rs1048661 was included, the AUC showed lower values (around 0.80), indicating that *LOXL1*_rs2165241 was a better predictor than *LOXL1*_rs1048661. It is worth noting that the two SNPs were highly correlated with each other (Pearson's test, *p*-, r = 0.66), suggesting that they are part of the same genetic signal. Previous studies have reported high linkage disequilibrium (LD) between *LOXL1*_rs2165241 and *LOXL1*_rs1048661 [17]. The present study revealed a significant correlation between *LOXL1*_rs2165241 and *LOXL1*_rs1048661, indicating that they were part of the same genetic signal. Based on the results, it is likely that both SNPs need not be included in clinical models. The research further indicates that *LOXL1*_rs2165241 has the highest AUC values among the SNPs and, therefore, would be the most appropriate option for inclusion in the models.

This study examined two distinct SNPs, namely *LOXL1*_rs2165241 and *LOXL1*_rs1048661, which were selected based on previous research that linked them to visual field progression in patients with exfoliation glaucoma [8]. Another SNP, *LOXL1*_rs3825942, was identified in earlier studies involving Scandinavian populations which was strongly linked to exfoliation and exfoliation glaucoma [17,18]. Prior research investigated allele frequencies between healthy individuals and exfoliation glaucoma patients (case-control studies), revealing highly skewed frequencies of *LOXL1*_rs3825942. Specifically, the A allele of *LOXL1*_rs3825942 was found in only 0.4% of glaucoma patients but 17.9% of healthy individuals, consistent with previous findings [7,17]. Due to the limited sample size and low frequency of *LOXL1*_rs3825942 in glaucoma patients, it was not included in the current study.

Our study aimed to evaluate the progression of glaucoma in patients using visual fields, which is widely regarded as the most accurate method. We selected two parameters to assess the outcomes—mean deviation (MD) and visual field index (VFI). Although MD is a traditional technique that allows for comparison with previous studies, it has limitations as other eye conditions apart from glaucoma may also impact the MD values. For example, cataract development alters the MD values. Previous studies have evaluated visual field deterioration using the "pointwise" linear regression method [19,20]. The pointwise method correlates well with the VFI method [21]. The reason for evaluating visual field deterioration using VFI in our study is clinical. In Sweden, most ophthalmologists prefer using VFI to evaluate glaucoma progression as it is a more effective measure. VFI is a recalculation of the MD that emphasizes the central portions of the visual fields that are primarily affected by glaucoma [22].

It should be noted that this study has certain limitations to be considered. Firstly, this study only included patients diagnosed with MD between 0 and −16 dB, excluding cases of advanced glaucoma to avoid "ceiling effects" in the visual fields. Therefore, this study's findings are only applicable to early and moderate glaucoma patients according to Hodapp's classification [23]. Secondly, this study only involved patients with exfoliation glaucoma, limiting the generalizability of the results to other types of glaucoma. Thirdly, all patients in this study were recently diagnosed with glaucoma, meaning that disease progression was high, although the treatment received would slow down the disease. Fourthly, all patients included in this study were born in Scandinavia, and, given the significant role of genetics in exfoliation glaucoma, other ethnic groups may respond differently. Fifthly, this study only examined the *LOXL_1* gene and did not consider other genes or other SNPs located in the *LOXL_1*. Sixthly, the analysis conducted in this study cost around USD 200 per patient, totaling USD 20000. This study took place in Sweden, a wealthy country. Although the prices for genetic analysis are decreasing, they may still be unaffordable in poorer countries. Finally, disease progression was evaluated solely using visual fields, without anatomical measurements like optical coherence tomography (OCT).

5. Conclusions

The present study investigated the effectiveness of three distinct strategies for evaluating visual field deterioration. To achieve this, this study focused on analyzing the impact of genetics on the accuracy of risk factor models. Through the analysis of two specific genetic factors, *LOXL1*_rs2165241 and *LOXL1*_rs1048661, this study found that including genetic information significantly increased the accuracy of risk factor models. Furthermore, this study recommends that future research explore other genes related to EXFG to provide a more comprehensive understanding of the factors contributing to visual field deterioration. By expanding our knowledge of the genetic factors, we can better diagnose and manage visual field deterioration, improving the quality of life for individuals affected by this condition.

Supplementary Materials: The following supporting information can be downloaded at: https://www.mdpi.com/article/10.3390/biomedicines12061225/s1, Table S1: STROBE check-list.

Funding: This research received no external funding.

Institutional Review Board Statement: The Institutional Review Board at the University of Gothenburg granted approval. Approval number: DNR: 119-12. This study was conducted in accordance with the Declaration of Helsinki.

Informed Consent Statement: Informed consent was obtained from all subjects involved in this study.

Data Availability Statement: Dataset available on request from the author.

Conflicts of Interest: The author declares no conflicts of interest.

References

1. Tham, Y.C.; Li, X.; Wong, T.Y.; Quigley, H.A.; Aung, T.; Cheng, C.Y. Global prevalence of glaucoma and projections of glaucoma burden through 2040: A systematic review and meta-analysis. *Ophthalmology* **2014**, *121*, 2081–2090. [CrossRef] [PubMed]
2. Aström, S.; Stenlund, H.; Lindén, C. Incidence and prevalence of pseudoexfoliations and open-angle glaucoma in northern Sweden: II. Results after 21 years of follow-up. *Acta Ophthalmol. Scand.* **2007**, *85*, 832–837. [CrossRef] [PubMed]
3. Schlotzer-Schrehardt, U. Molecular pathology of pseudoexfoliation syndrome/glaucoma--new insights from LOXL1 gene associations. *Exp. Eye Res.* **2009**, *88*, 776–785. [CrossRef] [PubMed]
4. Aboobakar, I.F.; Johnson, W.M.; Stamer, W.D.; Hauser, M.A.; Allingham, R.R. Major review: Exfoliation syndrome; advances in disease genetics, molecular biology, and epidemiology. *Exp. Eye Res.* **2017**, *154*, 88–103. [CrossRef]
5. Founti, P.; Haidich, A.B.; Chatzikyriakidou, A.; Salonikiou, A.; Anastasopoulos, E.; Pappas, T.; Lambropoulos, A.; Viswanathan, A.C.; Topouzis, F. Ethnicity-Based Differences in the Association of LOXL1 Polymorphisms with Pseudoexfoliation/Pseudoexfoliative Glaucoma: A Meta-Analysis. *Ann. Hum. Genet.* **2015**, *79*, 431–450. [CrossRef] [PubMed]
6. Greene, A.G.; Eivers, S.B.; Dervan, E.W.J.; O'Brien, C.J.; Wallace, D.M. Lysyl Oxidase Like 1: Biological roles and regulation. *Exp. Eye Res.* **2020**, *193*, 107975. [CrossRef]
7. Ayala, M.; Zetterberg, M.; Skoog, I.; Zettergren, A. Association of Single Nucleotide Polymorphisms Located in LOXL1 with Exfoliation Glaucoma in Southwestern Sweden. *Genes* **2021**, *12*, 1384. [CrossRef] [PubMed]
8. Ayala, M.; Zetterberg, M.; Zettergren, A. Single nucleotide polymorphisms in LOXL1 as biomarkers for progression of exfoliation glaucoma in Sweden. *Acta Ophthalmol.* **2023**, *101*, 521–529. [CrossRef] [PubMed]
9. Leske, M.C.; Heijl, A.; Hussein, M.; Bengtsson, B.; Hyman, L.; Komaroff, E. Factors for glaucoma progression and the effect of treatment: The early manifest glaucoma trial. *Arch. Ophthalmol.* **2003**, *121*, 48–56. [CrossRef]
10. Ernest, P.J.; Schouten, J.S.; Beckers, H.J.; Hendrikse, F.; Prins, M.H.; Webers, C.A. An evidence-based review of prognostic factors for glaucomatous visual field progression. *Ophthalmology* **2013**, *120*, 512–519. [CrossRef]
11. Chan, T.C.W.; Bala, C.; Siu, A.; Wan, F.; White, A. Risk Factors for Rapid Glaucoma Disease Progression. *Am. J. Ophthalmol.* **2017**, *180*, 151–157. [CrossRef] [PubMed]
12. von Elm, E.; Altman, D.G.; Egger, M.; Pocock, S.J.; Gotzsche, P.C.; Vandenbroucke, J.P.; Initiative, S. The Strengthening the Reporting of Observational Studies in Epidemiology (STROBE) Statement: Guidelines for reporting observational studies. *Int. J. Surg.* **2014**, *12*, 1495–1499. [CrossRef] [PubMed]
13. Ayala, M. Risk Factors and Frequency of Examinations for Detecting Visual Field Deterioration in Patients Newly Diagnosed Exfoliation Glaucoma in Sweden. *J. Glaucoma* **2024**, *33*, 168–175. [CrossRef]
14. Ayala, M. Estimating functions for visual field progression in newly diagnosed exfoliation glaucoma patients in Sweden. *Sci. Rep.* **2023**, *13*, 20979. [CrossRef]
15. Heijl, A.; Alm, A.; Bengtsson, B.; Bergstrom, A.; Calissendorff, B.; Lindblom, B.; Linden, C.; Swedish Ophthalmological Society. The Glaucoma Guidelines of the Swedish Ophthalmological Society. *Acta Ophthalmol. Suppl.* **2012**, *90*, 1–40. [CrossRef] [PubMed]

16. Nguyen, A.T.; Greenfield, D.S.; Bhakta, A.S.; Lee, J.; Feuer, W.J. Detecting Glaucoma Progression Using Guided Progression Analysis with OCT and Visual Field Assessment in Eyes Classified by International Classification of Disease Severity Codes. *Ophthalmol. Glaucoma* **2019**, *2*, 36–46. [CrossRef]
17. Thorleifsson, G.; Magnusson, K.P.; Sulem, P.; Walters, G.B.; Gudbjartsson, D.F.; Stefansson, H.; Jonsson, T.; Jonasdottir, A.; Jonasdottir, A.; Stefansdottir, G.; et al. Common sequence variants in the LOXL1 gene confer susceptibility to exfoliation glaucoma. *Science* **2007**, *317*, 1397–1400. [CrossRef] [PubMed]
18. Lemmelä, S.; Forsman, E.; Onkamo, P.; Nurmi, H.; Laivuori, H.; Kivelä, T.; Puska, P.; Heger, M.; Eriksson, A.; Forsius, H.; et al. Association of LOXL1 gene with Finnish exfoliation syndrome patients. *J. Hum. Genet.* **2009**, *54*, 289–297. [CrossRef] [PubMed]
19. Mahmoudinezhad, G.; Nishida, T.; Weinreb, R.N.; Baxter, S.L.; Eslani, M.; Micheletti, E.; Liebmann, J.M.; Fazio, M.A.; Girkin, C.A.; Zangwill, L.M.; et al. Impact of Smoking on Visual Field Progression in a Long-term Clinical Follow-up. *Ophthalmology* **2022**, *129*, 1235–1244. [CrossRef]
20. Asano, S.; Murata, H.; Matsuura, M.; Fujino, Y.; Miki, A.; Tanito, M.; Mizoue, S.; Mori, K.; Suzuki, K.; Yamashita, T.; et al. Validating the efficacy of the binomial pointwise linear regression method to detect glaucoma progression with multicentral database. *Br. J. Ophthalmol.* **2020**, *104*, 569–574. [CrossRef]
21. De Moraes, C.G.; Ghobraiel, S.R.; Ritch, R.; Liebmann, J.M. Comparison of PROGRESSOR and Glaucoma Progression Analysis 2 to Detect Visual Field Progression in Treated Glaucoma Patients. *Asia Pac. J. Ophthalmol.* **2012**, *1*, 135–139. [CrossRef] [PubMed]
22. Bengtsson, B.; Heijl, A. A visual field index for calculation of glaucoma rate of progression. *Am. J. Ophthalmol.* **2008**, *145*, 343–353. [CrossRef] [PubMed]
23. Hodapp, E.; Parrish, R.K.; Anderson, D.R. *Clinical Decisions in Glaucoma*; Mosby: St. Louis, MO, USA; London, UK, 1993.

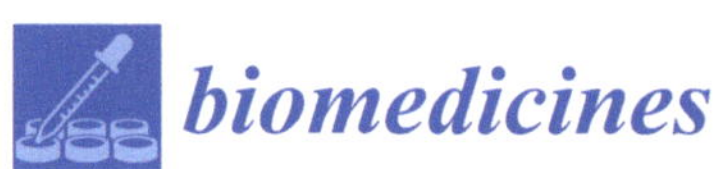 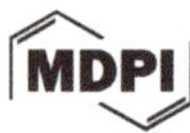

Article

Possible Causal Association between Type 2 Diabetes and Glycaemic Traits in Primary Open-Angle Glaucoma: A Two-Sample Mendelian Randomisation Study

Je Hyun Seo [1,*,†] and Young Lee [1,2,†]

[1] Veterans Medical Research Institute, Veterans Health Service Medical Center, Seoul 05368, Republic of Korea; lyou7688@gmail.com
[2] Department of Applied Statistics, Chung-Ang University, Seoul 06974, Republic of Korea
* Correspondence: jazmin2@naver.com; Tel.: +82-2-2225-1445
† These authors contributed equally to this work.

Abstract: Existing literature suggests a controversial relationship between type 2 diabetes mellitus (T2D) and glaucoma. This study aimed to examine the potential causal connection between T2D and glycaemic traits (fasting glucose [FG] and glycated haemoglobin [HbA1c] levels) as exposures to primary open-angle glaucoma (POAG) in multi-ethnic populations. Single-nucleotide polymorphisms associated with exposure to T2D, FG, and HbA1c were selected as instrumental variables with significance ($p < 5.0 \times 10^{-8}$) from the genome-wide association study (GWAS)-based meta-analysis data available from the BioBank Japan and the UK Biobank (UKB). The GWAS for POAG was obtained from the meta-analyses of Genetic Epidemiology Research in Adult Health and Aging and the UKB. A two-sample Mendelian randomisation (MR) study was performed to assess the causal estimates using the inverse-variance weighted (IVW) method, and MR-Pleiotropy Residual Sum and Outlier test (MR–PRESSO). Significant causal associations of T2D (odds ratio [OR] = 1.05, 95% confidence interval [CI] = [1.00–1.10], $p = 0.031$ in IVW; OR = 1.06, 95% CI = [1.01–1.11], $p = 0.017$ in MR–PRESSO) and FG levels (OR = 1.19, 95% CI = [1.02–1.38], $p = 0.026$ in IVW; OR = 1.17, 95% CI = [1.01–1.35], $p = 0.041$ in MR–PRESSO) with POAG were observed, but not in HbA1c (all $p > 0.05$). The potential causal relationship between T2D or FG and POAG highlights its role in the prevention of POAG. Further investigation is necessary to authenticate these findings.

Keywords: primary open-angle glaucoma; mendelian randomisation; type 2 diabetes; fasting glucose; single-nucleotide polymorphisms

Citation: Seo, J.H.; Lee, Y. Possible Causal Association between Type 2 Diabetes and Glycaemic Traits in Primary Open-Angle Glaucoma: A Two-Sample Mendelian Randomisation Study. *Biomedicines* **2024**, *12*, 866. https://doi.org/10.3390/biomedicines12040866

Academic Editor: Da-Wen Lu

Received: 26 February 2024
Revised: 3 April 2024
Accepted: 12 April 2024
Published: 15 April 2024

1. Introduction

Glaucoma is a major cause of permanent vision loss. It is a progressive condition that affects the optic nerve, leading to the deterioration of the retinal ganglion cells and their axons [1]. Primary open-angle glaucoma (POAG) is the predominant form of glaucoma subtype [2]; however, its pathogenesis remains unclear due to the role of multiple factors in its pathophysiology [3–6]. The proposed risk factors for glaucoma include ageing, elevated intraocular pressure (IOP), vascular factors, genetic factors, systemic disorders (such as diabetes), and environmental factors [3,5–10]. Thus, the identification of POAG causal risk factors may facilitate the early detection and prevention of glaucoma; therefore, these studies form the basis for eye and vision research.

Type 2 diabetes (T2D) is an increasingly prevalent chronic metabolic disorder [11,12] that affected approximately 415 million people in 2015 worldwide [13]. This representative systemic illness is frequently regarded as a systemic risk factor, along with systemic hypertension, for glaucoma prevention. However, in contrast to IOP and ageing in POAG, epidemiological findings regarding the effects of T2D on POAG development remain controversial [14–18]. The Blue Mountains Eye Study suggested a substantial correlation between T2D and POAG and considered it a risk factor [15]. Subsequently, several studies have examined the relationship between T2D and POAG, indicating that T2D may be a risk factor for POAG development with increasing IOP related to glycaemic traits [16–18]. However, the Rotterdam Study and Baltimore Eye Survey raised concerns regarding the non-significant association between T2D and POAG [19,20]. Additionally, recent studies have reported an insignificant association [21–24] or negative point estimate [20,25,26] between the two.

A large-scale study using the Korean National Health Insurance Data demonstrated that the hazard ratio of glaucoma for T2D was 1.80 (95% confidence interval [CI], 1.58–2.04) with adjustment [27]. Another meta-analysis suggested that upon comparing patients with and without diabetes, the pooled relative risk for glaucoma was 1.48 (95% CI, 1.29–1.71), with significant heterogeneity (I^2 = 82.3%, $p < 0.001$) [28]. Due to this heterogeneity, it is unclear whether T2D is a risk factor for POAG. In addition, this retrospective association analysis was unable to prove the causality, thus, the nature of the association remains unclear.

Mendelian randomisation (MR) is a genetic epidemiological technique that employs genetic variants linked to potential exposures as the instrumental variables (IVs) to assess their causal impact on disease outcomes [29,30]. A previous study using MR analysis suggested variable evidence for an association between T2D and POAG (odds ratio [OR] = 1.97, 95% CI 1.01–1.15) in individuals with European ancestry [31]. However, a recent MR study of the Japanese population demonstrated that glycaemic traits such as fasting glucose (FG), glycated haemoglobin (HbA1c), and C-peptide levels did not display a significant correlation with POAG [32]. Although POAG prevalence differs between ethnic groups [7], it is a representative common complex disease in terms of genetics and multi-ethnic group analysis and is reliable if the subject pool is large enough for MR analysis [33,34]. Furthermore, a study on the two-sample MR analysis methodology using large cohorts, such as the UK Biobank (UKB), reported that the MR-Egger bias did not affect the inverse-variance weighted (IVW) and weighted median [35]. Moreover, the results of the MR analysis may vary based on the selection of IVs for T2D. Therefore, large datasets combining the meta-analysis of the Biobank Japan (BBJ) and UKB [36] are expected to generate more substantial results. To this end, this study aimed to conduct a two-sample MR analysis to investigate the possible causal effects of T2D and glycaemic traits (FG, and HbA1c levels) on POAG based on the BBJ and UKB meta-analyses [36], as well as the Genetic Epidemiology Research in Adult Health and Aging (GERA) and UKB meta-analyses [37].

2. Materials and Methods

2.1. Study Design

The study protocol was approved by the Institutional Review Board of the Veterans Health Service Medical Centre (IRB No. 2022-03-004), and the need for informed consent was waived because of its retrospective study design. The research was conducted in accordance with the tenets of the Declaration of Helsinki.

2.2. Data Sources

Figure 1 is a schematic of the analytical study design. To examine the potential causal effects of T2D and glycaemic traits (FG and HbA1c) on the risk of POAG, the following datasets were selected: (1) exposure data from the summary statistics of the genome-wide association study (GWAS)-based meta-analysis of the BBJ and UKB for the multi-ethnic population (n = 667,504 for T2D [84,224 cases vs. 583,280 controls], n = 448,252 for FG, and n = 415,403 for HbA1c) (Table 1) [36]; and (2) outcome data from the summary statistics of the POAG GWAS data from the meta-analysis (n = 240,302; [12,315 cases vs. 227,987 controls]) of the GERA and UKB [38]. POAG is defined by the International Classification of Diseases-9 diagnosis code of POAG or normal-tension glaucoma, excluding other subtypes of glaucoma (e.g., pseudoexfoliation, pigmentary, etc.) [38]. Table 1 enlists the datasets used for the summary statistics.

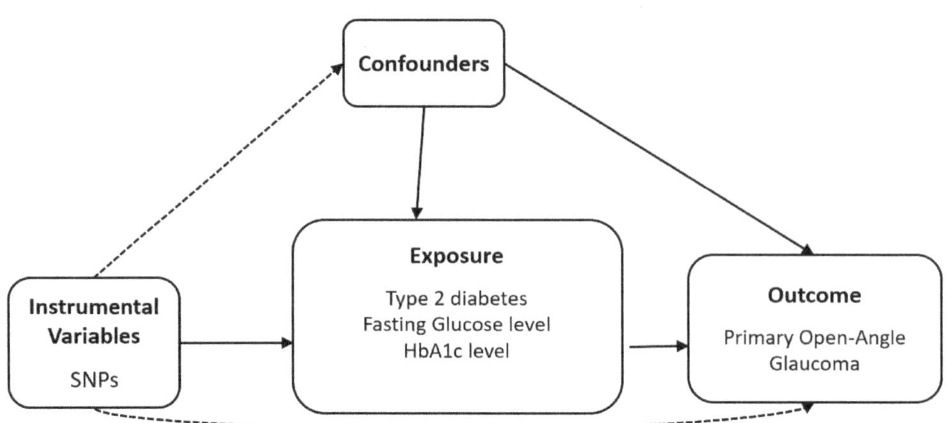

Figure 1. Diagram of two-sample Mendelian randomisation analysis. Abbreviation: HbA1c, glycated haemoglobin; SNP, Single nucleotide polymorphism.

Table 1. Statistical measures summarizing the data source.

Traits	Data Source	Subjects Number	Population	Variants Number	Reference
T2D	BBJ Project + UKB	667,504 (84,224 cases + 583,280 controls)	East Asian + European	25,845,091	[36]
FG	BBJ Project + UKB	448,252	East Asian + European	20,535,873	[36]
HbA1c	BBJ Project + UKB	415,403	East Asian + European	20,525,742	[36]
Glaucoma	GERA cohort + UKB	240,302 (12,315 cases + 227,987 controls)	Multi-ethnic: 214,102 European 5103 African unspecified 3571 Other admixed ancestry 1847 African American or Afro-Caribbean 5189 Hispanic or Latin American 5370 East Asian 5120 South Asian	7,760,820	[37]

Abbreviations: T2D, type 2 diabetes; BBJ, BioBank Japan; UKB, UK Biobank; FG, fasting glucose; HbA1c, glycated haemoglobin; GERA, Genetic Epidemiology Research in Adult Health and Ageing.

2.3. Selection of the Genetic IVs

Single-nucleotide polymorphisms (SNPs) associated with each exposure at the GWAS threshold $p < 5.0 \times 10^{-8}$ were used as IVs. To verify that each IV was independent of the other, the SNPs were pruned based on linkage disequilibrium (LD; $r^2 = 0.001$, clumping distance = 10,000 kb). The 1000 Genomes Phase III Dataset (European population) was used as the reference panel to compute the LD for the clumping procedure. The F-value was determined using the formula $F = R^2(n-2)/(1-R^2)$, where n is the sample size and R^2 is the proportion of exposure variance by genetic variance [39]. F-values > 10 indicate the absence of a weak instrument bias [40].

2.4. Mendelian Randomisation

The MR analysis was conducted based on the following three presumptions concerning IVs: (1) they have to show a significant association with the exposure, (2) they must be unrelated to the confounding variables, and (3) they should solely affect the outcomes via exposure, indicating the absence of a directional horizontal pleiotropy effect. We employed the inverse variance-weighted (IVW) MR method with random effects as the major strategy [33,40,41]. The Cochran's Q-test was used to evaluate the heterogeneity among SNPs in the IVW technique [41]. The presence of heterogeneity was shown by a *p*-value of less than 0.05 for Cochran's Q-test. Heterogeneity may suggest the potential existence of horizontal pleiotropy. The effectiveness of IVW analysis is maximized when all genetic variations satisfy the three assumptions for IVs [42]. We conducted a sensitivity analysis to test the validity and reliability, taking into consideration potential concerns such as instrumental bias or pleiotropy. The weighted median approach [43], MR-Egger regression (with or without adjustment using the Simulation Extrapolation [SIMEX] method) [44,45], and the MR pleiotropy residual sum and outlier (MR-PRESSO) [46] were employed for sensitivity analysis. The weighted median approach yields reliable estimates, even when as many as 50% of the IVs are inaccurate [42]. The MR-Egger approach provides estimates of appropriate causal effects, even when pleiotropic effects are present, by taking into account a nonzero intercept that denotes the mean horizontal pleiotropic impacts and a slope that serves as an estimate of the causal impact [43]. If there is a violation of the assumption that there is no measurement error ($I^2 < 90\%$), bias can be addressed by employing MR-Egger regression with SIMEX [45]. The heterogeneity of the MR-Egger technique was assessed by the utilization of Rücker's Q′ statistic tests [47]. The MR-PRESSO method is an expansion of the IVW with the objective of mitigating the presence of pleiotropic outliers [46]. The MR–PRESSO global test was employed to assess the presence of directional horizontal pleiotropy [46]. When the MR-PRESSO global test gives a *p*-value below 0.05, the MR-PRESSO outlier test is utilized to detect the presence of particular horizontal pleiotropic outlier variations [46]. As a consequence, the findings were interpreted in accordance with the suitable technique for MR analysis [48]. All analyses were conducted using the TwoSampleMR and SIMEX packages in R version 3.6.3 (R Core Team, Vienna, Austria).

3. Results

3.1. Genetic IVs

In total, 180 IVs were identified at the significance threshold values of $p < 5.0 \times 10^{-8}$ for T2D (Table 2). In addition, 108 and 303 IVs were identified at the significance limit of $p < 5.0 \times 10^{-8}$ for FG and HbA1c, respectively. The mean F-statistics for T2D, FG, and HbA1c (176.16, 111.30, and 119.61, respectively) used for MR were > 10, demonstrating a low likelihood of weak instrument bias (Table 2 and Supplementary Table S1). Detailed information on the IVs is provided in Supplementary Table S1.

Table 2. Heterogeneity and horizontal pleiotropy of instrumental variables.

Exposure				Heterogeneity			Horizontal Pleiotropy			
				Cochran's Q Test from IVW	Rucker's Q′ Test from MR-Egger	MR-PRESSO Global Test	MR-Egger		MR-Egger (SIMEX)	
	N	F	I^2 (%)	*p*-Value	*p*-Value	*p*-Value	Intercept, β (SE)	*p*-Value	Intercept, β (SE)	*p*-Value
T2D	180	176.16	95.57	<0.001	<0.001	<0.001	0.001 (0.004)	0.720	0.001 (0.004)	0.771
FG	108	111.30	97.76	<0.001	<0.001	<0.001	0.005 (0.004)	0.179	0.005 (0.004)	0.191
HbA1c	303	119.61	97.63	<0.001	<0.001	<0.001	−0.001 (0.002)	0.565	−0.001 (0.002)	0.548

Abbreviation: N, number of instruments; F, mean F statistic; IVW, inverse-variance weighted; MR, Mendelian randomisation; PRESSO, pleiotropy residual sum and outlier; SIMEX, simulation extrapolation; β, beta coefficient; SE, standard error; T2D, type 2 diabetes; FG, fasting glucose; HbA1c, glycated haemoglobin.

3.2. Heterogeneity and Horizontal Pleiotropy of IVs

To evaluate the quality of the IVs, we computed the I^2 and p values for Cochran's Q statistic using IVW, Rücker's Q′ statistic using MR-Egger, and the MR-PRESSO global test, as displayed in Table 2. The Cochran's Q test from IVW demonstrated that the IVs for T2D, FG, and HbA1c (all $p < 0.001$) were heterogeneous (Table 2); therefore, a random-effects IVW approach was used. Additionally, the Rücker's Q′ test from the MR-Egger demonstrated heterogeneity between the IVs (all $p < 0.001$). Although heterogeneity suggests genetic variations could indicate pleiotropy, the MR-Egger regression intercepts did not show horizontal pleiotropy ($p > 0.05$) in all tests, regardless of the SIMEX correction (Table 2). In the MR-PRESSO global test for T2D, FG, and HbA1c, which showed substantial horizontal pleiotropic effects (all $p < 0.001$), the MR-PRESSO results were considered the primary outcomes based on prior research [48].

3.3. Mendelian Randomisation for the Possible Causal Association between T2D and POAG

T2D demonstrated a significant and probable causal association with glaucoma using the IVW method (MR OR = 1.05, 95% confidence interval (CI): 1.00–1.10 $p = 0.031$), weighted median method (MR OR = 1.08, 95% CI: 1.01–1.16, $p = 0.026$), and MR-PRESSO (MR OR = 1.06, 95% CI: 1.01–1.11 $p = 0.017$) (Figure 2). The genetic correlation between T2D and glaucoma for each SNP was a significant positive correlation in scatter plots (Figure 3).

T2D

Method	Number of SNPs	OR (95% CI)	*p* value
IVW	180	1.05 (1.00, 1.10)	0.031
Weighted median	180	1.08 (1.01, 1.16)	0.026
MR Egger	180	1.04 (0.94, 1.14)	0.478
MR Egger (SIMEX)	180	1.04 (0.94, 1.15)	0.464
MR PRESSO	179	1.06 (1.01, 1.11)	0.017

0.7 0.97 1.24 1.51

Figure 2. Forest plot of causal associations of T2D on glaucoma. Abbreviations: T2D, type 2 diabetes; IVW, inverse-variance weighted; SIMEX, Simulation Extrapolation; MR–PRESSO, MR- pleiotropy residual sum and outlier test; OR, odds ratio; CI, confidence interval.

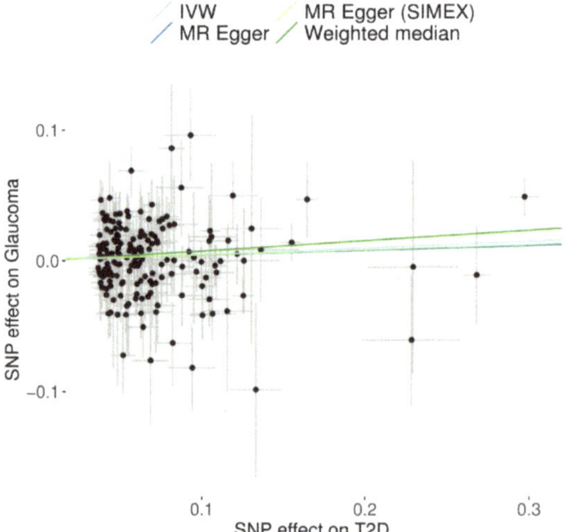

Figure 3. Scatter plots of MR tests assessing the effect of T2D on glaucoma. Abbreviations: T2D, type 2 diabetes; IVW, inverse-variance weighted; SIMEX, Simulation Extrapolation; MR, Mendelian randomisation. Light blue, light green, dark blue, and dark green regression lines represent the IVW, MR–Egger (SIMEX), MR–Egger, and weighted median estimate, respectively.

3.4. Mendelian Randomisation for the Possible Causal Association of FG and HbA1c with POAG

FG demonstrated a significant causal association with POAG using the IVW method (MR OR = 1.19, 95% CI: 1.02–1.38 p = 0.026) and MR-PRESSO (MR OR = 1.17, 95% CI: 1.01–1.35, p = 0.041) (Figure 4). However, HbA1c did not demonstrate a significant causal association with POAG (all $p > 0.05$, all MR methods; Figure 4). Scatter plots indicate the genetic association between FG and HbA1c and that with POAG for each SNP (Figure 5).

FG

Method	Number of SNPs	OR (95% CI)	p value
IVW	108	1.19 (1.02, 1.38)	0.026
Weighted median	108	1.06 (0.87, 1.30)	0.565
MR Egger	108	1.02 (0.78, 1.33)	0.887
MR Egger (SIMEX)	108	1.02 (0.78, 1.34)	0.880
MR PRESSO	107	1.17 (1.01, 1.35)	0.041

0.5 0.93 1.36 1.79

HbA1c

Method	Number of SNPs	OR (95% CI)	p value
IVW	303	1.05 (0.96, 1.14)	0.302
Weighted median	303	1.08 (0.95, 1.23)	0.219
MR Egger	303	1.09 (0.93, 1.27)	0.299
MR Egger (SIMEX)	303	1.09 (0.93, 1.28)	0.292
MR PRESSO	298	1.05 (0.97, 1.14)	0.227

0.6 0.96 1.32

Figure 4. Forest plot of causal associations of FG and HbA1c on glaucoma. Abbreviations: FG, fasting glucose; IVW, inverse-variance weighted; SIMEX, Simulation Extrapolation; MR–PRESSO, MR-pleiotropy residual sum and outlier test; OR, odds ratio; CI, confidence interval, HbA1c, glycated haemoglobin.

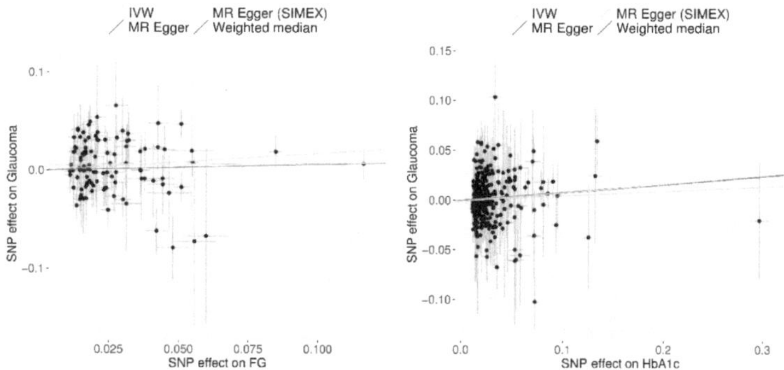

Figure 5. Scatter plots of MR tests assessing the effect of FG and HbA1c on glaucoma. Abbreviations: FG, fasting glucose; IVW, inverse-variance weighted; SIMEX, Simulation Extrapolation; HbA1c, glycated haemoglobin; MR, Mendelian randomisation. Light blue, light green, dark blue, and dark green regression lines represent the IVW, MR–Egger (SIMEX), MR–Egger, and weighted median estimate, respectively.

4. Discussion

Our study demonstrated a possible causal association between T2D and POAG. Moreover, FG levels, which are popular glycaemic traits to diagnose T2D and prediabetes conditions, demonstrated a potential causal association with POAG. In contrast, HbA1c levels did not demonstrate a causal association with POAG.

Several observational studies have reported an association between T2D and glaucoma [15,49,50]. In addition, a meta-analysis has suggested that upon comparing individuals with and without diabetes, the pooled OR for POAG was 1.50 (95% CI, 1.16–1.93) [51]. However, several studies have reported an insignificant association [21–24] or negative point estimate [20,25,26]. Therefore, a large-scale study is required to address the disparities between these findings. A large meta-analysis, including 47 studies with 2,981,341 individuals, suggested that T2D is associated with POAG, indicating a pooled relative risk of 1.48 (95% CI: 1.29–1.71) [28]. In addition to an association, an MR analysis method was used to analyse these causal associations. Our study is consistent with the findings of an MR study, which reported on the possible causal relationship between POAG and T2D in Europeans (body mass index [BMI]-unadjusted: OR = 1.07, 95% CI, 1.01–1.14, and $p = 0.028$; BMI-adjusted: OR = 1.07, 95% CI, 1.01–1.15, and $p = 0.035$) [31] (Table 3). In our study, considering the possibility of pleiotropy due to the use of multi-ethnic genome-wide data, we conducted additional analyses using data composed of individuals of European descent (Additional File S1). As a result, we confirmed that T2D has a robust causal effect on POAG. The mechanistic consideration of the causality of T2D in POAG is necessary, and there is evidence from other studies that the presence of T2D causally contributes to an increase in IOP [52]. However, one previous study showed the possible causality between T2D and POAG was absent in the analysis of East Asian ancestry (BMI-unadjusted: OR = 1.01, 95% CI, 0.95–1.06, and $p = 0.866$; BMI-adjusted: OR = 1.00, 95% CI, 0.94–1.05, and $p = 0.882$) [31]. This difference can be attributed to the inclusion of approximately 46,000 East Asians in the outcome data, as well as the limited sample size, resulting in the possibility that the result may have been insignificant.

Table 3. Comparison of previous studies using MR on type 2 diabetes and glycaemic traits on glaucoma.

Ethnicity	Exposure Dataset	Outcome Dataset	Instrumental Variables	Causal Association with Glaucoma	References
EUR	339,224	8591 cases, 210,201 controls	BMI: $n = 64$ WC: $n = 36$ WHR: $n = 29$	BMI: Significant WC: Significant WHR: NS	[52]
EUR	BMI: $n = 339{,}224$ WC and HC $n = 224{,}459$	1824 cases, 93,036 controls	BMI: $n = 31$ WC: $n = 33$ HC: $n = 24$	BMI: Significant WC: NS HC: Significant	[53]
EUR/EAS	T2D: EUR 74,124 cases, 824,006 controls EAS 77,418 cases, 356,122 controls FG and HbA1c EUR: 196,991 EAS: 36,584	182,702 EUR (15,229 cases, 177,473 controls)	T2D: $n = 165$ FG: $n = 58$ HbA1c: $n = 60$	T2D: Significant FG: NS HbA1c: NS	[31]
		46,523 EAS (6935 cases, 39,588 controls)	T2D: $n = 129$ FG: $n = 11$ HbA1c: $n = 15$	T2D: NS FG: NS HbA1c: NS	
EAS	FG: $n = 17{,}289$ HbA1c: $n = 52{,}802$ C-peptide: $n = 1666$	22,795 (3980 cases, 18,815 controls)	FG: $n = 34$ HbA1c: $n = 43$ C-peptide: $n = 17$	FG: NS HbA1c: NS C-peptide: NS	[32]
Multi-ethnicity	T2D: 667,504 FG: 448,252 HbA1c: 415,403	240,302 (12,315 cases, 227,987 controls)	T2D: $n = 180$ FG: $n = 108$ HbA1c: $n = 303$	T2D: Significant FG: Significant HbA1c: NS	This study

Abbreviations: EUR, Europeans; EAS, East Asians; BMI, body mass index; WC, waist circumference; WHR, waist hip ratio; HC, hip circumference; T2D, type 2 diabetes; FG, fasting glucose; HbA1c, glycated haemoglobin; NS, not significant.

FG levels are often used for screening and evaluating prediabetes and T2D [54,55]. Elevated blood glucose levels, an important feature of T2D, are expected to be a reasonable indicator to evaluate the association between T2D and POAG. An observational study using 374,376 individuals from the Korea National Health Insurance data reported a positive association between FG levels and the incidence of glaucoma, with a hazard ratio of 2.022 (95% CI: 1.494–2.736) [56]. Similarly, we observed a strong association between FG and glaucoma using the MR analysis, which is a more stringent validation technique. Despite being a distinct genetic dataset, our results suggesting the causality of FG in POAG are substantial because they are novel and significant, compared with those of a previous study that used an MR analysis (Table 3). A hypothesis to explain this possibility may be that higher plasma FG is associated with higher glucose levels in the aqueous humour, which increases trabecular fibronectin levels and is associated with elevated IOP [57]. These hypotheses are supported by recent meta-analyses that suggest a pooled average increase of 0.09 mmHg in the IOP associated with a 10 mg/dL increase in the FG [28]. However, the association between diabetic retinopathy and glaucoma has been inconsistently demonstrated in several studies [58].

Clinically, HbA1c levels are associated with diabetic microvascular complications, which in turn are associated with long-term glycaemic control [59]. Researchers recommend maintaining a target HbA1c < 48 mmol/mol (6.5%) for the general population with T2D [60–62]. Regarding HbA1c and glucose levels, the Singapore Malay Eye Study demonstrated an elevated but insignificant trend, whereas a case-control study in Europe demonstrated a statistically significant association between elevated HbA1c levels and glaucoma [16]. However, HbA1c levels were not causally associated with POAG in our study, consistent with previous results (Table 3). Although we used 303 IVs in this study, heterogeneity and horizontal pleiotropy may have affected our results. An MR study using a large dataset demonstrated that HbA1c indicated marginal significance ($p = 0.064$); however, combined with the UKBB and FinnGen project dataset, the HbA1c indicated a possible causal association (OR: 1.28 95% CI, 1.01–1.61) [63]. A previous study had shown that the dose-response relationships between glucose metabolism markers and glaucoma prevalence are hockey-stick-shaped for HbA1c, and J-shaped for FG [18]. HbA1c quantifies glycaemic control over a period of 2 to 3 months, whereas FG assesses acute blood glucose levels. Consequently, FG is more sensitive to diseases as compared to HbA1c [64]. These different sensitivities in FG and HbA1C may lead to the different causal effects on POAG.

The chief strength of our study was the use of a relatively large cohort dataset, which suggested a possible causal association between T2D, and FG in glaucoma. However, this study had a few limitations. First, we did not have access to individual-level data; thus, we were unable to explain the presence of numerous confounding factors using summary statistics based on two-sample MR. Second, the test procedures to validate the MR hypotheses do not provide complete validation. The violations of MR assumptions can lead to invalid conclusions, thus warranting a cautious interpretation of the results. Third, few genome datasets include ophthalmic phenotype data; thus, it was difficult to separate and summarise a meta-analysis that included a portion of the UKB. However, considering the research results according to the large-cohort MR analysis methodology [35], the IVW and weighted median remain unaffected, which in turn influences the bias of MR-Egger. IVW and MR-PRESSO were the primary statistics in our study [48]; thus, the bias issue was minimised. In addition, there was no substantial difference between the MR methodologies, thus establishing the credibility of our results. Fourth, since our results contained heterogeneity issues, caution must be exercised when interpreting. The source of heterogeneity included the pleiotropy effect. As an alternative possibility, the samples used to estimate the SNP-exposure and SNP-outcome associations are not homogeneous; for example, a difference in the distribution of a covariate confounding the exposure-outcome relationship across samples could induce heterogeneity. In addition, the SNP-exposure and SNP-outcome relationships are not correctly specified—i.e., in the two-sample setting, the causal relationship between the exposure and the outcome is different in each of the samples [65]. Although we do not know the exact cause of heterogeneity, it was a multi-ethnic result, and since heterogeneity was not significant in the European race results that were additionally analysed (Additional File S1, [66]), it would be ideal to mention the possibility of heterogeneity due to heterogeneity in exposure and outcome data.

5. Conclusions

Our study demonstrated the possible causal association of T2D and FG on POAG development in European and East Asian populations using an MR analysis. The analysis of the European data set yielded consistent results, demonstrating the significance of POAG in T2D and enhancing the robustness and replicability of the findings. This potential causal relationship between T2D or FG and POAG highlights the significance of T2D in early detection and prevention of POAG, considering the high prevalence of T2D. Researchers should further clarify and investigate the association between T2D and POAG.

Supplementary Materials: The following supporting information can be downloaded at: https://www.mdpi.com/article/10.3390/biomedicines12040866/s1, Table S1. List of single-nucleotide polymorphisms used as instrumental variables. Additional File S1: Table S2. Summary statistics of data source. Table S3. Heterogeneity and horizontal pleiotropy of instrumental variables. Table S4. Estimates from MR methods for the association between type 2 diabetes and glaucoma. Figure S1. Forest plot for association of type 2 diabetes and glaucoma. Figure S2. Scatter plots of MR tests assessing the type 2 diabetes and glaucoma.

Author Contributions: J.H.S. and Y.L. designed the study, J.H.S. and Y.L. collected the data, Y.L. performed the statistical analysis, and J.H.S. drafted the manuscript. All authors have read and agreed to the published version of the manuscript.

Funding: This research was funded by the National Research Foundation of Korea (NRF) grant funded by the Korean Government (Ministry of Science and ICT) (No. 2022R1C1C1002929).

Institutional Review Board Statement: The study was conducted in accordance with the tenets of the Declaration of Helsinki and approved by the Institutional Review Board of the Veterans Health Service Medical Center (IRB No. 2022-03-004; 16 March 2022).

Informed Consent Statement: Informed consent was not required because anonymised and de-identified data were used in the analyses. The requirement for patient consent was waived owing to the retrospective nature of the study.

Data Availability Statement: The datasets used and/or analysed in the current study are available from Biobank Japan (BBJ https://pheweb.jp/, accessed on 30 July 2022) [36] and the GWAS catalogue (https://www.ebi.ac.uk/gwas/summary-statistics, accessed on 19 July 2022).

Acknowledgments: We would like to thank Biobank Japan (BBJ https://pheweb.jp/, accessed on 30 July 2022) [36], GWAS catalogue (https://www.ebi.ac.uk/gwas/summary-statistics, accessed 19 July 2022), and Genetic Epidemiology Research in Adult Health and Aging (GERA) cohort and UK Biobank (UKB) [37]. FinnGen (https://finngen.gitbook.io/documentation/v/r5/, accessed on 30 July 2023).

Conflicts of Interest: The authors declare no conflicts of interest.

References

1. Quigley, H.A. Glaucoma. *Lancet* **2011**, *377*, 1367–1377. [CrossRef] [PubMed]
2. Tham, Y.C.; Li, X.; Wong, T.Y.; Quigley, H.A.; Aung, T.; Cheng, C.Y. Global prevalence of glaucoma and projections of glaucoma burden through 2040: A systematic review and meta-analysis. *Ophthalmology* **2014**, *121*, 2081–2090. [CrossRef] [PubMed]
3. Jonas, J.B.; Aung, T.; Bourne, R.R.; Bron, A.M.; Ritch, R.; Panda-Jonas, S. Glaucoma. *Lancet* **2017**, *390*, 2183–2193. [CrossRef] [PubMed]
4. Bonomi, L.; Marchini, G.; Marraffa, M.; Bernardi, P.; Morbio, R.; Varotto, A. Vascular risk factors for primary open angle glaucoma: The Egna-Neumarkt Study. *Ophthalmology* **2000**, *107*, 1287–1293. [CrossRef] [PubMed]
5. Yanagi, M.; Kawasaki, R.; Wang, J.J.; Wong, T.Y.; Crowston, J.; Kiuchi, Y. Vascular risk factors in glaucoma: A review. *Clin. Exp. Ophthalmol.* **2011**, *39*, 252–258. [CrossRef] [PubMed]
6. Weinreb, R.N.; Aung, T.; Medeiros, F.A. The pathophysiology and treatment of glaucoma: A review. *JAMA* **2014**, *311*, 1901–1911. [CrossRef] [PubMed]

7. Shin, H.T.; Yoon, B.W.; Seo, J.H. Analysis of risk allele frequencies of single nucleotide polymorphisms related to open-angle glaucoma in different ethnic groups. *BMC Med. Genom.* **2021**, *14*, 80. [CrossRef]
8. Seo, J.H.; Kim, T.W.; Weinreb, R.N. Lamina cribrosa depth in healthy eyes. *Investig. Ophthalmol. Vis. Sci.* **2014**, *55*, 1241–1251. [CrossRef] [PubMed]
9. Jonas, J.B. Role of cerebrospinal fluid pressure in the pathogenesis of glaucoma. *Acta Ophthalmol.* **2011**, *89*, 505–514. [CrossRef]
10. Seo, J.H.; Kim, T.W.; Weinreb, R.N.; Kim, Y.A.; Kim, M. Relationship of intraocular pressure and frequency of spontaneous retinal venous pulsation in primary open-angle glaucoma. *Ophthalmology* **2012**, *119*, 2254–2260. [CrossRef]
11. International Expert Committee. International Expert Committee report on the role of the A1C assay in the diagnosis of diabetes. *Diabetes Care* **2009**, *32*, 1327–1334. [CrossRef] [PubMed]
12. American Diabetes Association. Diagnosis and classification of diabetes mellitus. *Diabetes Care* **2014**, *37* (Suppl. S1), S81–S90. [CrossRef] [PubMed]
13. Ogurtsova, K.; da Rocha Fernandes, J.D.; Huang, Y.; Linnenkamp, U.; Guariguata, L.; Cho, N.H.; Cavan, D.; Shaw, J.E.; Makaroff, L.E. IDF Diabetes Atlas: Global estimates for the prevalence of diabetes for 2015 and 2040. *Diabetes Res. Clin. Pract.* **2017**, *128*, 40–50. [CrossRef]
14. Ocular Hypertension Treatment Study Group; European Glaucoma Prevention Study Group; Gordon, M.O.; Torri, V.; Miglior, S.; Beiser, J.A.; Floriani, I.; Miller, J.P.; Gao, F.; Adamsons, I.; et al. Validated prediction model for the development of primary open-angle glaucoma in individuals with ocular hypertension. *Ophthalmology* **2007**, *114*, 10–19. [CrossRef] [PubMed]
15. Mitchell, P.; Smith, W.; Chey, T.; Healey, P.R. Open-angle glaucoma and diabetes: The Blue Mountains eye study, Australia. *Ophthalmology* **1997**, *104*, 712–718. [CrossRef] [PubMed]
16. Welinder, L.G.; Riis, A.H.; Knudsen, L.L.; Thomsen, R.W. Diabetes, glycemic control and risk of medical glaucoma treatment: A population-based case-control study. *Clin. Epidemiol.* **2009**, *1*, 125–131. [CrossRef] [PubMed]
17. Newman-Casey, P.A.; Talwar, N.; Nan, B.; Musch, D.C.; Stein, J.D. The relationship between components of metabolic syndrome and open-angle glaucoma. *Ophthalmology* **2011**, *118*, 1318–1326. [CrossRef] [PubMed]
18. Zhao, D.; Cho, J.; Kim, M.H.; Friedman, D.; Guallar, E. Diabetes, glucose metabolism, and glaucoma: The 2005-2008 National Health and Nutrition Examination Survey. *PLoS ONE* **2014**, *9*, e112460. [CrossRef] [PubMed]
19. Tielsch, J.M.; Katz, J.; Quigley, H.A.; Javitt, J.C.; Sommer, A. Diabetes, intraocular pressure, and primary open-angle glaucoma in the Baltimore Eye Survey. *Ophthalmology* **1995**, *102*, 48–53. [CrossRef]
20. de Voogd, S.; Ikram, M.K.; Wolfs, R.C.; Jansonius, N.M.; Witteman, J.C.; Hofman, A.; de Jong, P.T. Is diabetes mellitus a risk factor for open-angle glaucoma? The Rotterdam Study. *Ophthalmology* **2006**, *113*, 1827–1831. [CrossRef]
21. Quigley, H.A.; West, S.K.; Rodriguez, J.; Munoz, B.; Klein, R.; Snyder, R. The prevalence of glaucoma in a population-based study of Hispanic subjects: Proyecto VER. *Arch. Ophthalmol.* **2001**, *119*, 1819–1826. [CrossRef]
22. Leske, M.C.; Connell, A.M.; Wu, S.Y.; Hyman, L.G.; Schachat, A.P. Risk factors for open-angle glaucoma. The Barbados Eye Study. *Arch. Ophthalmol.* **1995**, *113*, 918–924. [CrossRef] [PubMed]
23. Tielsch, J.M.; Katz, J.; Sommer, A.; Quigley, H.A.; Javitt, J.C. Hypertension, perfusion pressure, and primary open-angle glaucoma. A population-based assessment. *Arch. Ophthalmol.* **1995**, *113*, 216–221. [CrossRef]
24. Kaimbo, D.K.; Buntinx, F.; Missotten, L. Risk factors for open-angle glaucoma: A case-control study. *J. Clin. Epidemiol.* **2001**, *54*, 166–171. [CrossRef]
25. Jonas, J.B.; Grundler, A.E. Prevalence of diabetes mellitus and arterial hypertension in primary and secondary open-angle glaucomas. *Graefes Arch. Clin. Exp. Ophthalmol.* **1998**, *236*, 202–206. [CrossRef] [PubMed]
26. Charliat, G.; Jolly, D.; Blanchard, F. Genetic risk factor in primary open-angle glaucoma: A case-control study. *Ophthalmic Epidemiol.* **1994**, *1*, 131–138. [CrossRef] [PubMed]
27. Jung, Y.; Han, K.; Park, H.L.; Park, C.K. Type 2 diabetes mellitus and risk of open-angle glaucoma development in Koreans: An 11-year nationwide propensity-score-matched study. *Diabetes Metab.* **2018**, *44*, 328–332. [CrossRef] [PubMed]
28. Zhao, D.; Cho, J.; Kim, M.H.; Friedman, D.S.; Guallar, E. Diabetes, fasting glucose, and the risk of glaucoma: A meta-analysis. *Ophthalmology* **2015**, *122*, 72–78. [CrossRef]
29. Burgess, S.; Thompson, S.G. Multivariable Mendelian randomization: The use of pleiotropic genetic variants to estimate causal effects. *Am. J. Epidemiol.* **2015**, *181*, 251–260. [CrossRef]
30. Burgess, S.; Thompson, S.G. Interpreting findings from Mendelian randomization using the MR-Egger method. *Eur. J. Epidemiol.* **2017**, *32*, 377–389. [CrossRef]
31. Hu, Z.; Zhou, F.; Kaminga, A.C.; Xu, H. Type 2 Diabetes, Fasting Glucose, Hemoglobin A1c Levels and Risk of Primary Open-Angle Glaucoma: A Mendelian Randomization Study. *Investig. Ophthalmol. Vis. Sci.* **2022**, *63*, 37. [CrossRef] [PubMed]
32. Hanyuda, A.; Goto, A.; Nakatochi, M.; Sutoh, Y.; Narita, A.; Nakano, S.; Katagiri, R.; Wakai, K.; Takashima, N.; Koyama, T.; et al. Association Between Glycemic Traits and Primary Open-Angle Glaucoma: A Mendelian Randomization Study in the Japanese Population. *Am. J. Ophthalmol.* **2022**, *245*, 193–201. [CrossRef] [PubMed]
33. Lee, Y.; Kim, Y.A.; Seo, J.H. Causal Association of Obesity and Dyslipidemia with Type 2 Diabetes: A Two-Sample Mendelian Randomization Study. *Genes* **2022**, *13*, 2407. [CrossRef] [PubMed]
34. Seo, J.H.; Lee, Y. Causal Association between Iritis or Uveitis and Glaucoma: A Two-Sample Mendelian Randomisation Study. *Genes* **2023**, *14*, 642. [CrossRef] [PubMed]

35. Minelli, C.; Del Greco, M.F.; van der Plaat, D.A.; Bowden, J.; Sheehan, N.A.; Thompson, J. The use of two-sample methods for Mendelian randomization analyses on single large datasets. *Int. J. Epidemiol.* **2021**, *50*, 1651–1659. [CrossRef] [PubMed]
36. Sakaue, S.; Kanai, M.; Tanigawa, Y.; Karjalainen, J.; Kurki, M.; Koshiba, S.; Narita, A.; Konuma, T.; Yamamoto, K.; Akiyama, M.; et al. A cross-population atlas of genetic associations for 220 human phenotypes. *Nat. Genet.* **2021**, *53*, 1415–1424. [CrossRef] [PubMed]
37. Choquet, H.; Paylakhi, S.; Kneeland, S.C.; Thai, K.K.; Hoffmann, T.J.; Yin, J.; Kvale, M.N.; Banda, Y.; Tolman, N.G.; Williams, P.A.; et al. A multiethnic genome-wide association study of primary open-angle glaucoma identifies novel risk loci. *Nat. Commun.* **2018**, *9*, 2278. [CrossRef] [PubMed]
38. Loh, M.; Zhang, W.; Ng, H.K.; Schmid, K.; Lamri, A.; Tong, L.; Ahmad, M.; Lee, J.J.; Ng, M.C.Y.; Petty, L.E.; et al. Identification of genetic effects underlying type 2 diabetes in South Asian and European populations. *Commun. Biol.* **2022**, *5*, 329. [CrossRef]
39. Burgess, S.; Thompson, S.G.; CRP CHD Genetics Collaboration. Avoiding bias from weak instruments in Mendelian randomization studies. *Int. J. Epidemiol.* **2011**, *40*, 755–764. [CrossRef]
40. Burgess, S.; Butterworth, A.; Thompson, S.G. Mendelian randomization analysis with multiple genetic variants using summarized data. *Genet. Epidemiol.* **2013**, *37*, 658–665. [CrossRef]
41. Bowden, J.; Del Greco, M.F.; Minelli, C.; Davey Smith, G.; Sheehan, N.; Thompson, J. A framework for the investigation of pleiotropy in two-sample summary data Mendelian randomization. *Stat. Med.* **2017**, *36*, 1783–1802. [CrossRef]
42. Burgess, S.; Davey Smith, G.; Davies, N.M.; Dudbridge, F.; Gill, D.; Glymour, M.M.; Hartwig, F.P.; Holmes, M.V.; Minelli, C.; Relton, C.L.; et al. Guidelines for performing Mendelian randomization investigations. *Wellcome Open Res.* **2019**, *4*, 186. [CrossRef] [PubMed]
43. Bowden, J.; Davey Smith, G.; Haycock, P.C.; Burgess, S. Consistent Estimation in Mendelian Randomization with Some Invalid Instruments Using a Weighted Median Estimator. *Genet. Epidemiol.* **2016**, *40*, 304–314. [CrossRef] [PubMed]
44. Bowden, J.; Davey Smith, G.; Burgess, S. Mendelian randomization with invalid instruments: Effect estimation and bias detection through Egger regression. *Int. J. Epidemiol.* **2015**, *44*, 512–525. [CrossRef] [PubMed]
45. Bowden, J.; Del Greco, M.F.; Minelli, C.; Davey Smith, G.; Sheehan, N.A.; Thompson, J.R. Assessing the suitability of summary data for two-sample Mendelian randomization analyses using MR-Egger regression: The role of the I2 statistic. *Int. J. Epidemiol.* **2016**, *45*, 1961–1974. [CrossRef] [PubMed]
46. Verbanck, M.; Chen, C.Y.; Neale, B.; Do, R. Publisher Correction: Detection of widespread horizontal pleiotropy in causal relationships inferred from Mendelian randomization between complex traits and diseases. *Nat. Genet.* **2018**, *50*, 1196. [CrossRef]
47. Greco, M.F.; Minelli, C.; Sheehan, N.A.; Thompson, J.R. Detecting pleiotropy in Mendelian randomisation studies with summary data and a continuous outcome. *Stat. Med.* **2015**, *34*, 2926–2940. [CrossRef] [PubMed]
48. Jin, H.; Lee, S.; Won, S. Causal Evaluation of Laboratory Markers in Type 2 Diabetes on Cancer and Vascular Diseases Using Various Mendelian Randomization Tools. *Front. Genet.* **2020**, *11*, 597420. [CrossRef] [PubMed]
49. Klein, B.E.; Klein, R.; Jensen, S.C. Open-angle glaucoma and older-onset diabetes. The Beaver Dam Eye Study. *Ophthalmology* **1994**, *101*, 1173–1177. [CrossRef]
50. Dielemans, I.; de Jong, P.T.; Stolk, R.; Vingerling, J.R.; Grobbee, D.E.; Hofman, A. Primary open-angle glaucoma, intraocular pressure, and diabetes mellitus in the general elderly population. The Rotterdam Study. *Ophthalmology* **1996**, *103*, 1271–1275. [CrossRef]
51. Bonovas, S.; Peponis, V.; Filioussi, K. Diabetes mellitus as a risk factor for primary open-angle glaucoma: A meta-analysis. *Diabet. Med.* **2004**, *21*, 609–614. [CrossRef] [PubMed]
52. Yuan, R.; Liu, K.; Cai, Y.; He, F.; Xiao, X.; Zou, J. Body shape and risk of glaucoma: A Mendelian randomization. *Front. Med.* **2022**, *9*, 999974. [CrossRef] [PubMed]
53. Lin, Y.; Zhu, X.; Luo, W.; Jiang, B.; Lin, Q.; Tang, M.; Li, X.; Xie, L. The Causal Association Between Obesity and Primary Open-Angle Glaucoma: A Two-Sample Mendelian Randomization Study. *Front. Genet.* **2022**, *13*, 835524. [CrossRef] [PubMed]
54. The Expert Committee on the Diagnosis; Classification of Diabetes Mellitus. Report of the expert committee on the diagnosis and classification of diabetes mellitus. *Diabetes Care* **2003**, *26* (Suppl. S1), S5–S20. [CrossRef]
55. Galicia-Garcia, U.; Benito-Vicente, A.; Jebari, S.; Larrea-Sebal, A.; Siddiqi, H.; Uribe, K.B.; Ostolaza, H.; Martin, C. Pathophysiology of Type 2 Diabetes Mellitus. *Int. J. Mol. Sci.* **2020**, *21*, 6275. [CrossRef] [PubMed]
56. Choi, J.A.; Park, Y.M.; Han, K.; Lee, J.; Yun, J.S.; Ko, S.H. Fasting plasma glucose level and the risk of open angle glaucoma: Nationwide population-based cohort study in Korea. *PLoS ONE* **2020**, *15*, e0239529. [CrossRef]
57. Sato, T.; Roy, S. Effect of high glucose on fibronectin expression and cell proliferation in trabecular meshwork cells. *Investig. Ophthalmol. Vis. Sci.* **2002**, *43*, 170–175.
58. Li, Y.; Mitchell, W.; Elze, T.; Zebardast, N. Association Between Diabetes, Diabetic Retinopathy, and Glaucoma. *Curr. Diab. Rep.* **2021**, *21*, 38. [CrossRef]
59. Kim, Y.A.; Lee, Y.; Seo, J.H. Renal Complication and Glycemic Control in Korean Veterans with Type 2 Diabetes: A 10-Year Retrospective Cohort Study. *J. Diabetes Res.* **2020**, *2020*, 9806790. [CrossRef]
60. UK Prospective Diabetes Study (UKPDS) Group. Intensive blood-glucose control with sulphonylureas or insulin compared with conventional treatment and risk of complications in patients with type 2 diabetes (UKPDS 33). *Lancet* **1998**, *352*, 837–853.
61. American Diabetes Association. 6. Glycemic Targets: Standards of Medical Care in Diabetes-2019. *Diabetes Care* **2019**, *42*, S61–S70. [CrossRef] [PubMed]

62. Diabetes Control and Complications Trial Research Group; Nathan, D.M.; Genuth, S.; Lachin, J.; Cleary, P.; Crofford, O.; Davis, M.; Rand, L.; Siebert, C. The effect of intensive treatment of diabetes on the development and progression of long-term complications in insulin-dependent diabetes mellitus. *N. Engl. J. Med.* **1993**, *329*, 977–986. [CrossRef] [PubMed]
63. Wang, K.; Yang, F.; Liu, X.; Lin, X.; Yin, H.; Tang, Q.; Jiang, L.; Yao, K. Appraising the Effects of Metabolic Traits on the Risk of Glaucoma: A Mendelian Randomization Study. *Metabolites* **2023**, *13*, 109. [CrossRef] [PubMed]
64. Ho-Pham, L.T.; Nguyen, U.D.T.; Tran, T.X.; Nguyen, T.V. Discordance in the diagnosis of diabetes: Comparison between HbA1c and fasting plasma glucose. *PLoS ONE* **2017**, *12*, e0182192. [CrossRef] [PubMed]
65. Hemani, G.; Bowden, J.; Davey Smith, G. Evaluating the potential role of pleiotropy in Mendelian randomization studies. *Hum. Mol. Genet.* **2018**, *27*, R195–R208. [CrossRef]
66. Jiang, L.; Zheng, Z.; Fang, H.; Yang, J. A generalized linear mixed model association tool for biobank-scale data. *Nat. Genet.* **2021**, *53*, 1616–1621. [CrossRef]

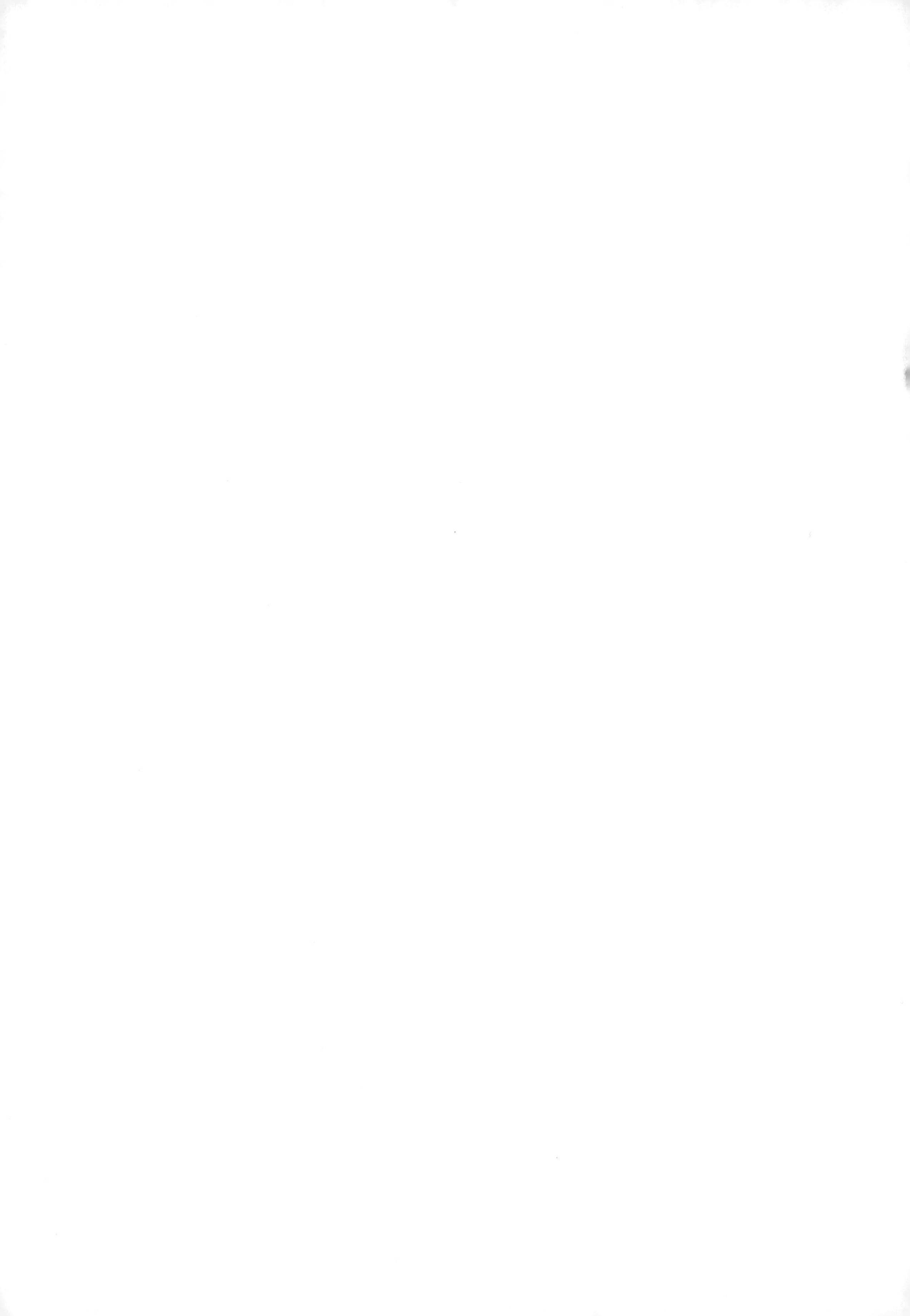

MDPI AG
Grosspeteranlage 5
4052 Basel
Switzerland
Tel.: +41 61 683 77 34

Biomedicines Editorial Office
E-mail: biomedicines@mdpi.com
www.mdpi.com/journal/biomedicines

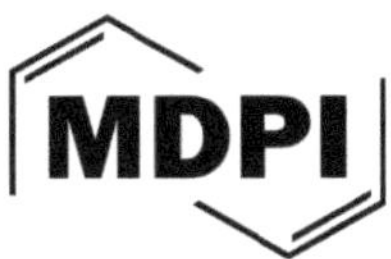

www.ingramcontent.com/pod-product-compliance
Lightning Source LLC
LaVergne TN
LVHW072359090526
838202LV00019B/2581

* 9 7 8 3 7 2 5 8 3 6 1 9 2 *